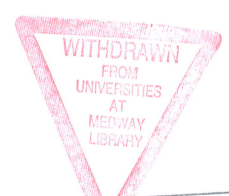

# Motor Speech Disorders

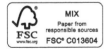

## COMMUNICATION DISORDERS ACROSS LANGUAGES

**Series Editors**: Dr Nicole Müller and Dr Martin Ball, *University of Louisiana at Lafayette, USA*

While the majority of work in communication disorders has focused on English, there has been a growing trend in recent years for the publication of information on languages other than English. However, much of this is scattered through a large number of journals in the field of speech pathology/ communication disorders, and therefore, not always readily available to the practitioner, researcher and student. It is the aim of this series to bring together into book form surveys of existing studies on specific languages, together with new materials for the language(s) in question. We also have launched a series of companion volumes dedicated to issues related to the cross-linguistic study of communication disorders. The series does not include English (as so much work is readily available), but covers a wide number of other languages (usually separately, though sometimes two or more similar languages may be grouped together where warranted by the amount of published work currently available). We have been able to publish volumes on Finnish, Spanish, Chinese and Turkish, and books on multilingual aspects of stuttering, aphasia, and speech disorders, with several others in preparation.

Full details of all the books in this series and of all our other publications can be found on http://www.multilingual-matters.com, or by writing to Multilingual Matters, St Nicholas House, 31-34 High Street, Bristol BS1 2AW, UK.

COMMUNICATION DISORDERS ACROSS LANGUAGES: 12

# Motor Speech Disorders

A Cross-Language Perspective

Edited by

## Nick Miller and Anja Lowit

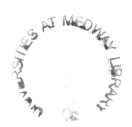

**MULTILINGUAL MATTERS**
Bristol • Buffalo • Toronto

**Library of Congress Cataloging in Publication Data**
A catalog record for this book is available from the Library of Congress.
Motor Speech Disorders: A Cross-Language Perspective/Edited by Nick Miller and Anja Lowit.
Communication Disorders Across Languages: 12
Includes bibliographical references.
1. Speech disorders. 2. Motor ability. I. Miller, Nick (Professor), editor of compilation.
II. Lowit, Anja, editor of compilation.
RC423.M6173 2014
616.85'5–dc23 2014009376

**British Library Cataloguing in Publication Data**
A catalogue entry for this book is available from the British Library.

ISBN-13: 978-1-78309-232-1 (hbk)

**Multilingual Matters**
UK: St Nicholas House, 31-34 High Street, Bristol BS1 2AW, UK.
USA: UTP, 2250 Military Road, Tonawanda, NY 14150, USA.
Canada: UTP, 5201 Dufferin Street, North York, Ontario M3H 5T8, Canada.

Website: www.multilingual-matters.com
Twitter: Multi_Ling_Mat
Facebook: https://www.facebook.com/multilingualmatters
Blog: www.channelviewpublications.wordpress.com

The policy of Multilingual Matters/Channel View Publications is to use papers that are natural, renewable and recyclable products, made from wood grown in sustainable forests. In the manufacturing process of our books, and to further support our policy, preference is given to printers that have FSC and PEFC Chain of Custody certification. The FSC and/or PEFC logos will appear on those books where full certification has been granted to the printer concerned.

Typeset by Deanta Global Publishing Services Limited.
Printed and bound in Great Britain by the CPI Group (UK Ltd), Croydon, CR0 4YY.

# Contents

## Part 2  Language Specific Profiles and Practices

# Contributors

**Ingrid Aichert** received her PhD in Speech Pathology from the University of Potsdam, Germany. She is a researcher at the Clinical Neuropsychology Research Group, City Hospital, Munich. Her main research interest is apraxia of speech. She also lectures on dyslexia and dysgraphia at the University of Munich and on aphasiology on different speech-language pathology courses.

**Simone dos Santos Barreto** is a professor in the Department of Speech, Language and Hearing Sciences of the Federal Fluminense University, Brazil. She has published book chapters and articles on dysarthria. Her research interests include motor speech disorders, language and cognition.

**Bettina Brendel** is a neurophonetician and a researcher at the Centre of Neurology in the University of Tübingen, Germany. Her research interests include apraxia of speech and dysarthria in adults. In addition, she is involved in investigating the organization of motor speech control in healthy speakers using functional magnetic resonance imaging.

**Alexandre Castro-Caldas** MD, PhD, is full professor of neurology and director of the Institute of Health Sciences at the Catholic University of Portugal. Among his many roles and accomplishments, he is past-president of the International Neuropsychological Society.

**Maysa Luchesi Cera** is a speech-language therapist at the Centre for Integrated Rehabilitation, State Hospital of Ribeirão Preto in Brazil and a PhD student in Human Communication Disorders at the Federal University of São Paulo. She has published a number of articles in the areas of language and speech in acquired neurological disorders.

**Kit Ying Chan** is an assistant professor of psychology at James Madison University, Harrisonburg, USA. Her research interests cover spoken word recognition and second language acquisition, with a focus on how foreign accents influence spoken word recognition and memory.

**Dora Colaço** is a speech and language therapist at the Hospital da Luz in Lisbon, Portugal. She is a PhD student at the Health Sciences Institute of the Catholic University of Portugal and a member of the cognitive neuroscience research group of the same university. Her main scientific interest is related to the cognitive neurosciences, specifically neurolinguistics, aphasia and clinical linguistics. She has published papers in this field. Recently, she won an award from the Foundation D. Pedro IV for one of her papers, published in *Clinical Linguistics and Phonetics*.

**Danielle Duez** was a senior scientist in linguistics and phonetics at the French National Research Centre (CNRS) and is now Research Director Emeritus at the Laboratoire Parole et Langage in Aix en Provence, France. Her domains of interest are the production and perception of speech with a special focus on prosody and speech sound patterns in different speech styles in normal and impaired speech. She has published research articles on a wide range of subjects including the temporal organization of speech, the patterns of reduction in speech sounds and parkinsonian speech disorders and their treatment effects.

**Carlos Gallego** is a professor of psychology of language and speech therapy at the Complutense University of Madrid. He is also the Dean of the Department of Psychology. He has published a number of books and articles in the areas of language processing, language development and language disorders.

**Rutherford Goldstein** is a member of the Cognitive Psychology Program at the University of Kansas, Lawrence, USA. He works in the Spoken Language Laboratory (director Dr Michael Vitevitch) studying spoken language processes. His recent research has explored how network science principles can be applied to the mental lexicon.

**Roel Jonkers** has worked in the Department of Linguistics and the Centre of Language and Cognition at the University of Groningen, the Netherlands, since 1993. His research interests include apraxia of speech and lexical disorders in aphasia and dementia. He was project leader on a project on the diagnosis and evaluation of therapy in apraxia of speech from which grew the Dutch Test for Apraxia of Speech (the DIAS; Feiken and Jonkers, 2012).

**Anja Kuschmann** is a British Academy postdoctoral fellow in the School of Psychological Sciences and Health, Strathclyde University, UK. Her research interests include intonation and prosody in developmental and acquired motor speech disorders, speech intelligibility and methodological frameworks for assessing disordered speech.

**Marina Laganaro** is an assistant professor at the University of Geneva, Switzerland, teaching the neuropsychology of language to students of psychology and speech and language pathology. Her research interests include lexical, phonological and phonetic processes in speech planning in healthy adults and in brain-damaged speakers.

**Anja Lowit** is a Reader in Speech and Language Therapy at Strathclyde University, UK. Her research interests include dysarthria, prosodic disorders, acoustic analysis of disordered speech, treatment effectiveness and the development of outcome measures.

**Joan K-Y. Ma** PhD is a lecturer in the Division of Speech and Hearing Sciences, Queen Margaret University, Edinburgh, UK. Her interests include the perception and production of tone and intonation in Cantonese, perceptual and instrumental analyses of motor speech disorders (with a particular interest in hypokinetic dysarthria), perceptual and acoustic correlates of speech intelligibility and motor control in speech and swallowing. She has published a number of articles on the interaction between tone and intonation in Cantonese and on motor speech disorders.

**Ben Maassen** is a professor of dyslexia and a clinical neuropsychologist, and has a background in cognitive neuropsychology and speech-language pathology. His previous affiliations were with the Max Planck Institute for Psycholinguistics; Radboud University Nijmegen, the Netherlands (PhD on intelligibility of the speech of the deaf); and Child Neurology, Radboud University Medical Center. Currently, he works in the Faculty of Arts and the University Medical Center, University of Groningen, the Netherlands. His main research areas are dyslexia and neurocognitive precursors of literacy; neurogenic speech disorders, in particular childhood apraxia of speech; perception-production modelling in speech development; and speech-related cognitive dysfunctions. He has been chair of the International Conference on Speech Motor Control (Nijmegen 2001, 2006; Groningen 2011).

**R. Manjula** is professor of speech pathology and currently heads the Department of Speech-Language Pathology at the All India Institute of Speech and Hearing, Manasagangothri, Mysore, India. Her areas of interest are motor speech disorders, augmentative and alternative communication, phonology and dysphagia, areas in which she has published numerous articles.

**María Teresa Martín-Aragoneses** is an assistant professor in the Faculty of Education at the National Distance Education University (UNED) and a member of the Laboratory of Cognitive and Computational Neuroscience in the Centre for Biomedical Technology (Technical University of Madrid and Complutense University of Madrid, Spain). Her research interests include language processing, language disorders and neurodegeneration of language, which are also the areas in which she has published.

**Natalia Melle** is a speech-language therapist at the University Hospital of the Infanta Elena and associate professor of the Speech-Language Therapy Programme at the Complutense University of Madrid, Spain. Her work has covered publications on motor speech disorders in Spanish speakers and neurogenic dysphagia.

**Nick Miller** is professor of motor speech disorders at Newcastle University, UK. His main research interests include apraxia, dysarthria and dysphagia and the psychosocial impact of neurogenic communication disorders.

**Ana Mineiro** gained her PhD in Linguistics from the University of Lisbon, Portugal. She is an associate professor and senior researcher at the Catholic University of Lisbon (UCP) where she is principal investigator on several scientific and developmental projects. She has published widely with an emphasis in recent years on research in clinical linguistics and sign language from biolinguistic and neurolinguistic perspectives. She directs the research group in sign language in UCP and co-coordinates the bachelor's and master's programmes in Portuguese Sign Language and deaf education as well as the master's programme in clinical linguistics.

**Masaki Nishio** is currently professor of the Department of Speech Language and Hearing Science at the Niigata University of Health and Welfare in Japan. He has published a number of books and articles in the field of motor speech disorders. He is the current president of the Japan Clinical Society of Dysarthria Research.

**Karin Zazo Ortiz** is a professor of speech pathology and audiology in the School of Medicine at São Paulo Federal University, Brazil. She has published books and articles on neurolinguistics in relation to aphasia, apraxia of speech, dysarthria and language disorders in Alzheimer's disease.

**Mia Le Roux** is a lecturer in the Department of Speech-Language Pathology and Audiology at the University of Pretoria, South Africa. She studied African languages and second language teaching before joining the Department of Speech-Language Pathology and Audiology. Her fields of interest are applied linguistics, phonetics and second language learning and teaching and she has published articles and contributed to books in these areas.

**Mary Overton Venet** is a bilingual speech-language therapist and aphasiologist. She works at the Faculty of Psychology and Educational Sciences, University of Geneva, Switzerland, as a lecturer and coordinator of the master's program in speech language therapy. Together with colleagues, she has published treatment studies on the topic of bilingual aphasia in the domains of acquired disorders of reading and oral language.

**Ellika Schalling** is a speech and language pathologist working at the Karolinska Institute in Stockholm, Sweden. Her main research interests include neurogenic communication disorders, especially in speech disorders in chronic, progressive neurological disease. She is presently programme director of the master's programme in speech and language pathology at the Karolinska Institute, where she also teaches courses primarily in the area of motor speech disorders and supervises doctoral students in the same area.

**Naresh Sharma** is senior lecturer in Hindi and Urdu at the School of Oriental and African Studies, University of London, UK. His interests lie in the field of applied linguistics, in particular second language acquisition.

**Hayo Terband** is a speech researcher collaborating with speech-language pathologists, neurologists, audiologists, psychologists and neurophysiologists. His research revolves around the developmental process of the speech production and perception system in both normal and disordered development, in which he combines behavioural experiments with neuro-computational modelling. Besides fundamental research, he also works on clinical applications and initiated the development and implementation of a process-oriented method for diagnostics and treatment planning of developmental speech disorders, a collaborative project between six Dutch university institutions.

**Martha E. Tyrone** is assistant professor in the Department of Communication Sciences and Disorders at Long Island University Brooklyn, USA, and senior research scientist at Haskins Laboratories. Her research interests include the phonetics of signed language, kinematic analyses of sign production and comparisons of typical and atypical signing.

**Anita van der Merwe** is professor of speech pathology in the Department of Speech-Language Pathology and Audiology at the University of Pretoria, South Africa. Her research interests are speech motor control, apraxia of speech and the treatment of apraxia of speech. She has developed a brain-behaviour model of speech sensorimotor control that explains the neurological control of normal speech production, characterizes pathological speech sensorimotor control and provides treatment guidelines for apraxia of speech. She has published a number of articles and book chapters in these fields.

**Michael S. Vitevitch** PhD is a professor of psychology at the University of Kansas, Lawrence, USA. His previous research examined the influence of phonotactic probability and phonological neighbourhood density on the retrieval of word-forms from the mental lexicon during the recognition and production of spoken words. His current research uses mathematical tools from the emerging field of Network Science to measure the structure that exists at multiple scales in the mental lexicon. These measures are combined with conventional tasks from psycholinguistics and computer simulations to examine how that lexical structure influences various language-related processes.

**Tara L. Whitehill** (1958–2013) was professor and head of speech and hearing sciences and director of the motor speech research laboratory at the University of Hong Kong. Sadly, she died before completion of this book, but we are privileged to have her contribution as a lasting memory. Her research focused on speech disorders related to cleft palate, dysarthria and oral cancer. She was especially interested in how disordered speech could be accurately judged, and in determining language-specific versus language-universal contributors to disordered speech. Her background as a Cantonese-speaker enabled her to conduct internationally recognized and influential cross-language, clinically grounded research work. Among her many honours, in 2008 she was elected a Fellow of the American Speech-Language-Hearing Association.

# 1 Introduction

## Nick Miller and Anja Lowit

## What is This Book All About?

This book is about motor speech disorders (MSDs), about aspects of their assessment and treatment, about understanding the underlying neurophysiological and neuropsychological disruptions that bring about disorders of speech motor control. More precisely, the book is about what we can find out about these disorders from a particular perspective – cross-language studies.

MSDs are a cover term for problems with voice production/phonation and articulation due to neurological damage that impairs the planning and execution of movements required to produce speech (we offer an introduction to the field later for those not familiar with it). Disruption may affect one or more of the processes and actions underlying speech production, for example dysfunction in the 'selection' of the sounds required to say a word, problems in the planning of the movements needed to produce those sounds. Disruption may alter the transmission of nerve impulses between parts of the brain involved in executing the planned movements, cause difficulties with transmission of these impulses between the brain and other parts of the central nervous system and/or problems with relaying the impulses out via the peripheral nervous system to the muscles involved in articulation. The muscles active in speech output range from the diaphragm and thorax involved in the control of in- and expiration, via the larynx for phonation and the velum for regulating the degree of nasality, to the tongue, lips and mandible. These disruptions may affect any or all of breathing, phonation, resonance and articulation and in turn the ability to produce a voice loud and clear enough to be heard, articulation precise enough to deliver intelligible speech and variations in stress and intonation patterns necessary to convey suprasegmental aspects of meaning for the language a person speaks.

There are countless tomes and myriad articles written on MSDs, and so we already know a great deal about them. But, there is one big proviso to most of what we have to say – what we know about MSDs, how to recognise them, how people classify them, their differential diagnosis and many of the clinical practices around their assessment and treatment, rest predominantly on studies of speakers of English (and within those mainly American speakers) and structurally and phonologically closely related Indo-European languages. Such a narrow perspective in the field of communication always runs the risk of producing theories and practices that may not be universally applicable and may even be wrong when applied beyond the narrow confines of the linguistic and social contexts in which they were developed. This provides the rationale for this book.

Studies of MSDs do exist in other languages, most notably Chinese, German, French and Japanese (see chapters later in the book). A cross-language dimension, though, has been largely lacking, especially when it has come to the development of theories around speech motor control and its breakdown, though studies of deaf sign language users who have different neurological conditions do provide a marked exception here, as elucidated in a later chapter. This book aims to redress some of that imbalance. It contains two sections. The first part provides an introduction to MSDs and related areas in a cross-language context. The first three chapters set the scene, defining what we mean by cross-language studies, providing background information on MSDs for those who are not that familiar with this group of communication impairments, and discussing the fundamentals of assessing and treating MSD in a cross-language context. These chapters are followed by selected topics that demonstrate the progress made in the understanding of MSDs and related areas from cross-language studies and the kinds of issues that need to be considered in further investigations in this area. The second half of the book gathers overviews from a range of languages around the world. Each chapter contains a summary of the segmental and suprasegmental features of the language that set it apart from English, and discusses assessments and treatment programmes that have been developed for this medium. In addition, they offer a flavour of the status of knowledge on MSDs in those languages and begin to look at the nature of similarities and differences between languages or types of language that could form the basis of future cross-language investigations to advance our understanding of MSDs and speech motor control in general.

There is one more dimension implicit in this book. Another angle from which researchers have viewed communication to gain insights into brain–language relationships, clues to how language and sound processing reflect neurological processing, has been the study of speech and language breakdown, whether in developmental disorders or in acquired disorders of language and speech after stroke, head injury or in other neurological conditions. By examining what breaks down, and in what ways, in association with lesions in which sites, researchers have sought clues to the central variables in speech motor control and how normal, healthy processing takes place.

It is this dual speech pathology and cross-language line of enquiry that forms the backbone of this book. On the one hand, what clues are there to universals of speech and how might these address issues in our knowledge and conceptualisation of MSDs?; on the other hand, what implications do language-specific manifestations and variations in the universal tendencies have for the support and management of people with MSDs? In more specific example terms, on the one hand, what does apraxia of speech or ataxic dysarthria look like in different languages, but on the other hand, does an examination of apraxic breakdown in diverse languages uncover clues to or settle theoretical arguments as to the precise nature of apraxia of speech? The perspective to the fore in this book is a clinical one. However, through this there is a much broader currency in terms of how findings from these fields might inform the development of neuropsychological and neurolinguistic theory, what they have to tell us about brain–language relationships and how they contribute to our overall understanding of language and speech.

# Part 1
# Setting the Scene

# 2 Introduction: Cross-Language Perspectives on Motor Speech Disorders

Nick Miller, Anja Lowit
and Anja Kuschmann

## The Rationale for Cross-Language Studies

As the name implies, such studies entail comparing and contrasting the appearance, behaviour, form and functioning of a given variable across different languages. Cross-language perspectives have long formed an important avenue for the advancement of theoretical and applied studies in language and sound structure, in the laboratory, classroom and clinic. In the sphere of language (as opposed to speech and voice) this has involved, for instance, studying how different languages signal past tense, how they mark negation, how certain areas of the lexicon are organised (e.g. colour naming, kinship terms, prepositions). More recently, researchers have examined neural correlates of possible divergences (Liu *et al.*, 2013). In relation to speech motor control, analyses have included the contrasting relationships between prosody and syntax; a comparison of vowel systems; specific variables such as voice onset time (Cho & Ladefoged, 1999), sensory-motor constraints on sound inventories (Lindblom, 2000; Lindblom *et al.*, 1983), motor control (Chakraborty, 2012), attempts to capture rhythmic variation across languages (Loukina *et al.*, 2011) and notions of language-specific articulatory settings (Gick *et al.*, 2005; Laver, 1978; Mennen *et al.*, 2010).

Through such scholarship, cross-language studies endeavour to derive theories of language functioning that are not tied to standard average European (SAE) or any other restricted language group, or they seek to test out theories and practices developed in one language to examine if they are equally applicable or require modification when applied to another language (Bozic *et al.*, 2013). In the 1930s, the American linguist Benjamin Whorf introduced the label SAE to refer to modern Indo-European languages that share a number of phonological and grammatical similarities and which constituted the vast majority of the languages on which theories of language form, function and processing were based at that time. He argued that over-reliance on SAE in investigations of language universals had lulled researchers into the false sense that these commonalities divulged natural or even universal properties of language, when in fact they were peculiarities of the SAE group. Whorf's studies of Hopi and other American indigenous languages amply illustrated the flaws in such argumentation. Admonitions regarding confounding surface forms with underlying properties persist to the present (Haspelmath, 2010, 2012).

Research along these lines has informed debates on the classification of language types and families, the development of linguistic theory, and has contributed to theories and practice in foreign language teaching and learning. One branch of the field has emphasised investigations into the differences between languages, into the different ways they function or are used. An arguably more potent line of enquiry in cross-language studies, however, has concerned the focus on commonalities across what on the surface might appear diverse and divergent systems, a focus not on the divides but on the shared. Among all the seemingly endless variety in sound, syntactic and semantic structures between languages, what clues are there to the fundamental, shared properties of the ways in which languages and sound systems are organised, operated and processed?

Studies have tackled issues around the general properties of syntax and morphology and the relationship between them, the semantic structure of utterances; closer to motor speech issues, scholarship has sought to establish the units of speech control that generalise across all languages, how do segmental and suprasegmental control relate, how are they integrated, what are the properties of syllables and concatenation of syllables, what light do comparisons throw on the debate around the phonology–phonetics division (or not). In this fashion the aim has been to construct theories concerning what aspects of language, and from the point of view of this book what aspects of speech motor control, reflect universal dimensions of how spoken languages work and insights into the brain systems that support them vs which aspects represent only language-specific adjustments to universal elements; what clues does this give to the unique properties of human language, and vitally, how do these underlying regularities reflect brain functioning, what insights do they deliver into neuropsychological, neurolinguistic and neurophysiological aspects of brain organisation and operation?

# Cross-Language Studies in Speech and Language Pathology

Before proceeding to introduce the field of cross-language studies in motor speech disorders (MSDs), this section offers selective examples from studies in germane areas of speech language pathology where cross-languages have been more prevalent for some time, to give a flavour of the directions and power of cross-language studies and illustrate the potential of cross-language insights to generate advances in knowledge and practice.

The field of aphasia provides a prime example. The understanding of agrammatic aphasia was revolutionised through cross-language comparisons (Bates *et al.*, 1991; Menn *et al.*, 1995, 1996; Paradis, 2001). Within English, it had been conceptualised, as its label reflects, as a breakdown in syntax, with characteristic 'telegrammatic' output from the omission of function words and difficulty with word order. How, though, would such a conceptualisation, if it was to be universally applicable, be manifest in a language where there are few or no function words, where grammatical relationships are signalled (primarily) via noun and verb inflection? How would word order difficulties be manifest in a language with largely free word order?

Within the same debate much was made in research prior to cross-language studies of agrammatism of the differences between passive and active sentence production and comprehension, or between 'do' questions and 'is' questions ('do dogs miau?', 'is it raining?'). If agrammatism represents a problem with syntax, then a more complex syntactic process (passives and 'do' questions in English were considered more complex than active voice and 'is' questions) should prove more problematic for speakers. Numerous studies purported to conclude this. What though of languages where the passive construction was actually less complex than or equally complex syntactically to the active structure or where different interrogative structures were formed in a variety of contrasting ways to English? Did the same divisions hold? In short, the answers were nowhere near as clear-cut as theories of agrammatic breakdown based on English would have led one to presume (Bates *et al.*, 1999; Wulfeck *et al.*, 1991).

The outcome of these cross-language studies in aphasia resulted in a radical reconceptualisation of what had been variously termed Broca's or agrammatic or non-fluent aphasia. New theories (e.g. Bastiaanse *et al.*, 2011; Bates *et al.*, 1991; Friedmann & Shapiro, 2003; Macwhinney, 1987; Menn & Duffield, 2013) were developed that sought to capture and explain the common denominators across languages in the types of breakdown seen after brain damage, that attempted to delve below purely surface syntactic manifestations and theories based on these. This has led to far deeper insights into universal aspects of syntactic processing and output and our understanding of aphasia.

Closer to speech output, the field of dysfluency research has provided further examples of the benefits of a cross-language approach. Irrespective of which language someone stutters in, the types of dysfluency that arise appear to be universal – there are blocks, hesitations and prolongations in

Russian just as in English or Hausa. However, what this surface similarity hides is that there is not equality across languages in the proportion of different stuttering moments (blocks to prolongations etc.), nor the loci of dysfluencies in terms of on what (kinds of) syllable or word or phrase they occur and where in the phrase they fall. Investigations into this variability have disclosed important aspects around the aetiology and manifestation of stuttering.

Taking just one illustration, a claim in the field of stuttering was that instances of dysfluency were strongly associated with stressed syllables (Wingate, 1979). Data from English appeared to support this contention. A key test would be whether the distribution of dysfluencies found in English would differ in languages that have decisively different patterns of stress placement and grammatical structure and whether the differing distribution paralleled the contrasts between English and other languages in word and sentence stress assignment. Some cross-language comparisons did appear to support the hypothesis. However, others did not, but opened up further possibilities for the apparent association and discrepancies between studies, e.g. locus of the word in a sentence, classes of words, lexical vs sentence stress, and syllable structure of words; and evolving change with age in preponderance of which word classes had higher dysfluency likelihood; and motor vs phonological determinants of dysfluency (Dworzynski *et al.*, 2003; Matsumoto-Shimamori & Ito, 2013; Natke *et al.*, 2004). Insights given by cross-language comparisons played a key role here.

Similar issues have emerged in relation to a germane condition, spasmodic dysphonia (SD). This is characterised by dystonic spasms that cause the vocal cords to suddenly lock in an open setting, leaving no or only whispered voice; or they suddenly close leading to what are heard as phonation blocks or dysfluencies similar to those in stuttering. The occurrence of dystonic ad- and abduction appears to be universal, though some individuals may show a bias towards greater prevalence of one or the other pattern. Based on studies with English speakers, various claims were made about the relative likelihood of ad- vs abductor events and what, therefore, the underlying impairment, or trigger, in SD must be. An important variable in triggering adductor spasms especially appears to be the presence of a voiced onset to a word or syllable. Adductor spasms are more liable to occur on these. This would predict that the likelihood of adductor spasms and the proportion of ad- vs abductor spasms would vary in relation to the balance of voiced vs voiceless syllable onsets across languages. Lorch and Whurr (2003) observed that the characterisation of SD varied between French (Klap *et al.*, 1993) and English. They analysed the utterances of six French speakers with SD and compared them to patterns found for English speakers. Pitch breaks so typical of English speakers were absent in French speakers; harsh and breathy voice quality not so prominent in English was marked in French. Lorch and Whurr (2003) argue that these differences are due to the contrasting phonological profiles in French and English, i.e. the proportion of ad- vs abductor spasms would vary in relation to the balance of voiced vs voiceless syllable onsets across the two languages, and especially vowel vs consonant onsets, given the propensity for vowels to elicit blocks compared to consonants.

Cross-language studies have also been prominent in addressing a number of issues in acquired dyslexia, such as the hypothesised distinction between deep and surface dyslexia. The latter is characterised by a reliance on letter by letter spelling/reading. This strategy succeeds so long as grapheme–phoneme correspondence remains regular. However, when irregular spellings are met, mispronunciation ensues. Thus, to quote the classic example, the person with surface dyslexia manages in English with 'mint' but fails on 'pint' (speaking it as a rhyme with mint). 'Belt, land, went' work well, but 'debt, choir and wand' do not. Is what has been described as surface dyslexia, though, purely an artefact of English, and other similarly structured orthographies, where there exist regular and irregular correspondences between spelling and pronunciation? Can one have surface dyslexia in a language with regular and transparent spelling?

Again, cross-language studies comparing reading in languages with regular and irregular orthographies were able to enlighten this debate and confirm that the surface-deep dyslexia distinction is universally valid (Davies et al., 2010; Erickson & Sachse, 2010; Robert & Fernando, 2005; Weekes et al., 2008), though compare Hricová and Weekes (2012). It is just that one has to search for manifestations in different places and different ways – coincidentally underlining implications for the assessment and management of dyslexic difficulties across different languages.

Another angle on reading and reading disorders has been afforded by studies within and between languages that have radically differing orthographic systems. Most notable here have been comparisons between phonemic, syllabic and ideographic spelling systems. Examples are provided by divergences between reading difficulties in English and Chinese or Japanese, or even more pertinently, within Japanese where contrasts between kana (syllabic characters representing sound combinations) and kanji (logographic characters similar to Chinese orthography representing whole words or morphemes) disclose even within single speakers the differential effects of lesions in different brain parts on reading skills depending on the demands of the code being employed (Huang et al., 2012; Sakurai et al., 2008; Sato et al., 2008). In this way, researchers have been able to develop theories not just of reading acquisition and breakdown, but also of the relationship between sound and visual aspects of reading and brain organisation for reading.

One more insight from reading studies provides an illustration of where cross-language studies have informed more general issues in phonological processing. In second language teaching and in clinical studies of children or adults with difficulties in speech output or reading, a common component of assessment entails tests of phonological or metaphonological awareness or manipulation. Speakers are asked to judge whether two words rhyme with each other or not; whether they have the same number of syllables; whether they have identical onsets/offsets or not; what would 'dog' sound like without the 'd' or 'sheepdog' without the 'dog'; what sounds does 'cat' consist of? The belief is that such tasks access components of phonological organisation and processing that are independent of language (e.g. Spanish, Cambodian) and of other language processes (e.g. morphology, reading). However, by comparing speakers who are or who are not literate in a language and from studying phonology or other linguistic variables in speakers of languages where there is no written form, it has been shown that these assumptions are far from true. Such studies favour arguments that many aspects claimed to be core, universal elements of phonological processing are in fact not. Rather, they may be by-products of learning to read and the methods through which one was taught (Chapter 8; Monzalvo & Dehaene-Lambertz, 2013; Nickels & Cole-Virtue, 2004; Tsegaye *et al.*, 2011).

The examples above begin to give some insights into the possibilities offered by cross-language studies. One might note that the implications of findings pertain not just to ivory tower theorisation on language functioning for the benefit of armchair theoreticians; they have decisive importance for practical, clinical issues. Establishing universal properties of speech systems should enable the development of assessment techniques and therapies that are applicable across all languages. Identifying where there are idiosyncrasies confined to particular languages, and which, therefore, may require language-specific techniques in assessment and therapy, will ensure that rehabilitation proceeds in a focused, targeted way. We now turn to the focus of this book, speech output and MSDs.

## Cross Language Perspectives on Speech Output and Motor Speech Disorders

Studies of MSDs in languages other than English are relatively infrequent. French, German, Japanese and Chinese probably number the most (see later chapters in this book). While some other languages are beginning to accumulate studies, the majority of languages in the world are not reported on at all. In addition, there is a significant lack of cross-language studies that investigate groups of speakers of different languages or examine the different languages of bi- and multilingual patients, with the aim of conducting a comparison of the breakdown in the respective languages to address an issue of theory or clinical importance.

One of the aims of this book is to stimulate work in that direction. One study that did take a cross-language perspective is Whitehill (2010). She emphasised the importance of performing cross-language studies in MSDs by reviewing studies on tone production and intonation in Mandarin and Cantonese Chinese speakers with cerebral palsy and Parkinson's disease and comparing them to the literature on English speakers. They noted, as might be surmised, that symptoms could be divided into language universals, i.e. features that were present across all the languages, and those that appeared to be determined by the phonology of the specific language, or more pertinently the tonal systems in this case. In view of the number of studies published about other languages, one would hope to already be able to perform more comparative studies from the existing literature. However, this task is hampered by the fact that there is a wide variety of research paradigms in use in the field of MSDs. Studies vary in the type and severity of MSD covered, the investigative parameter focused on (e.g. voice quality, intonation, vowel or consonant production, segment length, speech rate, rhythm, loudness and pitch features), the data collection tasks employed (e.g. single segment or word production, specifically structured phrases, reading, spontaneous speech, repetition) and the evaluation methods adopted (e.g. perceptual, acoustic, physiological). This renders transparent comparisons difficult at this stage.

In the absence of cross-language studies, or a sufficiently large pool of non-English language publications to base such comparisons on, the focus of this book is more towards an examination of the structural and operational differences across languages and how clinicians in those countries perform assessments, to inform future research in this area. However, by way of a more detailed introduction to cross-language studies in MSDs, the following section takes a look at the kinds of issues that arise in comparing speech across languages.

## Comparing speech output across languages

As already emphasised, while cross-language studies have not been absent from research into developmental and acquired communication disorders, within the narrower focus of MSDs there has been relative neglect. One reason for this disregard doubtless stems from the impression that speech motor control, and in parallel its dissolution, must already be universal and uniform across languages. It is easy to assume that controlling respiration, producing a vocal note, coordinating the tongue and lips must be the same for a speaker of Inuit as for a speaker of Maori, or any other language, and therefore impairment of respiration or other speech output processes must be identical across languages.

Why, for instance, should the underlying control of bringing the lips together for a /p/ or producing the vowel /i/ be any different in German to

Tamil? Are not the same muscles employed, presumably controlled by the same physiological networks irrespective of language context? Some sounds might exist in one language and not another, but the processes in planning and control, the muscles involved in producing the necessary movements must surely be invariable across languages? These assumptions are in many respects true, but with numerous qualifications, and the generalisation misses the vital point, that speech sounds never occur in isolation. They always exist and interact within a tightly structured speech sound system that in turn interacts with systematically structured semantic and morphosyntactic frameworks.

For the majority of people, the same left temporal–parietal–frontal axis of brain areas is engaged in language processing regardless of the language being spoken, but how disruptions in these networks manifest themselves are coloured by the filter of the structures employed in a given language. In parallel, control of movement operates identically across languages at the level of the neurophysiology and neuropsychology of control. However, the consequences of those breakdowns for disruption to the speaker's speech output and intelligibility interact with the sound structure of that language. The task of the researcher then is not only to view beyond the different surface characteristics of languages to discern the commonalities in control and execution, but also to understand how shared universal underlying impairments to speech output show themselves in the speech of someone from a given language.

Thus, whether one is a speaker of Yoruba, Sami, Navajo or Lardil, producing words with the correct sounds and with the appropriate stress and intonation patterns involves identical cortical motor planning and control regions, in tandem with subcortical inputs and reliance on nerve pathways between them and between them and the necessary muscles at the periphery. However, changes to articulator movement play into highly contrasting contexts and how that problem manifests itself in Greek compared to Malayalam is potentially quite dissimilar, differing in whether and where in speech it shows itself most prominently and whether or to what degree it creates a communication issue for speakers–listeners of a particular language.

Starting at a relatively superficial level, languages have different sound inventories, the sounds of French are not the same as Zulu or Vietnamese or Arabic. More importantly, there are differences in phonotactics, the distribution and combinatorial possibilities of sounds in different languages. In addition, the role of particular sounds and sound contrasts across languages differs. This variability is not restricted to segmental aspects. Languages contrast in the nature of their stress, intonation, rhythmic and durational structure, as well as their inventory, distribution and particularly the role of these suprasegmental features. The following paragraphs expand on some of these points and begin to highlight how a common underlying impairment may have divergent effects on different languages.

### Segmental sound contrasts

At the most superficial level, languages vary in what sounds they use. An English speaker with a MSD need not worry about implosives or clicks or unrounded high back vowels, German speakers do not have to deal with (inter)dental fricatives. What is more crucial though for understanding the relationship between an underlying disorder and its impact on intelligibility in different languages is the number of sounds a language uses and the distribution of their use, occurrence and contrasts.

Comparing two speakers of different languages, one may find, for instance, a comparable degree of impairment of tongue movement range, force, velocity and coordination for speech. One would, however, hypothesise that alterations in tongue placement accuracy will have a different impact in a language with a five-vowel contrast system (e.g. Spanish, Czech and Greek) compared to one with a contrast system well into the teens (e.g. Twi, German and Swedish) which demands much greater precision of tongue placement and coordination with lip positioning. Likewise, the repercussions of tongue movement alterations will vary across languages where there exists a two-way lingual contrast between velar and alveolar plosives vs languages that have a multiway (velar, palatal, palatal-alveolar, alveolar, dental) place distinction and maybe in addition manner distinctions at these places that require fine control to contrast blade, grooved, lateralised or retroflex articulations.

Equally vital for impact on intelligibility are differences in the distribution and combination of sounds. English and Swahili both have a /ŋ/ sound, but in English, unlike Swahili, this cannot occur in word initial positions. Both languages have /m/, /tʃ/ and /t/ sounds, but while the combinations /mtʃ/ (mchuzi, curry/sauce) and /mt/ (mtori, banana soup/porridge) at the start of a word are permissible in Swahili, they are not permissible in English. Such contrasts open the door for differential effects dependent on whether problems for instance affect syllable-initial or final sounds, or particular combinations of sounds within or across syllables.

A common consequence of MSDs concerns a difficulty with consonant to consonant transitions, whether within (**sk**i, i**nk**) or between syllables (hu**sk**y, i**nk**y). In turn the likelihood of whether transitions will be disrupted is subject to a number of factors (see Chapter 5) including syllable frequency and transitional probabilities – e.g. the sequence in English of /st-/ has a relatively high probability, which is more liable to confer relative robustness against derailment in the face of speech planning disturbances, while the sequence /sf/- in English is relatively infrequent and is expected to be more problematic where transitions are impaired.

Another aspect of sounds in combination is the phenomenon of coarticulation, the anticipation of elements of upcoming sounds in the movement/sound of earlier segments or the persistence of features of an earlier sound later in the string of movement/sound. Some of these are embodied in the spelling system – 'impatient' where an expected lingual 'n' sound is produced as a bilabial. Others pass by unnoticed by anyone apart from phoneticians – e.g. the different versions of /k/ in 'keep cool' (see below) influenced by upcoming front vs back vowels; the lip rounding on /s/ in 'swim' in anticipation of rounding for /w/. But alterations to coarticulatory processes are soon picked up by listeners in terms of their evaluation of formal vs informal talk, native vs foreigner or normal vs disordered speech. Consider the naturalness or reaction to, for instance, 'egg and bacon' that is uttered sounding every sound vs the more typical 'eggmbacon'; 'handbag' with every sound receiving equal emphasis vs the more usual 'hambag'; or 'swim' spoken with spread lips rather than rounded. Left to right coarticulation is probably determined by motor aspects, while right to left influences are more liable to represent phonological determinants. Importantly, though these coarticulatory processes look as if they are strongly dependent on local sound and movement factors at a relatively late stage in speech output control, they can actually vary significantly across languages. This suggests that aspects of a language's structure and execution (e.g. system of contrasts; rhythmic and timing qualities) play some role here and cross-language comparisons may have a lot to say (Manuel, 1999; Shin *et al.*, 2013).

The preceding paragraphs illustrate some key variations across languages in how sounds behave in sequence. However, the greatest differential effect of an impairment may be more likely to relate to the differing system of contrasts employed across languages. Even languages with the same or virtually the same sound inventory and combinatorial rules may well diverge in terms of what sounds contrast with which others to signal different meanings and, given that not all contrasts carry equal weight within and across languages, what consequences the loss of a particular distinction will have for speakers and listeners of that language.

Zulu and Hindi (see Chapters 9 and 14, respectively) offer an example. Both have aspirated and unaspirated versions of plosives. In standard British English these variations are determined by the position of a sound (e.g. /p/ aspirated in pit vs unaspirated in spit) or are secondary effects of more prominent contrasts (e.g. in English voiced /b/ has little aspiration vs heavily aspirated voiceless /p/). Although a problem with maintaining the aspirated–unaspirated distinction would lead listeners to hear an altered accent in English, it is unlikely to have major implications for understanding. Hindi, by contrast, employs a phonemic distinction between aspirated and unaspirated plosives and indeed the Hindi alphabet uses separate symbols for unaspirated–aspirated pairs of sounds. Aspirated vs unaspirated /k/ in Hindi are as different sounds to Hindi ears as /t ~ k/ is for English speakers, as shown in the contrast /kapi/ ('copy') vs /kʰapi/ ('meaningful'). A difficulty maintaining an aspirated–unaspirated distinction then is likely to be correspondingly more disruptive to Hindi speakers than to English ones.

Instances of where sound contrasts are linked to meaning contrasts in one language but not in another apply equally to vowel sounds. Vowel length provides a good example. In English, /i/ vs /i:/ as in leek vs league is determined by the following consonant – /li/ and /li:/ do not constitute different words in standard British English. In many languages though, this is precisely what happens, vowel length is phonemic, i.e. they attach meaning differences to short vs long vowels, see e.g. Japanese, Kannada, Czech, Finnish and even some varieties of English. Australian English, for example, is said to differentiate between ferry-fairy, cut-cart on the basis of vowel length rather than quality. Again, the consequences for intelligibility in speech disorders are clear. Difficulties maintaining length distinctions will have relatively little impact on understanding in English (though they may well have implications for naturalness or nativeness perception), but will do so in languages where such contrasts are an integral part of the sound contrast system.

These examples concern where one language attaches meaning change to a distinction, i.e. the contrast is phonemic, vs a language where the distinction is phonetic, without an accompanying meaning change. In other instances, two languages may both employ a given distinction to signal meaning change, but still be differentially impacted by an equivalent underlying impairment. For instance, one would expect soft palate problems that lead to difficulty maintaining nasality distinctions to impact differently in languages with an elaborate and extensive system of oral–nasal contrasts (French and Hindi for instance, see later chapters) compared to a language with few nasal contrasts (English); or a language with a rich system of contrasts between plosives and fricatives is liable to be more impacted by laxness of articulatory contacts than another language that does not maintain such a complex system. One further example would be akin to where e.g. in English the loss of the distinction between /Θ/ and /t/ or /Θ/ and /f/ is unlikely to be catastrophic for intelligibility – indeed many accents of English live quite happily without maintaining this distinction. However, loss of the contrast /s~t/ in English would be quite different, it being the basis of a highly productive contrast. In other words, it is not simply whether a particular language employs a given contrast, when it comes to cross-language differences in the effects of loss of that contrast it is more the frequency or centrality of that distinction to conveying meaning in that language.

## Suprasegmental sound contrasts

Divergent effects are not confined to segmental aspects of speech. Just as the inventory, distribution and system of contrasts around sound segments can be at variance across languages, so too they may differ in terms of inventory, distribution, use and realisation of stress and intonation patterns. There is the added dimension that in addition to lexical and grammatical meaning contrasts that might be signalled by stress and intonation differences, languages engage these features to also signal affective content variation and to lend prominence to certain words or syllables.

As regards lexical stress, some languages maintain highly predictable patterns – e.g. Polish on the penultimate syllable or Czech on the initial syllable in multisyllabic words. For others, Russian and English for instance, while there might be greater probability of stress falling at a particular locus, the predictability for any one word is far less clear. In some languages, stress is phonemic, i.e. used to signal meaning differences, as in Kinyambo, a Tanzanian Bantu language, or even Swedish (e.g. ['āndèn] (duck) vs ['āndê n] (spirit) – see Chapter 18). English has similar examples of phonemic stress contrasts such as 'object (as in 'a beautiful object' – noun) vs ob'ject (as in 'I object to this' – verb),' etc. However, as stress signals grammatical rather than lexical contrasts in English, i.e. the distinction between a noun and a verb or adjective, rather than two different nouns, misplacement of stress rarely has any impact on comprehensibility, as the context disambiguates the meaning. Moreover, in examples such as 'refuse/ re'fuse, 'content/con'tent, 'subject/sub'ject, there is also an alteration to vowel production as an automatic consequence of stress shift.

In languages where stress is phonemic, clearly MSDs associated with stress realisation difficulties will undermine conveying meaning. Even in languages where stress is not phonemic, assigning stress to the wrong syllable, stressing a syllable or word that would not normally receive prominence, not reducing a syllable that would typically be assigned less stress, can nevertheless lead to reduced intelligibility and/or reduced naturalness of speech (Martínez-Castilla & Peppé, 2010). Consider the phrase 'PEter moved the FURniture aROUND' spoken as 'PeTER moved THE furNIture Around'. To English listeners this would be perceived at least as out of the ordinary (and, depending on other clues in the environment, taken maybe as a foreign speaker of English or a speaker with a speech disorder). If inappropriate stress placement affects the perception of word boundaries, or results in changes in vowel quality, then comprehension may be affected.

Intonation entails a system of rising and falling movement in speech. Languages differ in their inventory of patterns. They also diverge in what degree of fall or rise is required by listeners to perceive an intended signal rise/fall. One language may require only a 25% rise in voice fundamental frequency to hear a rise, another a 50% rise. The degree of underlying impairment in pitch contour control will therefore have a correspondingly different effect across languages dependent on the language-specific parameters.

The exploitation of intonation variation is not confined to grammatical and affective contrasts. A very large proportion of languages in the world employ a system of tones to signal lexical meaning contrasts (Wong *et al.*, 2009). This topic is dealt with in detail in the chapters on Zulu and Tswana, Chinese and Japanese (Chapters 9, 10 and 15, respectively). Suffice it to say here that the system of tones that different languages employ is highly variable. They range from straightforward systems involving two- or three-way contrasts, e.g. between high and low or high, mid and low, to complex systems with five- or six-way contrasts entailing low and high rises, falls, combinations of rises and falls, as well as high vs low level realisation. Dependent on whether a language utilises tones and what system is involved, apraxia of speech and different kinds of dysarthria can be expected to exercise a differential effect.

In as far as stress and intonation patterns convey affective and social information, such changes can also exercise decisive differing consequences across languages in relation to the import and implications of given changes. Thus, flattening of intonation contours may lead to an impression of depression or indifference when none exists; reduced or excessive swings in intonation may be mistaken as indicating commands or doubt when these were not intended. Thus, even where intelligibility is not directly or appreciably compromised, these changes exert effects on activity limitation and participation (see below and Chapter 4). In as far as activity limitation and participation issues are strongly yoked to culture-specific conventions, once more the potential for cross-language divergence in effects is demonstrated.

## Phonation

Voice quality changes are a characteristic of most MSDs. Phonation may become more breathy where vocal cord approximation is too lax or excessively creaky where there is hypertonic approximation. When voice is affected it can lead to alterations in intelligibility, but even when this remains intact, changes can still lead to important differences in communication. Different voice qualities are employed to signal different affective states – reactions to someone speaking with a breathy tone are different to someone speaking with a modal or creaky tone. They indicate important gender, age and social messages. What precisely the nuances signal is of course language dependent, or even dependent on particular sub-speech communities within the overall language. Hence, once more, similar underlying changes in terms of physiological or acoustic parameters achieve differing effects depending on their impact on signalling crucial distinctions in a language.

Some languages, though, employ variations in voice quality phonemically. Zulu provides a good example (Chapter 9). Dinka (southern Sudan) too maintains a system of modal vs breathy vowels to distinguish meanings, as does Jalapa Mazatec (Mexico) and members of the Athabaskan family (USA), where creaky and breathy consonants contrast with each other. Similar to the impairments of segmental and suprasegmental speech production discussed above, changes to voice quality as a consequence of a neurological disorder can thus have an impact on communicative effectiveness, and more specifically the ability to signal meaning contrasts, in speakers of these languages.

## Broader implications

Without having delved into issues in any great detail, it is already possible to see how a cross-language perspective on MSDs may alter our understanding or beliefs around them. The Mayo classificatory system (Darley et al., 1975) that has held sway for several decades in the English-speaking world and has been adopted largely unquestioned into numerous other languages, rests on perceptual evaluations of American speech by a small number of American clinicians. Darley et al. classified different types of dysarthria according to the relative perceptual prominence of features such as imprecise consonants, hypernasality and monoloudness. It has been problematic to replicate the hierarchy of dimensions said to characterise different dysarthria types even in English, and even when employing the same recordings that Darley et al. utilised (Ludlow & Bassich, 1984; Zeplin & Kent, 1996; Zyski & Weisiger, 1987).

The reasons for this relate partly to well-attested listener perceptual artefacts and (mis)use of rating scales (Kreiman & Gerratt, 1998; Kreiman et al., 2007; Schiavetti, 1992), and underline the inter-listener variability that can occur even within one language. However, the cursory glance above at ways in which sound systems differ and the implications this has for how the same underlying impairments may manifest differently across languages illustrates that one might expect a different hierarchy of features and possibly even a different basis for perceptually distinguishing between putative subtypes of MSDs.

The same applies to the diagnosis of apraxia of speech, not just the classification of dysarthrias. Diagnosis of this disorder and its differentiation from types of dysarthria and from phonemic paraphasia has long been a bone of contention, as described in Chapter 3. Arguments have included what precisely are the pathognomonic features of apraxic speech; what features distinguish it from phonemic paraphasia, or for some, is there even a difference. Many of the debates centre on aspects of stress placement (e.g. are stressed or unstressed syllables more likely to be distorted or more difficult for apraxic speakers); the place in the syllable/word for maximum likelihood of derailment; rhythmic alterations; notions of increasing length and complexity; whether prosodic disturbance represents a primary symptom or is only secondary to other segmental disruptions. On the one hand, one may expect performances to differ across languages on these variables, but on the other hand such a comparison, across languages with fundamentally contrasting structures in these domains, should prove a decisive test for which features are distinctive, which are epiphenomena, which are unique to apraxia and which are shared with other MSDs.

These points apply not just to an evaluation of single sounds, syllables and words and distinctions between dysarthrias and the diagnosis of apraxia of speech. Cross-language evaluation of voice, even in speakers without disorders (Altenberg & Ferrand, 2006a; Gordon & Ladefoged, 2001; Hartelius et al., 2003; Scharff-Rethfeldt et al., 2008; Yamaguchi et al., 2003; Yiu et al., 2008), shows that although different languages exploit the same underlying parameters of pitch, loudness, voice quality, language- and cultural-specific filters act as powerful determinants of what will be judged as within or without normal variation. Such observations have implications for the assessment and interpretation of voice changes across languages. What in one language may constitute an undesirable level of hoarseness or an alteration to fundamental frequency may be perfectly acceptable in another, and not represent a target for intervention.

Furthermore, as was seen above, even before any listener perceptual effects become active, the very structure of a sound system may interact with an underlying disorder to produce a profile of change at variance with another language. People with Parkinson's disease may well evidence a reduced intonation and intensity envelope irrespective of which language they speak, or people with cerebellar lesions may experience alterations to the rhythmic qualities of their speech regardless of their native tongue. How these changes play themselves out across languages though can make decisive differences in terms of severity, profile, impact for the speaker and listener, and in turn implications for how and what (variables, items) one assesses and what the targets of intervention might be for speakers with Parkinson's disease or ataxia in the different languages. The example of SD above and the locus of dysfluency types portray these issues.

Finally, for similar reasons, given the different inventories of sounds across languages and, more centrally, given the different sound contrasts and the roles of those contrasts across languages, it would be no surprise that assertions and intelligibility tests based on English would not hold when applied to other languages. In terms of investigations of hierarchies of the fragility of sounds and sound contrasts in altering intelligibility, the order is likely to differ in association with the relative roles of those sounds, contrasts and combinations across different sound systems. Therefore, word and phrase tests, intelligibility items developed for one language that are simply translated into another language will lose all validity as well as their reliability (see comments in Chapter 12 vis-à-vis the shortcomings of an Intelligibility Test developed for French that was too closely tied to the original English items from which it was translated). Instead, what is required is the adaptation of items into other languages following underlying principles for test construction and assessment of a variable, but adjusted to the workings of the target language. Chapter 4 outlines methods to achieve this.

## Activity limitation and participation restriction

Attention so far has focused mainly on how impairment changes (i.e. changes in physiology, basic movement parameters) to speech may be manifest differently in diverse languages in association with between-language structural variations. There are though some crucial added dimensions that have already been hinted at, in which MSDs are liable to diverge across languages.

Arguments were presented for how similar underlying impairments may impact differentially across languages on perceived severity and intelligibility, and thereby differentially limit activities associated with speaking in that language. Turn-taking provides another example along these lines. It appears that there are universals in turn-taking patterns in conversations in terms of aiming for a minimal overlap of turns and a minimal gap between turns (Stivers et al., 2009). However, the mean gap tolerated between turns appears to vary across languages/cultures. What counts within the realm of acceptable for Danish or Lao (tolerant of relatively long lags) may be perceived as delayed or hesitant responses in languages with much shorter mean lags such as Tzeltal or Japanese. MSDs can alter the ability to initiate vocalisation, and therefore signal a start to a turn, either directly from motor factors or indirectly from cognitive-linguistic variables. Given the variance between languages in what length of lag is subjectively perceived as an immediate or delayed response, the door is opened for differential effects on interaction with the same underlying impairment across languages affecting getting into and staying in a conversation.

However, the impact of MSDs goes beyond these examples when it comes to activity limitation and participation restriction. It has also been alluded to that the same speech change in two speakers, even with speakers of the same language, may result in quite different issues in participation and impact. This relates to a complex knot of biopsychosocial factors.

This distinction and the non-linear relationship between the underlying impairment and its effects on activity, participation and impact has been formalised in the International Classification of Function (ICF) framework of disability. The framework has been applied in diverse fields of study and rehabilitation, including MSDs (Hartelius & Miller, 2011; Miller & Hartelius, 2011). The notion of different ICF levels (impairment, activity limitation, participation restriction) introduces the idea that cross-language differences are not focused simply on issues of phonology and phonetics, differences in kinematics, influences of different sounds inventories and combinations on speech output and perception and the like. Speaking activities do not occur in isolation. Speaking is a social activity; it is bound up with an intricate network of social and cultural values, views, conventions, attitudes and beliefs. Speech communities differ from the most subtle to the most marked ways in these dimensions.

Speech and language are intimately bound up with culture and society. Speech reflects our inner state, it transmits 'unspoken' conventions in interactions – empathy, deference, agreement, doubt, solidarity, distance, proximity, levels of formality, social and geographical origins, social and political sympathies, sexual orientation or intention, a whole range of affective states. In as far as conveying these messages rests on control of nuances in voice quality, prosody, rate of speech, loudness and articulatory precision, then MSDs impact on these levels of discourse as much as they do on movements of the tongue or vocal cords or on intelligibility. The associations between sound production and distortion and the social and psychological self and others exercise profound influences on what or who is perceived as disordered, on acceptability and on the subsequent place of an individual within a given speech community (Allard & Williams, 2008; Griffiths *et al.*, 2011; Jaywant & Pell, 2010; Miller *et al.*, 2006, 2008; Walshe & Miller, 2011).

However, what aspects of speech alteration disrupt what aspects of social discourse and in what manner and to what degree remain highly language, or more broadly, culture specific. Thus, a key additional perspective to cross-language studies of MSDs has to be the divergent relationship across languages between how different varieties of 'normal' speech and types and gradations of disordered speech are perceived by that speech community; what counts as a speech disorder in the first place; where the borderline lies between 'normality' and 'disorderedness'; along what dimensions judgements are made; what consequences that perception will have in terms of reception and perception of these speakers by their community, attitudes to them, how their roles and relationships will be altered; how their view of themselves as communicators may be affected. Such influences are well attested in the literature (Altenberg & Ferrand, 2006b; Bebout & Arthur, 1992; Fraas & Boyce, 2004; Ng *et al.*, 2012; Yiu *et al.*, 2008, 2011).

Given that the speech variables that signal social and psychological messages differ across languages, it follows that the same underlying motor speech impairment may be perceived as different across languages. Even where two languages share an articulatory or voice variable that signals social or psychological status, the threshold at which listeners perceive a difference arises is likely to vary.

At an even wider level, beliefs around speech and its control influence ideas on the cause and course of speech disorders and in turn visions of what should be done to remedy changes and who should or is able to accomplish that (Allard & Williams, 2008; Bebout & Arthur, 1992; Fredman, 2001; Mshana et al., 2008).

In conclusion, we see that the manifestation and consequences for intelligibility of a given underlying neuromuscular or speech motor control impairment can vary across languages dependent on the divergent structural elements of those languages. However, discussion of MSDs within a wider ICF levels model illustrates how the presentation and, more pertinently, the perception and reception of possible impairments impact on the position of the speaker within their speech community.

The focus of this book is more towards an examination of the structural and operational differences across languages and how clinicians in different countries perform assessments, it is towards investigating possible cross-language differences and seeking lessons for our understanding of MSDs. Discussion of activity limitation and participation matters are not given centre stage. However, we emphasise that a deep understanding of MSDs will never ensue without a full appreciation of these factors. Pursuance of this dimension represents a seriously neglected field, but it is hoped that the coming years will overturn that state of affairs. The next two chapters give an overview of what MSDs are and how they are managed from a speech-language pathology perspective. These provide an introduction for the more detailed chapters that follow.

## References

Allard, E.R. and Williams, D.F. (2008) Listeners' perceptions of speech and language disorders. *Journal Communication Disorders* 41, 108–123.

Altenberg, E.P. and Ferrand, C.T. (2006a) Fundamental frequency in monolingual English, bilingual English/Russian, and bilingual English/Cantonese young adult women. *Journal of Voice* 20, 89–96.

Altenberg, E.P. and Ferrand, C.T. (2006b) Perception of individuals with voice disorders by monolingual English, bilingual Cantonese-English, and bilingual Russian-English women. *Journal of Speech, Language and Hearing Research* 49, 879–887.

Bastiaanse, R., Bamyaci, E., Hsu, C.-J., Lee, J., Duman, T.Y. and Thompson, C.K. (2011) Time reference in agrammatic aphasia: A cross-linguistic study. *Journal of Neurolinguistics* 24, 652–673.

Bates, E., Wulfeck, B. and Macwhinney, B. (1991) Cross-linguistic research in aphasia – an overview. *Brain and Language* 41, 123–148.

Bates, E., Devescovi, A. and D'Amico, S. (1999) Processing complex sentences: A cross-linguistic study. *Language and Cognitive Processes* 14, 69–123.

Bebout, L. and Arthur, B. (1992) Cross-cultural attitudes toward speech disorders. *Journal of Speech and Hearing Research* 35, 45–52.

Bozic, M., Szlachta, Z. and Marslen-Wilson, W.D. (2013) Cross-linguistic parallels in processing derivational morphology: Evidence from Polish. *Brain and Language* 127, 533–538.

Chakraborty, R. (2012) Invariant principles of speech motor control that are not language-specific. *International Journal of Speech-Language Pathology* 14, 520–528.

Cho, T. and Ladefoged, P. (1999) Variation and universals in VOT: Evidence from 18 languages. *Journal of Phonetics* 27, 207–229.

Davies, R., Cuetos, F. and Rodriguez-Ferreiro, J. (2010) Recovery in reading: A treatment study of acquired deep dyslexia in Spanish. *Aphasiology* 24, 1115–1131.

Dworzynski, K., Howell, P. and Natke, U. (2003) Predicting stuttering from linguistic factors for German speakers in two age groups. *Journal of Fluency Disorders* 28, 95–113.

Erickson, K. and Sachse, S. (2010) Reading acquisition, AAC and the transferability of English research to languages with more consistent or transparent orthographies. *Augmentative and Alternative Communication* 26, 177–190.

Fraas, M. and Boyce, S. (2004) Perception of Spanish, Parkinsonian speech by English listeners. *The Journal of the Acoustical Society of America* 115, 2465–2466.

Fredman, M. and Miller, N. (2001) Communication disorders in multilingual populations. *Special edition Folia Phoniatrica* 53, 119–184.

Friedmann, N. and Shapiro, L.P. (2003) Agrammatic comprehension of simple active sentences with moved constituents: Hebrew OSV and OVS structures. *Journal of Speech Language and Hearing Research* 46, 288–297.

Gick, B., Wilson, I., Koch, K. and Cook, C. (2005) Language specific articulatory settings: Evidence from inter-utterance rest position. *Phonetica* 61, 220–233.

Gordon, M. and Ladefoged, P. (2001) Phonation types: A cross-linguistic overview. *Journal of Phonetics* 29, 383–406.

Griffiths, S., Barnes, R., Britten, N. and Wilkinson, R. (2011) Investigating interactional competencies in Parkinson's disease: The potential benefits of a conversation analytic approach. *International Journal of Language & Communication Disorders* 46, 497–509.

Hartelius, L., Theodoros, D., Cahill, L. and Lillvik, M. (2003) Comparability of perceptual analysis of speech characteristics in Australian and Swedish speakers with multiple sclerosis. *Folia Phoniatrica* 55, 177–188.

Hartelius, L. and Miller, N. (2011) The ICF framework and its relevance to the assessment of people with motor speech disorders. In A. Lowit and R. Kent (eds) *Assessment of Motor Speech Disorders* (pp. 1–20). San Diego, CA: Plural.

Haspelmath, M. (2010) Comparative concepts and descriptive categories in crosslinguistic studies. *Language* 86, 663–687.

Haspelmath, M. (2012) Escaping ethnocentrism in the study of word-class universals. *Theoretical Linguistics* 38, 91–102.

Hricová, M. and Weekes, B.S. (2012) Acquired dyslexia in a transparent orthography: An analysis of acquired disorders of reading in the Slovak language. *Behavioural Neurology* 25, 205–213.

Huang, K., Itoh, K., Kwee, I.L. and Nakada, T. (2012) Neural strategies for reading Japanese and Chinese sentences: A cross-linguistic fMRI study of character-decoding and morphosyntax. *Neuropsychologia* 50, 2598–2604.

Jaywant, A. and Pell, M.D. (2010) Listener impressions of speakers with Parkinson's disease. *Journal of the International Neuropsychological Society* 16, 49–57.

Klap, P., Marion, M.H., Perrin, A., Fresnel-Elbaz, E. and Cohen, M. (1993) Indications for botulinum toxin in laryngectomy. *Revue de Laryngologie Otologie Rhinologie* 114, 281–287.

Kreiman, J. and Gerratt, B.R. (1998) Validity of rating scale measures of voice quality, *Journal of the Acoustical Society of America* 104, 1598–1608.

Kreiman, J., Gerratt, B.R. and Ito, M. (2007) When and why listeners disagree in voice quality assessment tasks. *Journal of the Acoustical Society of America* 122, 2354–2364.

Laver, J. (1978) The concept of articulatory settings: An historical survey. *Historiographia Linguistica* 5, 1–14.

Lindblom, B. (2000) Developmental origins of adult phonology: The interplay between phonetic emergents and the evolutionary adaptations of sound patterns. *Phonetica* 57, 297–314.

Lindblom, B., MacNeilage, P. and Studdert Kennedy, M. (1983) Self-organizing processes and the explanation of phonological universals. *Linguistics* 21, 181–203.

Liu, C., Tardif, T., Wu, H., Monk, C.S., Luo, Y.-J. and Mai, X. (2013) The representation of category typicality in the frontal cortex and its cross-linguistic variations. *Brain and Language* 127, 415–427.

Lorch, M. and Whurr, R. (2003) Cross-linguistic study of vocal pathology: Perceptual features of spasmodic dysphonoia in French-speaking subjects. *Journal of Multilingual Communication Disorders* 1, 35–52.

Loukina, A., Kochanski, G., Rosner, B., Keane, E. and Shih, C. (2011) Rhythm measures and dimensions of durational variation in speech. *Journal of the Acoustical Society of America* 129, 3258–3270.

Ludlow, C. and Bassich, C. (1984) Relationships between perceptual ratings and acoustic measures of hypokinetic speech. In M. McNeil, J. Rosenbek and A. Aronson (eds) *The Dysarthrias: Physiology, Acoustics, Perception, Management* (pp. 163–195). San Diego, CA: College-Hill Press.

Macwhinney, B. (1987) Applying the competition model to bilingualism. *Applied Psycholinguistics* 8, 315–327.

Manuel, S. (1999) Cross-language studies: Relating language-particular coarticulation patterns to other language-particular facts. In W. Hardcastle and N. Hewlett (eds) *Coarticulation* (pp. 179–198). Cambridge: Cambridge University Press.

Martínez-Castilla, P. and Peppé, S. (2010) Cross-linguistic expression of contrastive accent: Clinical assessment in Spanish and English. *Clinical Linguistics & Phonetics* 24, 955–962.

Matsumoto-Shimamori, S. and Ito, T. (2013) Effect of word accent on the difficulty of transition from core vowels in first syllables to the following segments in Japanese children who stutter. *Clinical Linguistics & Phonetics* 27, 694–704.

Menn, L., O'Connor, M., Obler, L. and Holland, A. (1995) *Non-Fluent Aphasia in a Multilingual World*. Amsterdam: Benjamins.

Menn, L., Niemi, J. and Ahlsen, E. (1996) Cross-linguistic studies of aphasia: Why and how. *Aphasiology* 10, 523–531.

Menn, L. and Duffield, C.J. (2013) Aphasias and theories of linguistic representation: Representing frequency, hierarchy, constructions, and sequential structure. *Wiley Interdisciplinary Reviews: Cognitive Science* 4, 651–663.

Mennen, I., Scobbie, J.M., de Leeuw, E., Schaeffler, S. and Schaeffler, F. (2010) Measuring language-specific phonetic settings. *Second Language Research* 26, 13–41.

Miller, N., Noble, E., Jones, D. and Burn, D. (2006) Life with communication changes in Parkinson's disease. *Age Ageing* 35, 235–239.

Miller, N., Noble, E., Jones, D., Allcock, L. and Burn, D.J. (2008) How do I sound to me? Perceived changes in communication in Parkinson's disease. *Clinical Rehabilitation* 22, 14–22.

Miller, N. and Hartelius, L. (2011) Motor-speech disorders: Impact across the life span. In K. Hilari and N. Botting (eds) *The Impact of Communication Disability Across the Lifespan* (pp. 187–205). London: J&R Press.

Monzalvo, K. and Dehaene-Lambertz, G. (2013) How reading acquisition changes children's spoken language network. *Brain and Language* 127, 356–365.

Mshana, G., Hampshire, K., Panter-Brick, C., Walker, R. and Tanzanian Stroke Incidence Project Team (2008) Urban-rural contrasts in explanatory models and treatment-seeking behaviours for stroke in Tanzania. *Journal of Biosocial Science* 40, 35–52.

Natke, U., Sandrieser, P., van Ark, M., Pietrowsky, R. and Kalveram, K.T. (2004) Linguistic stress, within-word position, and grammatical class in relation to early childhood stuttering. *Journal of Fluency Disorders* 29, 109–122.

Ng, M.L., Chen, Y. and Chan, E. (2012) Differences in vocal characteristics between Cantonese and English produced by proficient Cantonese-English bilingual speakers—a long-term average spectral analysis. *Journal of Voice* 26, e171–e176.

Nickels, L. and Cole-Virtue, J. (2004) Reading tasks from PALPA: How do controls perform on visual lexical decision, homophony, rhyme, and synonym judgements?. *Aphasiology* 18, 103–126.

Paradis, M. (2001) The need for awareness of aphasia symptoms in different languages. *Journal of Neurolinguistics* 14, 85–91.

Robert, D. and Fernando, C. (2005) Acquired dyslexia in Spanish: A review and some observations on a new case of deep dyslexia. *Behavioural Neurology* 16, 85–101.

Sakurai, Y., Terao, Y., Ichikawa, Y., Ohtsu, H., Momose, T., Tsuji, S. and Mannen, T. (2008) Pure alexia for kana. Characterization of alexia with lesions of the inferior occipital cortex. *Journal of the Neurological Sciences* 268, 48–59.

Sato, H., Patterson, K., Fushimi, T., Maxim, J. and Bryan, K. (2008) Deep dyslexia for kanji and phonological dyslexia for kana: Different manifestations from a common source. *Neurocase* 14, 508–524.

Scharff-Rethfeldt, W., Miller, N. and Mennen, I. (2008) Unterschiede in der mittleren Sprechtonhöhe bei Deutsch/Englisch bilingualen Sprechern. *Sprache Stimme Gehör* 32, 123–128.

Schiavetti, N. (1992) Scaling procedures for the measurement of speech intelligibility. In R.D. Kent (ed.) *Intelligibility in Speech Disorders* (pp. 11–34). Amsterdam: Benjamins.

Shin, P., Warner, N.L., Hoffmann, M., McQueen, J. and Cutler, A. (2013) Perception of stressed vs unstressed vowels: Language-specific and general patterns. *The Journal of the Acoustical Society of America* 134, 4030.

Stivers, T., Enfield, N.J., Brown, P., Englert, C., Hayashi, M., Heinemann, T., Hoymann, G., Rossano, F., de Ruiter, J.P., Yoon, K.-E. and Levinson, S.C. (2009) Universals and cultural variation in turn-taking in conversation. *Proceedings of the National Academy of Sciences* 106, 10587–10592.

Tsegaye, M., De Bleser, R. and Iribarren, C. (2011) The effect of literacy on oral language processing: Implications for aphasia tests. *Clinical Linguistics & Phonetics* 25, 628–639.

Walshe, M. and Miller, N. (2011) Living with acquired dysarthria: The speaker's perspective. *Disability & Rehabilitation* 33, 195–203.

Weekes, B., Chan, A. and Tan, L. (2008) Effects of age of acquisition on brain activation during Chinese character recognition. *Neuropsychologia* 46, 2086–2090.

Whitehill, T. (2010) Studies of Chinese speakers with dysarthria: Informing theoretical models. *Folia Phoniatrica* 62, 92–96.

Wingate, M. (1979) The loci of stuttering: Grammar or prosody?. *Journal of Communication Disorders* 12, 283–290.

Wong, P.C.M., Perrachione, T.K., Gunasekera, G. and Chandrasekaran, B. (2009) Communication disorders in speakers of tone languages: Etiological bases and clinical considerations. *Seminars in Speech and Language* 30, 162–173.

Wulfeck, B., Bates, E. and Capasso, R. (1991) A cross-linguistic study of grammaticality judgments in Broca aphasia. *Brain and Language* 41, 311–336.

Yamaguchi, H., Shrivastav, R., Andrews, M.L. and Niimi, S. (2003) A comparison of voice quality ratings made by Japanese and American listeners using the GRBAS scale. *Folia Phoniatrica* 55, 147–157.

Yiu, E., Murdoch, B., Hird, K., Lau, P. and Ho, E. (2008) Cultural and language differences in voice quality perception: A preliminary investigation using synthesized signals. *Folia Phoniatrica* 60, 107–119.

Yiu, E., Ho, E., Ma, E., Verdolini Abbott, K., Branski, R., Richardson, K. and Li, N. (2011) Possible cross-cultural differences in the perception of impact of voice disorders. *Journal of Voice* 25, 348–353.

Zeplin, J. and Kent, R. (1996) Reliability of auditory perceptual scaling in dysarthria. In D. Robin, K. Yorkston and D. Beukelman (eds) *Disorders of Motor Speech* (pp. 145–154). Baltimore, MD: Brookes.

Zyski, B.J. and Weisiger, B.E. (1987) Identification of dysarthria types based on perceptual analysis. *Journal Communication Disorders* 20, 367–378.

# 3 Motor Speech Disorders: What are They?

## Anja Lowit, Nick Miller and Anja Kuschmann

There are numerous books and chapters that deal with all aspects of motor speech disorders (MSDs) (Duffy, 2013; Lowit & Kent, 2011; McNeil, 2008; Miller, 2010a; Yorkston *et al.*, 2010). This chapter provides a brief introduction to MSDs for the benefit of those who are not familiar with this type of communication breakdown. It also serves to define a number of concepts and highlight some of the controversies that exist in the MSD field which are mentioned in subsequent chapters. This introductory overview also outlines some of the approaches to management that are discussed in Chapter 4 and these will be picked up again at various points throughout the book. This chapter begins by expanding on the terms 'acquired', 'motor', 'speech' and 'disorder'. The principal division in MSDs is between dysarthria and apraxia of speech (AoS) and the middle part of the chapter takes a closer look at what these are said to represent in terms of taxonomies of MSDs and in terms of underlying pathological mechanisms. The broader social and neuropsychological contexts which are a precondition to a full understanding of MSDs are emphasised. We conclude with an exposition of a rationale for assessment and treatment.

## The Labels

As a prelude to examining the broad disorder types of dysarthria and AoS in more detail, this first section considers what lies behind the designation 'acquired motor speech disorder'.

*Acquired*: This denotes that the disorder arose at some point after normal speech development was underway or completed. It contrasts with congenital or developmental. While some have been tempted to draw parallels between developmental and acquired speech disorders, there are important contrasts. Consider, for instance, the contrasts between disruption to the emergence and establishment of a new, developing pronunciation system and the sensorimotor processes which support that vs the sudden or gradual breakdown of a system that has been fully up and running and the implications this has for what exactly is broken down or dysfunctioning. Consider too how impairment of a developing vs an already fully acquired system might interact differently with language, psychosocial and other factors that impact on the speaker and listener. Although there is clearly an area of overlap, both in theory and practice, the discussions in this book largely centre on instances where speech has been disrupted after it has been fully acquired.

*Motor*: Generally this term is used to contrast with structural (e.g. glossectomy; maxillofacial trauma) or psychogenic aetiologies (e.g. depression; functional speech disorders; feigning), and for some it contrasts with phonological and language disorders. But opinions vary on what is covered exactly by 'motor'. Does it only signify (alterations to) muscle tone, power and coordination? Does it extend to motor planning and control, or to sensory processes in control? The latter are certainly indispensable to motor functioning, and for this reason some prefer the term 'sensorimotor' disorder. In this book, we take motor to embrace planning and execution, including their sensory dimensions, as well as more purely neuromuscular aspects of underlying change. Of course, that raises multiple theoretical and practical issues when it comes to diagnosis and treatment. There is the issue of what exactly is planned, e.g. is it sound targets, space-time targets, phonemes, syllables or all or none of these? There are arguments around where does this planning take place – in the cortex, the subcortex or both? Debates over the relationship between planning and execution, phonology and phonetics, and so-called higher and lower levels in speech production enter here too – are phonological and motor planning one and the same; are they different but they interface; what is the nature of the interface? Many of these questions remain unanswered, and this work does not aim to settle them. However, we do aim to highlight where and how cross-language studies may be able to contribute to uncovering solutions to these issues.

*Speech*: 'Speech' signifies the medium, not the message, the means used to convey a message, not its content. It covers the production of speech segments as well as paralinguistic and suprasegmental aspects. Speech is generally contrasted with language, although as ever the boundary is blurred. There are the arguments about the motor vs language character of phonology. Certainly motor speech and language elements of communication may interact, e.g. processing costs or attention to the production of more complex syntactic and semantic structures can have a knock-on effect on articulatory accuracy; reduced breath and voice capacity may affect the length of utterances. In addition, speech changes may bear on pragmatic and discourse aspects of interaction, e.g. the ability to enter a conversation and maintain one's turn.

Speech performance also has an influence on listeners' perception of a person's psychosocial status. Quiet, slowed, monotonous, hesitant or slurred speech may be misconstrued by listeners as signs of depression, indifference, lack of motivation or cognitive incapacity.

Speech (associated with tongue, lip and jaw movements) is sometimes contrasted with voice (laryngeal or respiratory and laryngeal movements). In this book unless specifically stated, the tacit assumption is that both voice and speech will be affected.

*Disorders*: The word suggests something is wrong, not falling within the bounds of normal expectations. In terms of how far from 'normal' speech might be, there is a vast range – from speech being completely absent right through to changes hardly detectable by listeners or certain listeners may sometimes, under highly selective circumstances (when the speaker is tired, under emotional or time stress), feel they detect some mild distortion to some sounds. The big issue though concerns what counts as wrong, and where and what the bounds of normal expectations are. Notions of 'disorder', 'wrong' and 'normal bounds' all represent highly subjective, sociopolitically tendentious statements. Suffice it to say that there is not necessarily any one-to-one correspondence between scores on formal clinical tests, the clinician's opinion on the presence and degree of a disorder and the views of the individual speaker and their social circle. Whether a disorder exists or not and what the nature of that disorder might be ultimately rests on the perceptions of speakers and those who share their lives, and on societal attitudes and conceptions around speech disorders and people who show them. Furthermore, even within one community, one speaker or family might report no perceived communication problems in the face of very low scores on formal tests, while for another speaker the sense of change in their speech leads them to perceive a major disorder with wide-ranging implications for their whole lifestyle, despite test scores 'within normal limits'. Such individual differences have repercussions right the way through the diagnostic and rehabilitative process. Across languages too this underlines the fact that what in one language or speech community may be heard as disordered speech may in another be taken as unremarkable. This has clear implications for the development of assessment tools and the interpretation of results, especially evaluations that rely on the perceptual judgements of speakers or listeners as opposed to instrumental assessments of the acoustic or physiological dimensions of speech output.

The above gives a broad notion of what acquired, motor, speech and disorder might denote. What, though, are MSDs more specifically? As introduced previously the two broad categories of disorder normally linked to acquired MSDs are dysarthria and AoS. The following section takes a closer look at these labels.

## Dysarthria and AoS

*Dysarthria* denotes an articulatory disturbance which arises when neuromuscular impairment affects the working of any or all of the muscles of respiration, the larynx, velum, tongue, lips or jaw (Miller, 2010b). Neuromuscular disorders arise when central and/or peripheral nervous system damage (hence 'neuro') results in absent, diminished or abnormal innervation of the muscles (hence 'muscular'). Altered innervation changes muscle tone, power and coordination. Changes in tone may be in the direction of increased or decreased tone. Impairment of coordination comes from disturbance to the smooth alternation between the switching on and off of the contraction and relaxation of opposing muscle groups or disruption to the organisation of nerve impulses that determine the speed, direction, force and relative timing of movements.

The changes to tone, power and coordination in turn influence the speed, range, force and sustainability of movements, leading to loss or inaccuracy of articulatory movements. The resultant distortion or omission of sounds and syllables and the alterations to voice quality lead to what one hears as dysarthria.

For example, changes to lip and tongue movement may cause *tip* to be heard as *sip*, *hip* or *sieve*; *beach* to be heard as *eats*; *decide* as *sigh* or *say*. Changes in tone, power and coordination affecting the larynx alter the quality of phonation and the control of pitch and loudness. This may give an impression of loss of normal intonational rises and falls (sometimes termed monopitch) and blurring of contrasts between stressed and unstressed syllables (sometimes labelled monoloudness). Incoordination of movement can lead to other alterations of the normal flow of speech, of perceived changes in rhythm. Voice may be quiet or there may be inappropriate swings in pitch and loudness. Such changes can also be associated with changes to the respiratory function. The air needed to drive the articulators might be insufficient, or it is poorly regulated and/or escapes too quickly.

*AoS* (Miller & Wambaugh, 2011; Ziegler *et al.*, 2012) is defined in general as a problem with the volitional planning and control of movements for speech. Besides AoS, one can also find the equivalent terms articulatory dyspraxia, verbal dyspraxia and speech apraxia (and anarthria or cortical dysarthria in some French literature). In AoS, people describe their problem along the lines of: 'I know what I want to say, but I just can't say it. I tell my mouth to do one thing and it does another. Then when I don't want to say it I can do it'. In cases of isolated AoS, tone, power coordination, strength, sustainability and range of movement are all normal, thereby distinguishing it from dysarthria. The person knows what words they wish to say and can put them into grammatically well-formed sentences, hence dividing it from aphasia, a language disturbance affecting centrally syntax and semantics.

As suggested by 'volitional' in the definition, problems mount with the degree to which the person consciously thinks about speaking – the more they think about it, the more difficult it becomes. As a disorder of planning and control of speech actions, the central difficulty lies somewhere in the selection of target sounds and sound sequences and the movements required to produce them. Thus, apraxic speech can be described (note, not necessarily explained) by what sounds like false selection, or substitution, of sounds (*table* sounds like *cable*), false ordering (*Peter* sounds like *teper*), distortion (*tea* is heard as *tea* still, but it may sound very close to *Dee*, or the /t/ sound is very heavily aspirated) and apparent addition and omission of sounds (*street* sounds like *sptreet* or *seat*). Commonly, attempts to correct misdirected movements result in a visible or audible struggle and self-corrections. Apraxic speech is also typically characterised by the variability of sound realisation – on one occasion *tea* is produced like any other speaker would say it, but on others as *Dee, tsee, teat, ghee* or *ee*.

There is a long-standing debate on the differentiation between AoS and certain types of aphasia, both of which can result in the speech deviations mentioned for AoS above (Haley *et al.*, 2013; Miller & Wambaugh, 2011; Ziegler *et al.*, 2012). On the other hand, the distinction between dysarthria and AoS is generally considered to be much more certain, due to the presence of physiological impairment in the dysarthrias that is said to be lacking in (isolated) AoS.

These general characterisations offer a broad delineation of neuromuscular or dysarthric speech changes and apraxic, speech planning disorders. As already hinted, even this broad dichotomy is not without its challenges and controversies. Aside from the issues of speech vs language breakdown and what aspects of speech control constitute lower vs higher cortical dysfunction, MSDs can be described and classified from multiple perspectives, including site of lesion, acoustic or perceptual characteristics, physiological impairment types, neuropsychological presentation, psychosocial consequences and so forth. Furthermore, MSDs and the people who experience them are highly heterogeneous. They vary according to aetiology (stroke, tumour, head injury, many different neurological illnesses); nature of onset (sudden vs gradual) and course (unremitting decline, stepwise decline, gradual improvement to stable plateau of impairment or, exceptionally, to premorbid level). Some speakers may know they will not escape communication problems years before their onset (e.g. Friedreich's ataxia; Huntington's disease), for other families it is a bolt out of the blue. The speech picture may be accompanied by diverse disorders (language, swallowing, memory, attention, pain and many more difficulties). Underlying conditions may be amenable to surgical or medical amelioration or cure, while others have currently no effective cure. Medical and surgical interventions may or may not influence speech. The population embraces speakers with a flaccid neuromuscular condition, spasticity, ataxia, speakers with no neuromuscular disorder but instead difficulties planning movements for speech. Also to consider is the vast range of severity of speech-language impairment encountered, from no usable speech at all, to individuals who are indistinguishable from any other speaker except to their own mind's ear.

This holds decisive consequences for the assessment and management of MSDs. Although descriptions on any level are equally valid, their usefulness is dictated by what question one wants to answer, be it a clinical one, a research one, focused on underlying neurology, directed at psychosocial consequences or whatever. The relationship between levels of analysis is not linear and descriptions on one level are not explanations of changes on another. Further, what this also stresses is that it is probably rather artificial to isolate components of speech from each other (e.g. tongue movement from laryngeal function and breathing; breathing and respiration from signalling emotional content through prosody) and speech from the whole communication chain (phonation, listener perception and so forth). One can try and abstract various components for closer scrutiny, but in everyday life the production of the speech signal is intimately bound up not just with the planning and control of movement, but also with the syntactic and semantic message, the environment in which the message is conveyed, its perception by the listener and the attitudes of society. As a result, speech should not be understood merely by attending to (extracted elements of) the signal. It should be understood through the interaction of the message and the medium, of the speaker and the listener and in the interaction between the feelings of the speaker and the attitudes of society.

However, there are added issues. If classification into subtypes of disorder is to be anything more than totally arbitrary, there must be some support and a rationale stating why and on what basis one arrives at a given division. Typically this is through recourse to theoretical models, be they models of brain functioning, of neurophysiology, of linguistics, of self-perception and social interaction, of speech perception and production and their relationship and so on. The problem for the understanding of MSDs is that within any perspective for classification there are contrasting and competing theoretical claims.

The classification of AoS provides a classic example. On just about every level its definition and classification are disputed (Miller & Wambaugh, 2011; Ziegler *et al.*, 2012). Is it a language or a speech disorder; a phonological or phonetic disorder; a planning or an execution problem; a purely motor or a sensorimotor disturbance? If it is a phonological disorder, which approach gives the best account – linear, non-linear; generative, articulatory? If it is a planning disorder, where and how is the line drawn between planning and execution; can it in fact be drawn; what is planned and how; in what way do the units defined by psycholinguistic arguments relate to neurophysiological processes?

The issues are endless, but the arguments are not idle speculations for ivory tower theoreticians. They have fundamental implications for assessment and treatment. The answers to queries dictate the assessment tasks used to tease out behaviours that typify apraxia and differentiate it from other disorders, and lead to predictions about which techniques should work in therapy. So, a classification of AoS as a disorder of individual phoneme selection would entail assessment tasks that tap this function and therapy would be directed at elicitation and stabilisation of single sounds. Alternatively, if one classifies it as a problem in the selection and concatenation of syllables, assessment and treatment approaches would alter accordingly.

Much research has been generated and directed at these issues. The vast majority has entailed work focused on one language. However, using cross-language data that compare speakers with different language backgrounds and investigations into bilingual speakers with MSDs have the potential to provide decisive enlightenment on many of these issues. Such information can assist in uncovering which speech attributes relate to underlying neuropathology regardless of language, and which are determined by e.g. the phonological structure of a particular language. Common patterns associated with particular types of disorders might be more readily recognisable if they can be shown to exist across different languages; an underlying impairment might be better distinguishable from compensatory behaviours employed by a speaker to overcome underlying difficulties when one observes patterns of compensation across different languages.

## The Speaker's Perspective

We have discussed ways in which MSDs might be described and classified. However, there is another dimension that was hinted at when we expanded the notion of what counts as a speech disorder – the perspective, role and experience of the speaker. Descriptions of neuromuscular dysfunction, the range and speed of movement of the articulators, the perceived level of nasality, the rate of speech, omissions, distortions and so forth, all provide some information about a person's speech. The vital missing ingredient though is that they do not tell us whether any of this constitutes a problem for the speaker and their social circle, and if so, in what way, why and how severe. A further way therefore of describing MSDs (and for that matter any disorder) is in terms of the individual's own perspective. Do they perceive that a problem exists, in what ways are their daily activities limited because of the changes they perceive, what restrictions does that put on their participation in life, what impact does it have on them as a person and on their social circle?

These distinctions have been formalised by the World Health Organisation (WHO) in their classification of disability (Hartelius & Miller, 2011; Miller & Hartelius, 2011; Wambaugh & Mauszycki, 2010). The classification speaks of the impairments that affect body structures and systems, activity limitation and participation restriction (earlier WHO formulations spoke of impairment, disability and handicap which divided along slightly different lines).

In the context of MSDs, *impairment* refers to the loss or abnormality of the body structures or systems that support speech production, e.g. recurrent laryngeal nerve palsy and consequent vocal cord immobility; facial nerve conductivity and the consequent effects on power, speed and range of movement of facial muscles.

*Activity limitation* focuses on the way that a person's daily living activities are changed as a result of structural and systemic anatomical and physiological pathologies. Activities may be limited in terms of the nature and range of activities that the person can now perform, i.e. they cannot carry out all the things they used to. Further limitations can occur with regard to the quality of those activities in comparison with what might be acceptable for someone of a similar age, gender and social circumstances, i.e. they can still carry out activities, but not to the extent that they used to or need to. Furthermore, the duration of those activities can be affected, i.e. the person can still achieve satisfactory levels of functioning in certain activities, but only for short periods.

Regarding the nature and range of speech activities, one might consider for instance whether the person's ability to make themself understood (intelligibility) is altered, and in what ways this limits their ability to communicate in different situations (face-to-face; over the phone; in a group, etc.). Is the individual maybe intelligible, able to carry out the same range of activities as previously, but the quality of those activities is reduced? Speech and voice may no longer sound as natural or acceptable to listeners as previously, and this for its part may limit activities. As part of an assessment, one also needs to consider that other aspects of a disorder may limit a person's communication activities. This might arise from a lack of eye movement or visual acuity and perception, hearing loss, problems in using assistive or augmentive means of communication because of impaired arm function, or because of cognitive impairments undermining the intellectual capacity to acquire new skills.

Under *participation restriction*, one considers whether activity limitation has changed an individual's pattern of participation in society, their involvement in life situations, e.g. work, leisure, the family and the wider community. Note that here more than in the domains of impairment and activity limitation the focus is very much two way. The role of the interlocutor, laws, attitudes and customs in society and the physical environment in which a person exists can all determine the degree of participation restriction, in both a facilitatory and a hindering direction. The individual's personal reaction to the situation and internal and external adjustments they make also play a role.

In the past decade or so it has at last become adequately appreciated that a full appraisal of the implications of illness or change must address all these spheres of effect – impairment, limitations, restrictions, impact, the speaker, their family and friends (Baylor *et al.*, 2013; Hartelius *et al.*, 2008; Walshe *et al.*, 2009). A narrow focus on impairment description and classificatory labels and the speaker alone deliver a very blinkered view. Equally, ideas for rehabilitation derived from an impairment point of view are likely to be constrained, even misconceived or misdirected. This restricted view ignores the full implications of changes for all, and denies the richness of people's past, present and future existence, precluding a full understanding of what an individual and their family may or may not want from rehabilitation.

Many argue even further than that. Description and classification are irrelevant. The starting point, indeed the central and maybe only point, in understanding MSDs is the experience, the perception, the hopes and wishes of speakers themselves. Only through insight into a person's experience of their situation, of their past, their present and what it means for the person's vision for the future, can one even begin to appreciate what acquired MSD really means to the individual (Brady *et al.*, 2011; Miller *et al.*, 2006; Walshe & Miller, 2011; Yorkston *et al.*, 2008). Medically oriented models of illness dehumanise a very living experience. Pathologising changes heard in the listener's (clinician's) ear or indicated by instruments as fundamental frequency deviations, spirantisation, hypernasality and the like force the speaker into the role of object to be manipulated, to be rehabilitated to some notional norm.

This book is not the forum to elaborate on the debate between social and medical models, on which approach should be taken in classifying or managing someone's speech disorder. Nevertheless, the issues should be central to every clinician's understanding of acquired MSDs and their attitudes to individual speakers whom they label as having a speech 'disorder'. They are particularly crucial in decisions of what, where, when, how and why 'intervention' might be instigated.

Once more a cross-language perspective has much to offer in this respect. This is especially so since activity limitation, participation and impact are fundamentally influenced in general by culture and in particular by sociolinguistic aspects of language use, in which accent, pronunciation and changes to speech play a prominent role (Llamas & Watt, 2010; Wodak *et al.*, 2010). Culture defines what is taken as deviating from some social norm, and why that should pose a problem in the particular speech community. It defines what social consequences and impact there will be for the individual and their family and the individual's access to and participation in the ambient society. This is turn colours what might be the target of rehabilitation and the methods employed to achieve this. A narrower focus on variables in speech and voice output can highlight which features are crucial for attention in rehabilitation for a given speech community, but also show how this might vary across cultures. In Chapter 2, we noted how mean fundamental frequency and perceived pitch level, as well as differences in perceived voice quality can be evaluated differently by listeners from different cultures (even between different communities within the same language) (Altenberg & Ferrand, 2006; Hartelius *et al.*, 2003; Scharff-Rethfeldt *et al.*, 2008; Yiu *et al.*, 2008, 2011). In the same Chapter, we noted how the level of perceived nasality, degree of dysfluency, rate of speech, length of pauses and particular pronunciations of specific sounds are also candidates for investigations of cross-language differences of impact on activity and participation.

Wider societal and sociolinguistic issues furthermore become crucial when it comes to developing measures of impact of MSDs. Simple translation of instruments into another language is unlikely to suffice (Karimi *et al.*, 2011; McKenna & Doward, 2005; Stevelink & van Brakel, 2013; Wild *et al.*, 2005). Not only are the gradations of impact associated with given social, psychological and interactional variables and/or repercussions of given speech changes likely to diverge, the likelihood is that the very issues that are central to the perception and experience of impact will be decisively different across languages; views on why someone develops a speech disorder, what that says about their character and place in society, what one should do to remedy the believed departure from norms all will bear heavily on assessment and management here. These issues are straying somewhat from the central emphasis of this book, but certainly constitute matters that cannot be ignored and are further mentioned in relation to management in Chapter 4.

## A Rationale for Management

How do the foregoing sections help form our attitudes to the management of acquired MSDs? We have described the diversity of pictures that fall under the label of acquired neurogenic MSDs and the multitude of perspectives from which they might be described or explained. Among other things, this rich variability speaks against any blanket solutions for assessment and rehabilitation of the disorders. We have tried to emphasise that, especially as regards clinical management, MSDs happen to people, and a disorder constitutes a problem when it is perceived as impacting on that person's ability to function in life as they would wish. The starting point is the speaker-defined problem and goals. Outcomes for speech intervention will be measured against whether speaker-defined goals are attained. Between these points, a variety of assessment and rehabilitation approaches may be valid, but which, when and in what combination are driven by individual circumstances and aims, not by some set menu of management.

Obviously, other perspectives on MSDs and their assessment are relevant, rather than merely psychosocial and perceptual issues. We argue, though, that other assessment, especially of impairment variables, only becomes relevant and comprehensible once the wider context has been established. In rehabilitation, too, the focus on impairment, on acoustics, kinematics and physiology can only be fully understood, capitalised on and integrated into intervention when their relationship to speaker-led functional communicative aims is clearly defined. A cross-language perspective can assist in uncovering these issues. More broadly though, any language-specific analyses and cross-language comparisons have to be viewed in the wider sociolinguistic and sociocultural milieu. The next chapter now looks at some principles of management of MSDs in view of our discussion above.

## References

Altenberg, E.P. and Ferrand, C.T. (2006) Perception of individuals with voice disorders by monolingual English, bilingual Cantonese-English, and bilingual Russian-English women. *Journal of Speech, Language and Hearing Research* 49, 879–887.

Baylor, C., Yorkston, K., Eadie, T., Kim, J., Chung, H. and Amtmann, D. (2013) The Communicative Participation Item Bank (CPIB): Item bank calibration and development of a disorder-generic short form. *Journal of Speech, Language, and Hearing Research* 56, 1190–1208.

Brady, M., Clark, A., Dickson, S., Paton, P. and Barbour, R. (2011) The impact of stroke-related dysarthria on social participation and implications for rehabilitation. *Disability & Rehabilitation* 33, 178–186.

Duffy, J. (2013) *Motor Speech Disorders*. St Louis, MO: Mosby Elsevier.

Haley, K.L., Jacks, A. and Cunningham, K.T. (2013) Error variability and the differentiation between apraxia of speech and aphasia with phonemic paraphasia. *Journal of Speech, Language, and Hearing Research* 56, 891–905.

Hartelius, L., Theodoros, D., Cahill, L. and Lillvik, M. (2003) Comparability of perceptual analysis of speech characteristics in Australian and Swedish speakers with multiple sclerosis. *Folia Phoniatrica* 55, 177–188.

Hartelius, L., Elmberg, M., Holm, R., Lövberg, A. and Nikolaidis, S. (2008) Living with dysarthria: Evaluation of a self-report questionnaire. *Folia Phoniatrica* 60, 11–19.

Hartelius, L. and Miller, N. (2011) The ICF framework and its relevance to the assessment of people with motor speech disorders. In A. Lowit and R. Kent (eds) *Assessment of Motor Speech Disorders* (pp. 1–19). San Diego, CA: Plural.

Karimi, H., Nilipour, R., Shafiei, B. and Howell, P. (2011) Translation, assessment and deployment of stuttering instruments into different languages: Comments arising from Bakhtiar et al., Investigation of the reliability of the SSI-3 for preschool Persian-speaking children who stutter [J. Fluency Disord. 35 (2010) 87/–91]. *Journal of Fluency Disorders* 36, 246–248.

Llamas, C. and Watt, D. (eds) (2010) *Language and Identities*. Edinburgh: Edinburgh University Press.

Lowit, A. and Kent, R. (eds) (2011) *Assessment of Motor Speech Disorders*. San Diego, CA: Singular.

McKenna, S.P. and Doward, L.C. (2005) The translation and cultural adaptation of patient-reported outcome measures. *Value in Health* 8, 89–91.

McNeil, M. (ed.) (2008) *Clinical Management of Sensorimotor Speech Disorders*. New York: Thieme.

Miller, N. (2010a) Motor speech disorders. In J. Gurd, U. Kischka and J. Marshall (eds) *Handbook of Clinical Neuropsychology* (pp. 251–273). Oxford: Oxford University Press.

Miller, N. (2010b) Dysarthria. In J. Stone and M. Blouin (eds) *International Encyclopedia of Rehabilitation*. Buffalo, NY: Center for International Rehabilitation Research Information and Exchange (CIRRIE). See http:www.cirrie.buffalo.edu/encyclopedia/article.php?id=242&language=en (accessed March 2014).

Miller, N., Noble, E., Jones, D. and Burn, D. (2006) Life with communication changes in Parkinson's disease. *Age Ageing* 35, 235–239.

Miller, N. and Hartelius, L. (2011) Motor-speech disorders: Impact across the life span. In K. Hilari and N. Botting (eds) *The Impact of Communication Disability Across the Lifespan* (pp. 187–205). London: J&R Press.

Miller, N. and Wambaugh, J. (2011) Apraxia of speech: Nature, assessment, treatment. In I. Papathanasiou, P. Coppens and C. Potagas (eds) *Aphasia and Related Neurogenic Communication Disorders* (pp. 431–457). Boston, MA: Jones & Bartlett.

Scharff-Rethfeldt, W., Miller, N. and Mennen, I. (2008) Unterschiede in der mittleren Sprechtonhöhe bei Deutsch/Englisch bilingualen Sprechern. *Sprache Stimme Gehör* 32, 123–128.

Stevelink, S. and van Brakel, W. (2013) The cross-cultural equivalence of participation instruments: A systematic review. *Disability and Rehabilitation* 35, 1256–1268.

Walshe, M., Peach, R. and Miller, N. (2009) Dysarthria impact profile: Development of a scale to measure the psychosocial impact of acquired dysarthria. *International Journal of Language and Communication Disorders* 44, 693–715.

Walshe, M. and Miller, N. (2011) Living with acquired dysarthria: The speaker's perspective. *Disability and Rehabilitation* 33, 195–203.

Wambaugh, J.L. and Mauszycki, S.C. (2010) Application of the WHO ICF to management of acquired apraxia of speech. *Journal of Medical Speech-Language Pathology* 18, 133–140.

Wild, D., Grove, A., Martin, M., Eremenco, S., McElroy, S., Verjee-Lorenz, A. and Erikson, P. (2005) Principles of good practice for the translation and cultural adaptation process for patient-reported outcomes (PRO) measures: Report of the ISPOR task force for translation and cultural adaptation. *Value in Health* 8, 94–104.

Wodak, R., Johnstone, B. and Kerswill, P. (eds) (2010) *Handbook of Sociolinguistics*. London: Sage.

Yiu, E.M.L., Murdoch, B., Hird, K., Lau, P. and Ho, E. (2008) Cultural and language differences in voice quality perception: A preliminary investigation using synthesized signals. *Folia Phoniatrica* 60, 107–119.

Yiu, E., Ho, E., Ma, E., Verdolini, K., Abbott, R., Branski, K., Richardson, R. and Li, N. (2011) Possible cross-cultural differences in the perception of impact of voice disorders. *Journal of Voice* 25, 348–353.

Yorkston, K.M., Kuehn, C.M., Johnson, K.L., Ehde, D.M., Jensen, M.P. and Amtmann, D. (2008) Measuring participation in people living with multiple sclerosis: A comparison of self-reported frequency, importance and self-efficacy. *Disability and Rehabilitation* 30, 88–97.

Yorkston, K.M., Beukelman, D.R., Strand, E.A. and Hakel, M. (2010) *Management of Motor Speech Disorders in Children and Adults*. Austin, TX: Pro-Ed Inc.

Ziegler, W., Aichert, I. and Staiger, A. (2012) Apraxia of speech: Concepts and controversies. *Journal of Speech, Language and Hearing Research* 55, 1485–1501.

# 4 Motor Speech Disorders: Issues in Assessment and Management

Anja Kuschmann, Nick Miller and Anja Lowit

This chapter provides an overview of some issues in the management of motor speech disorders (MSDs), though with the focus lying more on assessment, given the paucity of treatment efficacy studies in general, and in a cross-language context in particular. As briefly mentioned in the preceding chapter, assessment of MSDs is ideally aligned with the International Classification of Functioning, Disability and Health (ICF) framework. This chapter is structured along those lines. It starts with some observations around evaluating impairment changes in relation to speech and voice, followed by an appraisal of their impact and participation restriction. The chapter presents general notions and suggestions about how such assessment be conducted based on research from the English language literature, but in each case will make reference to cross-language issues where appropriate. A special focus is given to general principles and factors that should be considered when attempting to adapt existing assessments to languages other than that which they were devised for. More detailed information of this sort with specific examples of published assessments appears for selected languages in the second part of the book.

## Impairment of Body Function

Clinically, once all parties have agreed that there is an issue with speech status, assessment commences with a diagnostic intelligibility examination to ascertain which segmental and non-segmental aspects of the speaker's output are influencing communication success and to what degree (Hustad, 2006; Miller, 2013). Following this, though, one is likely to need to apply targeted assessments of underlying physiological function to establish why particular contrasts (plosives vs fricatives; tongue tip vs dorsum, etc.) are impaired (see summaries in Aronson & Bless, 2009; Duffy, 2013; Lowit & Kent, 2011 and McNeil, 2008). This may uncover problems with e.g. range and/or rate of movement. Then, one wishes to understand why these variables are below par (e.g. due to hypertonia, bradykinesia), what implications this has for treatment (methods that tackle the underlying impairment situation, e.g. tone-reducing therapies would be inappropriate in cases of hypotonia) and what compensatory mechanisms might be available.

This is generally achieved through the use of speech motor tasks such as sequential and alternating repetition of single syllable words (e.g. pea, tea, key), producing words of increasing length and complexity (e.g. tie-tidy-tidily; ace-lace-place-placed), producing words with contrasting stress and intonation (e.g. a BIG dog vs a big DOG; 'yes' with rising vs falling intonation) and similar. Ability may be tested at habitual and maximum levels of performance and elicitation typically contrasts output to imitation with spontaneous speech, and single words with connected speech. There is debate concerning the degree to which the performance on such tasks relates to actual speech movements. Current consensus suggests verbal but non-speech tasks such as repetitions of /pa/, /ta/, /ka/ provide insights into underlying neuromuscular physiological impairment, but for closer correlation with natural speech, then real words are required. Certainly, if the tasks involve no speech element (i.e. they are non-verbal, e.g. stick out tongue, blow out cheeks) then the relevance to speech assessment is tenuous (McCauley et al., 2009; Powell, 2008; Weismer, 2006; Ziegler & Ackermann, 2013).

Through such assessments, one aims to disclose important information regarding differential diagnosis between underlying programming and neuromuscular disorders and subtypes within the broader categories. As this is not principally a book on the assessment of MSDs, we do not go into great detail here regarding speech motor assessment. Ample other dedicated books and chapters cover this (Aronson & Bless, 2009; Duffy, 2013; Lowit & Kent, 2011; McNeil, 2008; Yorkston et al., 2010).

As regards cross-language perspectives, since physiological function is language independent, there should be no specific considerations to attend to in terms of a speaker's language background – increased muscle tone or slowness of movement is increased tone or slowness whatever language one speaks. However, as emphasised before, cross-language variation starts to encroach when one considers the relative importance of (disturbances to) various speech subsystems and articulatory variables in different languages. Issues around resonance, for instance, are unlikely to be as disruptive to intelligibility in English compared to French; difficulties with consonant clusters probably do not exert as much influence on communication in languages with a predominantly CV syllable structure compared to ones with rich cluster possibilities; tongue dorsum movement should prove less of a hurdle in languages with fewer vs greater numbers of contrasts involving velar and pharyngeal contact/approximations. At least, these would be the assumptions. The definitive comparisons remain to be conducted.

# Activity Limitation

At this level, assessment focuses primarily on intelligibility and naturalness. As part of that process, segmental articulation and prosody are investigated for their appropriateness for individual speakers and to ascertain how far changes in these features impact on the ability of the person to make themself understood. The outcome of the examination here is an indication of whether, how far and which aspects of voice quality, intensity; speech rate, aspects of prosody; and loss of ability to (consistently) signal particular segmental contrasts are responsible for the curtailed activity. Bearing in mind that this volume is not a general textbook on the evaluation of MSDs, the challenges and practices of conducting such assessments are not detailed here, but are amply aired elsewhere (e.g. De Bodt *et al.*, 2002; Hustad, 2006; McHenry & Parle, 2006; Miller, 2013; Ziegler & Zierdt, 2008). The intention is to provide a brief overview of considerations that need to be taken when constructing suitable materials to use as diagnostic or explanatory intelligibility assessment in different languages.

## Constructing a diagnostic intelligibility assessment

An important consideration of assessment is that it should be diagnostic, i.e. not only should it highlight the presence, type and severity of the presenting disorder, but it should also provide the clinician with detailed information on what particular features contribute to the reduction in intelligibility and naturalness and where treatment should be targeted. In the case of intelligibility, this has been referred to as Explanatory or Diagnostic Intelligibility Testing (DIT) (Kent *et al.*, 1989; Yorkston & Beukelman, 1981). It should provide answers to questions such as:

- Which sounds does the person have difficulty producing/the listener have difficulty perceiving?
- More crucially, since sound systems and the transmission of information through speech are not built up on a system of sounds in isolation but rather sounds in contrast, which sound contrasts do the speaker and/or listener have difficulty discerning?
- In what syllable structures, syllable positions and words do problems arise?
- Which alterations to sound production have the greatest consequences for intelligibility, and therefore stand out as prime targets for intervention?

The boundary between intelligibility and naturalness of speech is blurred when it comes to alterations of non-segmental speech dimensions such as changes to e.g. loudness, pitch, intonation, rate or struggle behaviour, as these can have an impact on both factors. For reasons of simplicity, we will discuss all of these aspects under the heading of DIT for the remainder of this chapter.

## Evaluations of intelligibility

In terms of stimuli on which evaluations are based, there are principally two ways of assessing intelligibility – in single words and in connected speech. In terms of rating intelligibility, this may be based on rating scales of one kind or another or on word recognition and transcription tasks (again with different variations on this theme). Full details of the arguments around which (combinations of) methods deliver the optimum outcome for clinical assessment are aired elsewhere (Miller, 2013). The following outlines some of these issues in passing but focuses more on general design principles for DIT that can be applied across languages.

Connected speech assessments make use of sentences, reading passages and spontaneous speech samples. The latter has the greatest face validity due to its closeness to everyday speech production; however, it is also the most difficult to evaluate reliably, especially across time, and has little diagnostic value in terms of highlighting exactly which speech impairments result in the reduction of communication efficiency. Although reading passages are slightly better suited for such an analysis as at least the target production is known to the clinician, there are too many influencing factors involved in passage reading that are different to spontaneous speech to produce a clear picture of how segmental and non-segmental factors contribute to intelligibility. DIT is thus better done on the basis of single words, or well-controlled sentences, if connected speech is the focus of assessment (see below for suggestions). Evaluation of larger speech samples such as reading and spontaneous speech is of course essential in addition to DIT.

There is a wide range of literature covering aspects that need to be considered in the evaluation methods of such data (Borrie et al., 2011, 2012; Hustad, 2008; Lansford et al., 2011; Miller, 2013), and we will therefore not go into too many details at this point. Suffice to say that the clinician needs to choose the most reliable evaluation method possible. In terms of pinpointing therapeutic targets, rating scales do not provide any insights. They are also susceptible to a range of listener, speaker and speech tasks confounds that render them rather unreliable even for the overall task of rating the severity of intelligibility impairment (see references above). Recognition of unstructured (e.g. according to sound content, syllable structure and so forth) word lists is also an unreliable path to follow for reliable diagnostic purposes. In addition, any speech evaluation, even for well-constructed and applied diagnostic intelligibility tests, be it for single words or connected speech, will be more realistic if the listener judges the sample under adverse, and thus more natural listening conditions, e.g. in the presence of background noise, or if the speaker has been asked to produce the speech sample under dual-tasking conditions (Adams *et al.*, 2010; Bunton & Keintz, 2008; Dromey & Shim, 2008). Listener familiarity also needs to be taken into account, both with the speaker and the speech material, and it would be advantageous to collect evaluations from several types of judges, e.g. the clinician as well as the close family or carer.

Specific impairments of non-segmental aspects are equally difficult to judge from larger segments of speech, hence they are often grouped under the term naturalness and evaluated on the basis of scales or percentages. In addition, speech rate, pausing, overall volume and on occasion rhythm will be evaluated separately. Features such as intonation and stress placement are best assessed in shorter utterances in structured tasks such as contrastive stress exercises or question/answer minimal pairs.

When assessing connected speech, one should ensure that the speech material is representative of the speaker's language. Abberton (2005) advises that any text of about 1000 phonemes that is easy to read will be sufficient for a voice assessment. To investigate MSDs, more requirements should be fulfilled. In particular, reading passages should be phonetically balanced and include to the greatest extent the full range of a language's phonemes and representative range of sound combinations, all as far as possible in proportion to their occurrence in a language. To achieve complete phonetic balance, some more unusual words might have to be identified in order for the phoneme to occur in all possible positions (hence e.g. the inclusion of 'zest' in the Grandfather passage).

In addition, it is important that a range of utterance lengths is included to be able to gauge the speaker's breath support and pausing patterns, and that some prosodic contrasts are included. English language assessments frequently make use of the Grandfather passage (Reilly & Fisher, 2012) or the Rainbow passage (Fairbanks, 1960). Another prolific passage that can be found across a wide range of languages is 'The North Wind and the Sun' (International Phonetic Association, 1949) – though note that the International Phonetic Association version has simply translated the original into other languages, and not adapted the passage to the sound characteristics of those other languages. Abberton (2005) highlights this issue well in her comparison of different language versions of 'The North Wind and the Sun' where she found, for instance, different proportions of obstruents and sonorants which could potentially lead to different evaluations of speaker impairment.

More recent passages such as the Cherry Tree passage by Lowit *et al.* (2006) or the Caterpillar passage by Patel *et al.* (2013) have the potential to provide a more naturalistic speech sample and have a number of prosodic contrasts built in, which widens their scope. Any passage in principle is appropriate, but the prose style should invite a broad range of prosodic variation in addition to the representativeness of the segmental sound and syllable structure content. In the absence of any specifically developed reading passages in a given language, clinicians are advised to find a text, or design their own, that includes the above-mentioned features. Choosing a dialogue between speakers can aid with this, producing question-answer pairs, and allowing the inclusion of contrastive stress.

A major confound in connected speech intelligibility evaluation concerns the influence of semantic and syntactic clues to sounds. Solutions to this have encompassed devising lists of very low predictability sentences (McHenry & Parle, 2006), or sentences where identifying a target word still depends on sound processing and not syntactic or semantic cues (e.g. It's a picture of the bees/peas in the garden; that's my friend Don/John standing in the line/Rhein). Others have used story formats with scores for information accuracy to complement the speech analyses (Hustad, 2008).

Reading passages capture the performance on individual sounds and sound combinations in connected speech. Crucially, they also permit a detailed examination of prosodic and voice quality variables such as mean fundamental frequency, range and standard deviation; the same for intensity, and speech and articulation rate and rhythm (Kuschmann et al., 2011; Patel, 2011; White et al., 2011).

## Single-word intelligibility testing

Single-word intelligibility tests, or word recognition tests, have always been an important part of speech assessments. A speaker is given a list of words to produce (read; repeat; name pictures). The examiner or other listener counts the number of words or sounds correctly recognised, giving what appears to be a valid measure of intelligibility. The procedure generally achieves greater inter-rater reliability than the scaling methods or percentage judgements used for connected speech evaluation (Miller, 2013; Schiavetti, 1992). But, there are several factors in the construction and evaluation of some published lists that make the technique less than ideal as a valid and reliable measure of intelligibility and rather directionless when it comes to defining intervention targets.

Among early published lists, such as those from Robertson's (1982) *Dysarthria Profile* or Enderby's (1983) *Frenchay Dysarthria Assessment* and even some items in Yorkston and Beukelman's (1981) *Assessment of Intelligibility of Dysarthria Speech* (ASSIDS), there is typically little control of syllable structure, word length and familiarity, and sound contrasts covered. As a result, one might arrive at a more or less reliable quantification of percentage intelligibility (i.e. number of words correctly recognised). However, one cannot tell why the particular intelligibility level pertains; and one remains none the wiser about specific therapy goals. Such information is only provided by DIT, which, if well constructed, allows the examiner to gain insights into which aspects of speech production disturbance are leading to misunderstandings. The basic rationale is that intelligibility rests not so much on the production of isolated sounds out of context, but of being able to signal/hear sound contrasts in different word and phrase contexts. A speaker may not be able to pronounce /s/ accurately, but if listeners still discern a contrast between it and say /t/ or /ʃ/, even if they would not pass their phonetics exam with it, then this deviation from the norm may not be so important, as the speaker remains functionally intelligible. If, however, the ability of the speaker to produce and the listener to perceive a contrast is impaired, then a problem with intelligibility may exist.

In creating word lists for DIT, sets of words are chosen that oblige the speaker to make, and the listener to hear, distinctions between sound contrasts vital for the language they speak. Sets are constructed containing items that differ in terms of place of articulation, manner of articulation, syllable structure, stress pattern and so forth. So, items might be derived by systematically building up sets that depend on discriminating +/– voice (pear bear), +/– oral (mare bear), +/– obstruent (pear fair), tongue tip vs dorsum contact (key tea); differentiating them in varying positions in the word (pat-bat, pat-pad; seek-teak, case-Kate), in different syllable structures (skate state spate) and different lengths of word (lie-rye, light-right, flight-fright, flying-frying; A's-aid, raise-raid, raising-raiding, braising-braiding).

In this way, one might arrive at a set such as *main, wane, vein, feign, pain, bane, sane, Shane, Dane, Teign, lane, rain, Jane, chain, cane, gain* as one of the items to look at word initial place and manner contrasts for English. One important issue to consider when constructing the word list is not just to arrive at pools of similar sounding words such as the above, but that the options presented to the listener encompass phonologically important contrasts for the language. This is an important distinction between e.g. the Multiword Intelligibility Test (MWIT) (Kent *et al.*, 1989) and the ASSIDS (Yorkston & Beukelman, 1981). In the MWIT, the choice of the wrong target word by the listener will inform the examiner about what phonetic contrast is impaired, whereas the ASSIDS word pools are insufficiently controlled in that way and serve purely to ensure that listeners do not become familiar with the word set the patient produces.

Note, not all of the contrasts necessarily comply with the strictest phonetic definition of a minimal pair. For instance, *bear* and *pear* in English differ not only in voice onset time, but also in aspiration. Nevertheless, the aim is to examine contrasts that are functionally significant for listeners and speakers of a language. The issue of functional significance is a very important consideration when DIT lists are collated. Besides English language DIT versions, other tests have been developed for languages along similar lines, e.g. German (Ziegler & Hartmann, 1993), Danish (Petersen, 1997) and French (Gentil, 1992). Although these tests are constructed with the same principles, they contain different sets of phonetic contrasts, as briefly discussed above. German, for example, has a wider variety of fricatives than English, which need to be considered; French has the oral/nasal distinction; and Chinese will need to take account of tones in addition to segmental contrasts. Equally, there might be contrasts that are unimportant for English but that have significance in another language, either because a particular phoneme does not exist, because it is phonotactically not appropriate in the particular contexts, or because listeners are less likely to identify fault with a production because the two sounds might be in complementary distribution in certain dialects in the language. This is particularly prominent in vowel contrasts.

Ideally, DIT word lists should thus be properly validated via research studies. Despite recent developments (Fraas, 2002; Lillvik *et al.*, 1999; Miller *et al.*, 2012; and see Chapters 12, 17 and 18), few such tools exist for languages other than English. The clinician who is faced with a lack of standardised methods and needs to construct their own DIT should ensure to take the following factors into account when choosing the phonetic contrasts to be included in their list or when weighing up the worth of lists compiled by someone else. The following lists some desiderata for the construction of intelligibility tests:

- Do the items adequately reflect the range of sounds, vowels included, found in the local language/accent?
- More importantly, do items reflect as closely as possible the relative frequency with which particular sounds and sound contrasts occur and the positions in which they come. A list overladen with /t~Θ/ initial or /n~ŋ/ final contrasts will give a very distorted impression of someone's intelligibility for English.
- Does the list cover the range of syllable structures and word lengths found in the language and reflect their approximate relative frequency? A list of all CVC for English will give as biased a reading as a list made up exclusively of complex 4+ syllable words. It should be noted, however, that the sound structure of English is relatively favourable when it comes to selecting minimal pairs, even in two-syllable words. For other languages this is not the case.
- Do the levels of difficulty cover the range of disability likely to be met?
- Are there sufficient items to make the test valid and sensitive? One can hardly achieve a representative list of sounds, positions and syllable structures in 10 or even 20 items.

- Are the targets and foils balanced across common and less frequent words? If the target is always the high-frequency member of a set (always *key, joke, teacher* rather than varying with *ghee, yoke* and *teaser*), a false reading may arise simply because listeners tend to choose familiar items in single-word recognition tests.
- Do the foils represent the kinds of contrasts which listeners mistake and the kinds of contrasts that speakers may find difficult? Items searching the ability to contrast /m~k/ are not required for English, whereas one will most likely need several to look at contrasts of /s~t~ts~st/ in varying syllable positions.
- Are the contrasts that are used valid for the local accent? The following may be minimal pairs in standard received pronunciation (RP) British English, but not in the bracketed places – *grader-grater* (New York, Belfast), *tin-thin* (Dublin), *fin-thin* (London), *bike-bake* (Wellington), *chalk-choke* (Todmorden), *him-hem* (Glasgow). Conversely, homophones in one dialect may be minimal pairs elsewhere. *Saw-sore* are homophones in Sydney and London, but not in English accents where /r/ is pronounced; *dew-jew* sound the same in British RP accent but not in Edinburgh, Leicester or Toronto; in some accents *hood* pairs with *hoot* in others with *hut*.
- Avoid items in the test that are problematic to pick up (on sound recording) even when spoken by speakers without motor speech problems (e.g. CVm ~ CVn ~ CVng; f~th; s~th). This adds another item to the desiderata, that there is control data for the word lists based on speakers of similar age and background and scored via the same methods (live, from recordings, etc.) employed in the test administration.

The following boxes are ideas for four items from a test. These sets highlight just four possibilities. A full test would comprise sets looking at many more variables appropriate for a given language.

*Vowel contrasts (for a non-rhotic accent)*

| hit | het | hid | hoot | height | hood |
|-----|------|-------|------|--------|-------|
| hurt | hot | heat | hard | hat | heart |
| hut | head | heard | hide | hod | heed |

*Place and manner of articulation for final consonants in VC words*

| ache | ate | aim | ape | aid | ale |
|-------|-------|-----|-----|-----|-----|
| aigue | aitch | a | age | ace | ain |

*Consonant clusters word initial and final*

| scream | seem | seemed | creams | reams | screamed |
|--------|-------|---------|---------|-------|----------|
| seams | cream | creamed | screams | ream | scree |

*Word medial/second syllable onset manner and place contrasts, with coincidental w~r contrast word initially*

| raping | waiting | rating | raking | whaling | raving |
|--------|---------|--------|--------|---------|--------|
| raiding | raining | raging | waking | wading | railing |
| waving | waging | raising | weighing | waning | racing |

In order to score a DIT, listeners judge which word they think they heard, either by circling the word from among the particular minimal pair set (or word pool) on a score sheet (termed closed response form), or they make a free choice from all words in the language (open response form). There is little to indicate whether circling a word from a restricted choice or free recognition gives a more valid or reliable picture, but differences in outcomes can be expected depending on the severity of the speaker and the evaluation method chosen. Closed scoring methods appear to add more sensitivity in the severe range, open scoring in the milder range (Vigouroux & Miller, 2007; Yorkston & Beukelman, 1978).

Clearly, it is not practical to administer interminable word lists designed to cover every last sound, sound combination and position. More typically, DITs are based on a fair range of contrasts and number of items from which one can judge whether a speaker/listener has difficulties with a particular variable. To then confirm this, clinicians construct probe tests of say 30 items around the specific feature (e.g. place of articulation in word final position, oral~nasal distinction in word initial position, high~mid vowels) to gain greater insight into whether the distinction really does present a problem, much in the same fashion that one might carry out supplementary naming tests focusing just on word frequency or imageability variables.

Intelligibility and naturalness (of voice, rate and so forth) provide a vital piece in the jigsaw of assessment. What impairment-directed speech motor assessments and activity limitation intelligibility and naturalness tests do not tell one is whether, and if so how or why a given speech profile impacts on the life of the speaker and their social circle. It is well recognised that MSDs also impact on lifestyle, employment and social networks, and carers can be similarly affected, with further repercussions for well-being (Bloch & Wilkinson, 2009; Brady *et al.*, 2011; Dickson *et al.*, 2008; Hartelius *et al.*, 2008; Miller *et al.*, 2006, 2011; Walshe & Miller, 2011). On top of this, it is also well attested that the clinical severity of the MSD does not bear a linear relationship to the level or nature of impact. It is perfectly common to find speakers who have, from formal clinical testing a severe speech disorder, but for whom social intercourse and feelings about self as a communicator have scarcely altered; conversely, some speakers with changes to their speech and voice that are barely perceptible to listeners may experience major social and psychological consequences because of them (Baylor *et al.*, 2013; Miller *et al.*, 2008; Yorkston *et al.*, 2007). We now turn to some issues in the evaluation of these factors.

# Impact and Participation Restriction

Assessment of the impact of a communication disorder on a person is a relatively new field, and accordingly, few profiles have been established for that purpose, especially ones with a sound psychometric base (Eadie *et al.*, 2006). Impact assessment essentially tries to establish to what degree a communication disorder affects a person's communication-related, health-related, and general quality of life [QOL]. QOL is a multifaceted concept which encompasses personal as well as external factors. These encompass changes in identity and self-esteem, including the person's role in the family and their relationship with others. Often, such changes lead to associated changes such as depression or anxiety. As alluded to in the previous chapter, the consequences of MSDs can include anger and frustration about how speech has changed, fear of communication, a negative self-image and feelings of isolation and loneliness. Capturing such a wide range of factors is a complex endeavour and a range of tools might have to be used to gather a holistic picture of how the individual is affected by their communication problem.

Several measures have been developed, including Baylor *et al.* (2013), Hartelius *et al.* (2008) and Walshe *et al.* (2009) and reviews appear in Miller and Hartelius (2011) and Walshe (2011). In contrast to the fixed question format of Walshe *et al.* and Hartelius *et al.*, the Communicative Participation Item Bank (CPIB) (Baylor *et al.*) takes an item-specific, patient-reported, outcome measure information system approach that is built on research with particular speaker groups to include communication situations specifically identifed by them as posing issues in communication. The specificity of the CPIB for particular types of disorders highlights the need to tailor the sensitivity of impact and participation profiles to the needs of individual speakers. This not only applies across different types of MSD, but it is also likely to apply to speakers with different language and cultural backgrounds.

Speech, its roles, its nuances and its uses are intimately tied up with cultural conventions and norms. Again, taking a cross-language perspective predicts that impact and participation measures devised for one culture are unlikely to apply wholesale to speakers in another culture – even for subcultures of speakers of the same language. The role(s) of speech, what is conveyed and how, in daily living are likely to differ The roles and responsibilities channelled through speech may well vary. Beliefs about why speech changes arise and what should be done about them and who that should be may differ from culture to culture, alongside attitudes to and beliefs about disability in general. Family roles and responsibilities might be different and in turn determine the relative impact of an MSD on an individual and their family. Olivares and Altarriba (2009) refer to notions such as 'familismo', pervasive in Hispanic communities in the USA, dictating that decision-making favours the whole family instead of having the patient's best interest at heart (Brice, 2002), and this in turn may be in conflict with the health professional's clinical decision-making structures.

Self-perception can also be significantly affected by the attitudes of those close to the individual (Allard & Williams, 2008; Bebout & Arthur, 1992; Overby et al., 2007; Walshe & Miller, 2011). Bebout and Arthur (1986) for example found that listeners born outside North America were more likely to think that a person with a communication disorder was emotionally disturbed or could do better if they tried harder, than those born in North America. Altenberg and Ferrand (2006) report that bilingual English–Chinese and English–Russian listeners (most of whom were born outside the USA) perceived the same level of voice disorder more negatively than monolingual English listeners, and differed in terms of their assignment of personality traits such as 'lovable or clean'. Altenberg and Ferrand (2006) interpret this as showing different levels of acceptance of the disorder across cultures, a fact which might have significant implications for the individual's self-perception and confidence and the support they receive from those around them.

In short, even with an assessment as apparently generic as QOL or impact scales, it is not appropriate to employ an assessment developed for one language and with individuals from one cultural background with persons from another milieu. In the absence of profiles specifically devised for a particular language, the development of new or parallel tools can follow the methodology of other instruments (e.g. DIP, Dysarthria Impact Profile). Part of this entails starting at the very beginning in terms of establishing the dimensions along which impact and participation vary in the culture of the speakers that the tool is intended for; setting items and the tool overall within the cultural attitude and belief systems of the culture around disability in general and communication and speech changes in particular. Even where instruments appear relatively culture independent and where it seems justified to simply translate from one language to another, there are still recognised ways of translating  and checking that the items are still valid in the target language/culture (Karimi et al., 2011; Stevelink & van Brakel, 2013; Wild et al., 2005). Unchecked and culturally unadjusted translation is never an option.

The components of the assessment process will have established if there is a problem around speech and voice; and if so, what kind of problem, with respect not only to the underlying causes but also in relation to the impact on a person's life. Assessment details what variables are affecting communication for the speaker and their social circle, what they want to do about it and what avenues will be used to arrive at their goals and thereby lay the foundations for intervention.

It is not within the scope of this book to give a detailed exposition of the management of the many problems that people with MSDs present with. There are ample textbooks available on this (see references at the start of the chapter). As with many other disorders, establishing conclusive evidence for the effectiveness of these techniques remains a work in progress. We conclude this chapter with brief comments on the role cross-language studies might play in advancing the field of treatment.

Cross-language studies of the efficacy of particular treatments outside of English are presently scarce. Some techniques, such as methods to improve breath control or alter voice quality may show positive generalisation outside of the original language in which they were devised. However, it does not always follow that they will always be equally successful in another language. The case of rate control provides a case in point. Rate control can improve intelligibility in English. In Chapter 15, we see how certain methods of rate control are exquisitely suited to the rhythmic quality of Japanese and attain gains beyond what many have found for English. A study by Lee and McCann (2009) demonstrated that phonation therapy was more effective in improving intelligibility in Mandarin Chinese than English for two speakers with dysarthria. Although this study was based on limited participant numbers, it highlights the fact that certain techniques have the potential to be more effective in one language than another.

The more a treatment focuses on variables specific to a particular language as opposed to more universal aspects of speech motor control, the less one would expect it to apply equally well across languages. At least, that would be the prediction from Chapter 2 – this speculation is in need of confirmation by many more studies in the field. Some evidence for the assumption is available in the germane field of cross-language and bilingual studies of aphasia therapy, but at the same time this evidence points to issues being somewhat more complex than simply language specific vs language universal. A similar literature needs to develop in the MSD arena.

Treatment programmes do not take place in isolation from the culture in which they are conceived. One might therefore also expect that a therapy approach with a strong cultural bias in terms of how it is implemented, even if it has a strong evidence base for success in one language, may not realise the same degree of success in another setting. An example is provided by the Lee Silverman Voice Treatment (LSVT) programme (Sapir et al., 2011). There is no reason to doubt that the basic technique (attention to effort, think loud) would be applicable and successful irrespective of language. However, its implementation as described in the LSVT manual and training courses is strongly biased towards US cultural norms, practices and values. Experience demonstrates that these pose challenges to therapy fidelity even in the same language but a different culture, let alone across languages and cultures. Beyond that, there are obviously matters concerning the huge range of service delivery models across the globe which may not suit the programme either.

Use and provision of alternative and augmentative communication (AAC) devices (aside from financial and technological barriers) represent another area where cross-language investigations are liable to contribute significantly, for instance in speech recognition, text to speech and speech to text technologies and so forth.

# Conclusion

This chapter has focused on how to assess MSDs, indicating important aspects for consideration when developing equivalent materials for other languages. Although MSDs arise in association with impaired physiological function, we have highlighted the importance of having well-developed tools at one's disposal to describe performance status on other levels and how language-specific issues are likely to impact on the development of these tools. The same assumptions may apply to therapy techniques and materials. Even where therapy techniques appear eminently suited to other languages, therapists should nevertheless monitor treatment outcomes closely when adapting techniques that have been researched in other languages.

The second part of this book will not only present what kind of assessments are available in a selection of languages, but also provide basic information on the phonology of each language, to provide readers with information on its important features as well as differences to English, which should allow them to construct DITs themselves if no published resources are available.

## References

Abberton, E. (2005) Phonetic considerations in the design of voice assessment material. *Logopedics, Phoniatrics, Vocology* 30, 175–180.

Adams, S.G., Winnell, J. and Jog, M. (2010) Effects of interlocutor distance, multi-talker background noise, and a concurrent manual task on speech intensity in Parkinson's disease. *Journal of Medical Speech-Language Pathology* 18, 1–8.

Allard, E.R. and Williams, D.F. (2008) Listeners' perceptions of speech and language disorders. *Journal of Communication Disorders* 41, 108–123.

Altenberg, E.P. and Ferrand, C.T. (2006) Perception of individuals with voice disorders by monolingual English, bilingual Cantonese-English, and bilingual Russian-English women. *Journal of Speech, Language and Hearing Research* 49, 879–887.

Aronson, A. and Bless, D. (2009) *Clinical Voice Disorders* (4th edn). New York: Thieme.

Baylor, C., Yorkston, K., Eadie, T., Kim, J., Chung, H. and Amtmann, D. (2013) The Communicative Participation Item Bank (CPIB): Item bank calibration and development of a disorder-generic short form. *Journal of Speech, Language and Hearing Research* 56, 1190–1208.

Bebout, L. and Arthur, B. (1992) Cross-cultural attitudes toward speech disorders. *Journal of Speech and Hearing Research* 35, 45–52.

Bloch, S. and Wilkinson, R. (2009) Acquired dysarthria in conversation: Identifying sources of understandability problems. *International Journal of Language & Communication Disorders* 44, 769–783.

Borrie, S.A., McAuliffe, M.J., Liss, J.M., Kirk, C., O'Beirne, G.A. and Anderson, T. (2011) Familiarisation conditions and the mechanisms that underlie improved recognition of dysarthric speech. *Language and Cognitive Processes* 27, 1039–1055.

Borrie, S.A., McAuliffe, M.J. and Liss, J.M. (2012) Perceptual learning of dysarthric speech: A review of experimental studies. *Journal of Speech, Language and Hearing Research* 55, 290–305.

Brady, M.C., Clark, A.M., Dickson, S., Paton, G. and Barbour, R.S. (2011) Dysarthria following stroke – the patient's perspective on management and rehabilitation. *Clinical Rehabilitation* 25, 935–952.

Brice, A.F. (2002) *The Hispanic Child: Speech, Language, Culture, and Education*. Boston, MA: Allyn & Bacon.

Bunton, K. and Keintz, C. (2008) Use of dual task paradigm for assessing speech intelligibility in clients with Parkinson's. *Journal Medical Speech-Language Pathology* 16, 141–155.

De Bodt, M.S., Huici, M. and Van De Heyning, P.H. (2002) Intelligibility as a linear combination of dimensions in dysarthric speech. *Journal Communication Disorders* 35, 283–292.

Dickson, S., Barbour, R.S., Brady, M., Clark, A.M. and Paton, G. (2008) Patients' experiences of disruptions associated with post-stroke dysarthria. *International Journal of Language and Communication Disorders* 43, 135–153.

Dromey, C. and Shim, E. (2008) The effects of divided attention on speech motor, verbal fluency, and manual task performance. *Journal of Speech, Language, Hearing Research* 51, 1171–1182.

Duffy, J. (2013) *Motor Speech Disorders* (3rd edn). St Louis, MO: Mosby Elsevier.

Eadie, T.L., Yorkston, K.M., Klasner, E.R., Dudgeon, B.J., Deitz, J.C., Baylor, C.R. and Amtmann, D. (2006) Measuring communicative participation: A review of self-report instruments in speech-language pathology. *American Journal of Speech-Language Pathology* 15, 307–320.

Enderby, P. (1983) *Frenchay Dysarthria Assessment*. Austin, TX: ProEd.

Fairbanks, G. (1960) *Voice and Articulation Drillbook* (2nd edn). New York: Harper & Row.

Fraas, M. (2002) Intelligibility testing of native Spanish speaking adults. *Journal of the Acoustical Society of America* 112, 2359.

Gentil, M. (1992) Phonetic intelligibility testing in dysarthria for the use of French-language clinician. *Clinical Linguistics & Phonetics* 6, 179–189.

Hartelius, L., Elmberg, M., Holm, R., Lovberg, A.S. and Nikolaidis, S. (2008) Living with dysarthria: Evaluation of a self-report questionnaire. *Folia Phoniatrica* 60, 11–19.

Hustad, K. (2006) Estimating the intelligibility of speakers with dysarthria. *Folia Phoniatrica* 58, 217–228.

Hustad, K.C. (2008) The relationship between listener comprehension and intelligibility scores for speakers with dysarthria. *Journal of Speech, Language, Hearing Research* 51, 562–573.

International Phonetic Association (1949) *The Principles of the International Phonetic Association*. London: International Phonetic Association.

Karimi, H., Nilipour, R., Shafiei, B. and Howell, P. (2011) Translation, assessment and deployment of stuttering instruments into different languages: Comments arising from Bakhtiar et al., Investigation of the reliability of the SSI-3 for preschool Persian-speaking children who stutter [J. Fluency Disord. 35 (2010) 87–91]. *Journal of Fluency Disorders* 36, 246–248.

Kent, R., Weismer, G., Kent, J. and Rosenbek, J. (1989) Toward phonetic intelligibility testing in dysarthria. *Journal of Speech and Hearing Disorders* 54, 482–499.

Kuschmann, A., Miller, N., Lowit, A. and Mennen, I. (2011) Assessment of intonation In A. Lowit and R. Kent (eds) *Assessment of Motor Speech Disorders* (pp. 253–268). San Diego, CA: Plural Publishing.

Lansford, K.L., Liss, J.M., Caviness, J.N. and Utianski, R.L. (2011) A cognitive-perceptual approach to conceptualizing speech intelligibility deficits and remediation practice in hypokinetic dysarthria. *Parkinson's Disease* 2011, 150962.

Lee, T. and McCann, C. (2009) A phonation therapy approach for Mandarin-English bilingual clients with dysarthria. *Clinical Linguistics & Phonetics* 23, 762–779.

Lillvik, M., Allemark, E., Karlstrom, P. and Hartelius, L. (1999) Intelligibility of dysarthric speech in words and sentences: Development of a computerised assessment procedure in Swedish. *Logopedics Phoniatrics Vocology* 24, 107–119.

Lowit, A., Brendel, B., Dobinson, C. and Howell, P. (2006) An investigation into the influences of age, pathology and cognition on speech production. *Journal Medical Speech-Language Pathology* 14, 253–262.

Lowit, A. and Kent, R.D. (eds) (2011) *Assessment of Motor Speech Disorders*. San Diego, CA: Plural Publishing.

McCauley, R.J., Strand, E., Lof, G.L., Schooling, T. and Frymark, T. (2009) Evidence-based systematic review: Effects of nonspeech oral motor exercises on speech. *American Journal of Speech Language Pathology* 18, 343–360.

McHenry, M.A. and Parle, A.M. (2006) Construction of a set of unpredictable sentences for intelligibility testing. *Journal Medical Speech-Language Pathology* 14, 269–271.

McNeil, M. (ed.) (2008) *Clinical Management of Sensorimotor Speech Disorders*. New York: Thieme.

Miller, N. (2013) Measuring up to speech intelligibility. *International Journal of Language and Communication Disorders* 46, 613–624.

Miller, N., Noble, E., Jones, D. and Burn, D. (2006) Life with communication changes in Parkinson's disease. *Age Ageing* 35, 235–239.

Miller, N., Noble, E., Jones, D., Allcock, L. and Burn, D.J. (2008) How do I sound to me? Perceived changes in communication in Parkinson's disease. *Clinical Rehabilitation* 22, 14–22.

Miller, N., Andrew, S., Noble, E. and Walshe, M. (2011) Changing perceptions of self as a communicator in Parkinson's disease: A longitudinal follow-up study. *Disability & Rehabilitation* 33, 204–210.

Miller, N. and Hartelius, L. (2011) Motor-speech disorders: Impact across the life span. In K. Hilari and N. Botting (eds) *The Impact of Communication Disability Across the Lifespan* (pp. 187–205). London: J&R Press.

Miller, N., Mshana, G., Msuya, O., Dotchin, C., Walker, R. and Aris, E. (2012) Assessment of speech in neurological disorders: Development of a Swahili screening test. *The South African Journal of Communication Disorders. Die Suid-Afrikaanse tydskrif vir Kommunikasieafwykings* 59, 27–33.

Olivares, I. and Altarriba, J. (2009) Mental health considerations for speech-language services with bilingual Spanish-English speakers. *Seminars in Speech and Language* 30, 153–161.

Overby, M., Carrell, T. and Bernthal, J. (2007) Teachers' perceptions of students with speech sound disorders: A quantitative and qualitative analysis. *Language Speech and Hearing Services in Schools* 38, 327–341.

Patel, R. (2011) Assessment of prosody. In A. Lowit and R.D. Kent (eds) *Assessment of Motor Speech Disorders* (pp. 75–96). San Diego, CA: Plural Publishing.

Patel, R., Connaghan, K., Franco, D., Edsall, E., Forgit, D., Olsen, L. and Russell, S. (2013) "The Caterpillar": A novel reading passage for assessment of motor speech disorders. *American Journal of Speech Language Pathology* 22, 1–9.

Petersen, E.F. (1997) Phonetic intelligibility testing in dysarthria. Validity and reliability of listeners' perceptions. *Logopedics Phoniatrics Vocology* 22, 105–117.

Powell, T.W. (2008) Epilogue – An integrated evaluation of nonspeech oral motor treatments. *Language Speech and Hearing Services in Schools* 39, 422–427.

Reilly, J. and Fisher, J.L. (2012) Sherlock Holmes and the strange case of the missing attribution: A historical note on "The Grandfather Passage". *Journal of Speech Language and Hearing Research* 55, 84–88.

Robertson, S. (1982) *Dysarthria Profile*. Bicester: Winslow.

Sapir, S., Ramig, L.O. and Fox, C.M. (2011) Intensive voice treatment in Parkinson's disease: Lee Silverman Voice Treatment. *Expert Review of Neurotherapeutics* 11, 815–830.

Schiavetti, N. (1992) Scaling procedures for the measurement of speech intelligibility. In R.D. Kent (ed.) *Intelligibility in Speech Disorders* (pp. 11–34). Amsterdam: Benjamins.

Stevelink, S.A.M. and van Brakel, W.H. (2013) The cross-cultural equivalence of participation instruments: A systematic review. *Disability and Rehabilitation* 35, 1256–1268.

Vigouroux, J. and Miller, N. (2007) Intelligibility testing: Issues in closed versus open format scoring. *Newcastle and Durham Working Papers in Linguistics* 12, 83–95.

Walshe, M. (2011) Psychosocial impact of acquired motor speech disorders. In A. Lowit and R.D. Kent (eds) *Assessment of Motor Speech Disorders* (pp. 97–122). San Diego, CA: Plural Publishing.

Walshe, M., Peach, R. and Miller, N. (2009) Dysarthria impact profile: Development of a scale to measure the psychosocial impact of acquired dysarthria. *International Journal of Language and Communication Disorders* 44, 693–715.

Walshe, M. and Miller, N. (2011) Living with acquired dysarthria: The speaker's perspective. *Disability & Rehabilitation* 33, 195–203.

Weismer, G. (2006) Philosophy of research in motor speech disorders. *Clinical Linguistics & Phonetics* 20, 315–349.

White, L.R., Liss, J. and Dellwo, V. (2011) Assessment of rhythm. In A. Lowit and R.D. Kent (eds) *Assessment of Motor Speech Disorders* (pp. 231–252). San Diego, CA: Plural Publishing.

Wild, D., Grove, A., Martin, M., Eremenco, S., McElroy, S., Verjee-Lorenz, A. and Erikson, P. (2005) Principles of good practice for the translation and cultural adaptation process for patient-reported outcomes (PRO) measures: Report of the ISPOR task force for translation and cultural adaptation. *Value in Health* 8, 94–104.

Yorkston, K.M. and Beukelman, D.R. (1978) A comparison of techniques for measuring intelligibility of dysarthric speech. *Journal of Communication Disorders* 11, 499–512.

Yorkston, K. and Beukelman, D. (1981) *Assessment of Intelligibility of Dysarthric Speech*. Tigard, OR: CC Publications.

Yorkston, K.M., Baylor, C.R., Klasner, E.R., Deitz, J., Dudgeon, B.J., Eadie, T. and Arntmann, D. (2007) Satisfaction with communicative participation as defined by adults with multiple sclerosis: A qualitative study. *Journal of Communication Disorders* 40, 433–451.

Yorkston, K.M., Beukelman, D.R., Strand, E.A. and Hakel, M. (2010) *Management of Motor Speech Disorders in Children and Adults* (3rd edn). Austin, TX: Pro-Ed Inc.

Ziegler, W. and Hartmann, E. (1993) The Munich Intelligibility Profile (Mvp) – Reliability and validity. *Nervenarzt* 64, 653–658.

Ziegler, W. and Zierdt, A. (2008) Telediagnostic assessment of intelligibility in dysarthria: A pilot investigation of MVP-online. *Journal of Communication Disorders* 41, 553–577.

Ziegler, W. and Ackermann, H. (2013) Neuromotor speech impairment: It's all in the talking. *Folia Phoniatrica* 65, 55–67.

# 5 Using English as a 'Model Language' to Understand Language Processing

## Michael S. Vitevitch, Kit Ying Chan and Rutherford Goldstein

## Introduction

In biological research, *model organisms* are non-human species that are extensively used to study phenomena that are difficult to study in humans for ethical or practical reasons. Model organisms are often chosen because, among other characteristics, they are readily available and amenable to experimental manipulation. Research with model organisms provides valuable insight into the mechanisms that underlie certain processes, and enables researchers to explore potential causes and treatments for human disease. However, care must be taken when generalising from one organism to another because small differences between organisms may have very large consequences. For example, the human and chimpanzee genomes are approximately 98% identical, but there are substantial differences between humans and chimpanzees with regard for instance to language use, culture and technology (The Chimpanzee Sequencing and Analysis Consortium, 2005).

In the language sciences, the analogue to a model organism might be a *model language*. One candidate for a model language is English. Consider that speakers of English are readily available in the form of undergraduate students enrolled in introductory courses of psychology, communication disorders and linguistics at several thousands of colleges and universities in the USA alone; students enrolled in such courses often have a 'research requirement' that can be fulfilled by participating in ongoing research projects. English is also amenable to experimental manipulation because of the many and extensive databases of information related to English words (e.g. word frequency counts of Kucera and Francis [1967]; Phonotactic Probability Calculator of Vitevitch and Luce [2004]; Child Mental Lexicon Calculator of Storkel and Hoover [2010]). Indeed, a search of the supplementary material archives of the journal *Behavior Research Methods* (http://springerlink.com/content/1554-351x/) using the keyword 'English norms' produced over 200 'hits' to word lists, pictures, word associations and other stimuli related to the English language.

Although psycholinguistic studies of English have provided much insight into the mechanisms that underlie both normal and disordered language processing, there are several characteristics of English (spoken as a first language by around 335 million people worldwide) that may limit how broadly studies using this model language can generalise to the other 6000 or so languages found in a diverse range of language families (e.g. Indo-European, Sino-Tibetan, Afro-Asiatic, Austronesian) spoken by the other six billion or so people on the planet.

In the present chapter, we will discuss several characteristics of English that are primarily phonological in nature – the phonemes that are found in the inventory of each language, the sequential constraints on those phonemes (sometimes referred to as *phonotactics*), syllable structures, the typical length of words, the phonological similarity among words and the frequency with which words occur in the language – and consider how these characteristics influence normal and disordered processing during the perception and production of speech in English. We will also explore these characteristics and their influence on normal and disordered processing in selected other languages. Finally, we will evaluate the implications of these findings for the assessment, treatment and understanding of motor speech disorders.

## Phonological Segments and Sequences

The number and type of phonemes found in the languages of the world can vary greatly. For example, English and Spanish have about the same number of consonants (although not exactly the same ones), but differ in the number of vowels used in each language. English uses about 20 vowels (e.g. /ɑ ɔ e ɛ ɪ i ʊ u o æ ʌ/), whereas Spanish uses only five vowels (/a e i o u/). For clinically oriented resources regarding the phoneme inventories of several commonly spoken languages, see http://www.asha.org/practice/multicultural/Phono.htm.

Being aware of potential differences that may exist among phoneme inventories has much clinical relevance when treating individuals who are bilingual, because it is well-known that phonemic contrasts that exist in a second language are difficult to perceive and produce if they do not exist in the native language (note, this difficulty is not a clinical condition). A classic example is the difficulty that native speakers of Japanese have in distinguishing the /r/–/l/ contrast in English, because no such contrast exists in Japanese (e.g. MacKain *et al.*, 1981). Note, however, that difficulty may not exist in both modalities (i.e. an individual can produce the contrast, but cannot perceive it) and may vary across word positions

(Sheldon & Strange, 1982). The use of high-variability training procedures, in which many different speakers produce the contrast in many different words and in many different positions across words has been shown to be effective in the training of non-native contrasts in second language learners, and may be useful in training other populations as well (Bradlow et al., 1999).

In addition to processing being influenced by *which* phonemes occur in a language, the *sequences* of phonemes that occur in words in a language, known as the phonotactics of a language, also influence processing. Certain sequences are 'legal' in a given language, such as the cluster /lb/ in the coda of English words (like the word 'bulb'), whereas other sequences, like /lb/ appearing in the onset of a word in English, are 'illegal' in a given language, making them difficult (if not impossible) to perceive or produce correctly (Berent et al., 2008).

Among the sequences of phonemes that are legal in a given language, there is still much variability in the frequency with which sequences occur in the language. For example, the sequence of phonemes /gʌ/ (found in words like *gull* and *gush*) is more common in English than the sequence of phonemes /ʃʌ/ (found in words like *shove* and *shun*). The frequency with which segments and sequences of segments occur in the language is known as *phonotactic probability* (Vitevitch et al., 1997). Although many studies in English have demonstrated that phonotactic probability influences word learning in typically developing children and in children with phonological disorders (Storkel, 2001, 2004), non-word repetition (Gathercole et al., 1999), word recognition in normal and hearing-impaired adults (Vitevitch & Luce, 1999; Vitevitch et al., 2002; for a *magnetoencephalographic* [MEG] component sensitive to phonotactic probabilities see Pylkkänen et al. [2002]) and word production in normal adults and in children who stutter (Anderson & Byrd, 2008; Vitevitch et al., 2004), comparatively less work has examined the influence of phonotactic probability on language processes in other languages (however, see Zamuner [2009] for work in Dutch).

Focusing just on processes related to speech production, it is typically found that words (and specially constructed non-words) comprising segments and sequences of segments that are commonly found in the language (i.e. they have high phonotactic probability) are produced more quickly and accurately than words (and specially constructed non-words) that have low phonotactic probability. For example, Vitevitch et al. (2004) used a picture-naming task – a task commonly used in psycholinguistic research to examine the processes involved in speech production in which participants see a black and white line drawing appear on a computer screen and must name the object they see (e.g. 'dog') as quickly and accurately as possible – and found that pictures named with words that had high phonotactic probability had faster response latencies than pictures named with words that had low phonotactic probability.

Another commonly used task is a repetition task, where a participant hears a word or a non-word and must repeat it as quickly and accurately as possible. This task is widely assumed to assess aspects of perceptual processing, but has also been used to assess other processes including short-term memory and speech production. For example, Gathercole *et al.* (1999) found that English-speaking children (7–8 years old) more accurately repeated non-words with high phonotactic probability than with low phonotactic probability. Consider now the results of Zamuner (2009), who asked Dutch-speaking children (approximately 2 years old) to engage in a non-word repetition task. Similar to the findings of Gathercole *et al.* (1999) with English-speaking children, Zamuner found that overall repetition was more accurate in Dutch non-words with high phonotactic probability than with low phonotactic probability.

With regard to measures of speech production, Munson *et al.* (2005) found that English-speaking children (ages 4–7 years) produced vowels with shorter durations in non-words with high phonotactic probability than in non-words with low phonotactic probability. Although this work was in children, there was no difference in vowel duration between the younger and older children, suggesting that this effect is not age dependent. Furthermore, phonotactic probability may have implications for various motor speech disorders in adults. Indeed, Lallini and Miller (2011) found in adults with speech impairment acquired after a stroke that repetition accuracy was greater for English words and non-words with high phonotactic probability than for words and non-words with low phonotactic probability.

## Syllable Frequency and Structure

Models of speech production (dating back to Fromkin [1971]) generally agree that multiple levels of representation and processing are involved in the production of speech. More controversial is what those levels of representation are, and whether those levels of representation interact in some way during processing (cf. Dell, 1986; Levelt *et al.*, 1999). Among the levels of representation involved in speech production, Levelt *et al.* (1999) proposed a mental syllabary, or a lexicon containing the gestural programs of commonly used syllables in a given language.

Motivation for a mental syllabary comes from several sources of evidence. Using corpus analyses, Levelt *et al.* (1999) reported that a small number of syllables are used in Japanese and Chinese, whereas Dutch and English use over 12,000 different syllables in the language. Given the frequency with which certain syllables are used, Levelt *et al.* suggested that processing effort could be reduced by simply retrieving precompiled gestural programs instead of generating anew for each syllable the required gestural program. Indeed, Levelt *et al.* further reported that in English about 80 different syllables accounted for about 50% of a speaker's output, and 500 syllables accounted for about 80% of a speaker's output. Gestural programs would only be generated 'on the fly' for novel or less common syllables in the language, which are not stored in the syllabary.

Given the apparent economy of retrieving precompiled gestural programs from the syllabary rather than generating anew gestural programs for each utterance, it is perhaps not surprising that influences of syllable frequency have been observed in a number of languages, including French (Laganaro & Alario, 2006), Spanish (Carreiras & Perea, 2004), Dutch (Levelt & Wheeldon, 1994) and German (Aichert & Ziegler, 2004). For example, Levelt and Wheeldon (1994) found faster naming latencies for words consisting of high-frequency syllables than words containing low-frequency syllables, even when word frequency was controlled for. It should also not be surprising that influences of syllable frequency have been observed in (German-speaking) individuals with apraxia of speech, who produced high-frequency syllables more accurately than low-frequency syllables (Aichert & Ziegler, 2004).

What is, perhaps, surprising is that influences of syllable frequency in the 'model language' of English have been somewhat elusive, leading some to question whether a syllabary is actually used during speech production. Recently, however, Cholin *et al.* (2011) found influences of syllable frequency in English. Consistent with the findings in other languages, high-frequency syllables in English were produced more quickly than low-frequency syllables in English.

Rather than casting doubt on the existence of the syllabary, the difficulty in finding syllable-frequency effects in English compared to the other languages investigated should instead raise questions about how English differs from the other languages that have been investigated (e.g. Spanish, Dutch, German, French). Cholin *et al.* (2011) observed that the previous languages investigated have relatively clear syllable boundaries in words, whereas the boundaries between syllables in English words are less clear. They suggested that such tendencies regarding syllable boundaries in words may influence the preferred planning scope during speech production within different languages. For languages with clear syllable boundaries (e.g. Spanish, Dutch, German, French), a syllable-size planning unit might be preferred when speaking, whereas in languages with less clear syllable boundaries (e.g. English) the preferred planning unit when speaking may be larger, or multisyllabic in nature.

Differences across languages in the way that syllables influence the process of word segmentation have been previously demonstrated (Cutler *et al.*, 1986), so in hindsight, it should not have been so surprising to find differences across languages in the way that syllables might be used during speech production. The prevalence of such cross-language differences in a variety of language-related processes further highlights the importance of keeping in mind the characteristics of the language spoken by a patient when considering assessment and treatment of various motor speech disorders.

Another factor to keep in mind when considering assessment and treatment of various motor speech disorders is the structure of the syllable. Syllables are said to consist of a nucleus (often a vowel, V) with optional sounds found in front of the nucleus (known as the onset, often consonants, C) or following the nucleus (known as the coda, and often a C as well; the nucleus and coda together are sometimes referred to as the rime). An open syllable does not have a coda (e.g. V, CV, CCV), whereas a closed syllable has a coda (e.g. VC, CVC, CVCC). Every syllable must have a nucleus (typically a V in most languages), but onsets and codas are optional in some languages.

Naturally occurring speech errors are one source of evidence that suggests abstract syllable structures are used during speech production. Corpora containing naturally occurring speech production errors typically contain the errors of English-speaking adults. For corpora of speech errors in English, French, Italian and German see the Max Planck Institute for Psycholinguistics (http://www.mpi.nl/cgi-bin/sedb/sperco_form4. pl), which maintains a collection of naturally occurring speech errors (some from the original collection of Vicki Fromkin, a pioneer in speech production research).

Analyses of naturally occurring speech production errors show that syllable structure is typically maintained in the errors in English (e.g. MacKay, 1972). That is, a consonant in the onset of one word will typically exchange with the consonant in the onset of a neighboring word, such as producing *h*eft *l*emisphere instead of *l*eft *h*emisphere. It is also possible, although less common, for a consonant cluster in the onset of one word to exchange with the consonant cluster in the onset of a neighboring word, such as producing *fl*eaky *squ*oor instead of *squ*eaky *fl*oor (Meyer, 1992). It is less common still (some would argue, not possible) for exchanges of segments (or clusters) across words to involve the onset of one word with the coda of another word, or an onset consonant to exchange with the medial vowel of another word. In addition, such exchanges typically occur in words that are adjacent or only a few words away from each other rather than being far away from each other in the utterance. These observations have often been taken as evidence that entire segments are exchanged during speech production errors, and that phonological segments are represented separately from abstract representations of the syllable during the planning of speech.

Evidence from psycholinguistic studies employing priming techniques also suggests that abstract representations of syllables (and separate phonemic representations) are used during speech production. Sevald *et al.* (1995) asked normal adults to repeat pairs of phonological words as often as possible in a four-second period. Across several experiments, they found that speakers had a faster speech rate when they produced stimuli that shared syllabic structure and phonemic content compared to a condition in which the phonemic content was repeated but the syllabic structure was not. Importantly, they found that there was no advantage to repeating both phonemic content and syllabic structure compared to repeating syllabic structure alone, further suggesting that phonological segments are represented separately from abstract representations of the syllable during the planning of speech. The separation of abstract syllable representations and phonological segments also highlights for the clinician that problems in producing speech may occur in the retrieval of information (e.g. phonological word forms, segments or syllable frames), or in the sequencing of information in some form of pre-articulation buffer (e.g. putting the phonological segments in the right spots in the syllable frames), in addition to during articulation itself.

It is also important to recall that the role of the syllable in the planning of speech may be somewhat language dependent. For example, the rate at which phonological exchanges occur in connected speech varies across languages (for Arabic see Abd-El-Jawad and Abu-Salim [1987] and for Japanese see Kubozono [1989]). This difference suggests that planning units of different size may be used in different languages, such as the mora in Japanese rather than the whole word or syllable (e.g. O'Seaghdha et al., 2010). Furthermore, using electromyographic measurements from the tongue, Mowrey and MacKay (1990) found that parts of segments (i.e. phonetic features) may be exchanged, suggesting that smaller units of representation may also be involved in the planning of speech.

## Word Length

Consider the Hawaiian word humuhumunukunukuāpua'a (the state fish of Hawaii), the word *fish* in English and the word *pez* in Spanish. Across the languages of the world, there is some variability in the typical length of a word. Indeed, comparing just English and Spanish, Vitevitch (2012; see also Bates *et al.*, 2003) found statistically significant evidence that English words are shorter than Spanish words (about six phonemes for English words compared to about nine phonemes for Spanish words). Looking within a given language there is also considerable and measurable variability in word length. For example, in English, monosyllabic content words are quite common, whereas in languages like Spanish and Italian, monosyllabic content words are rare.

Given such differences in word length among and within languages, one might ask how word length affects the process of speech production. Introspectively, the long Hawaiian word humuhumunukunukuāpua'a seems more difficult to produce than the roughly equivalent words in English (*fish*) or Spanish (*pez*). Evidence from the tip-of-the-tongue (TOT) phenomenon appears consistent with one's intuition. The TOT phenomenon describes a state during normal speech production where the speaker knows the word they are trying to say, but is temporarily unable to access the word from the lexicon (Brown & McNeill, 1966). Harley and Bown (1998) found that TOT states happen more often for longer words than for shorter words, suggesting that there is something about longer words that makes them more difficult to retrieve from the lexicon than shorter words during speech production. Some evidence also suggests that normal adults name pictures identified with longer words with longer latencies than pictures identified by short words (Johnson *et al.*, 1996).

It is important to note that the extent to which 'word length' influences speech production may depend on how word length is measured (number of phonemes or number of syllables). Furthermore, the influence of word length on speech production has been shown to vary across languages (Bates *et al.*, 2003). In an ambitious, large-scale project, Bates and colleagues from around the world had native-speaking participants of seven different languages (English, German, Spanish, Italian, Bulgarian, Hungarian and Chinese) name a common set of pictures. Among the relationships that were found in each language was a modest relationship between word length (in syllables and in characters) and response latency, such that pictures identified by shorter words were named more quickly than pictures identified by longer words, but this relationship varied in magnitude across languages.

Of greater concern is the fact that word length is correlated with a number of other variables that may also influence speech production (and other language-related processes). In the 1930s, George Kingsley Zipf observed a relationship between word length and the frequency with which a word is used in the language, such that shorter words are used more often than longer words. Also consider the two regularities observed by Paul Menzerath in the 1920s (see Altmann, 1980). First, as the length of a word increases (as measured by the number of syllables in the word), the average length of the syllable decreases (as measured by the number of phonemes in the syllable). Second, as the length of a word increases (as measured by the number of syllables in the word), the less variability there is in terms of syllable complexity. Fenk *et al.* (2006) found evidence for what has come to be known as Menzerath's law in a statistical analysis of 33 languages, and suggested that these relationships provide our limited cognitive capacities with a relatively constant flow of linguistic information (in the information-theory sense of the word 'information'). The correlation between word length and several other lexical characteristics highlights the importance of taking these characteristics and their interrelationships into account during assessment and treatment.

In highlighting the relationship between word length and other lexical characteristics, we do not mean to imply that word length does not have an independent influence on speech production. Indeed, Nickels and Howard (2004) showed that English-speaking patients with aphasia named shorter words more accurately than longer words as measured by the number of phonemes in the words. It is important to note that they statistically removed the influence of variables like number of syllables, syllable complexity (as measured by the number of consonant clusters in the syllable) and syllable frequency, and that none of these other variables significantly influenced production accuracy on their own. Thus, word length, as measured by the number of phonemes in the words, may influence speech production in languages, like English, that employ phonological segments in the planning or articulation process. Additional studies need to consider the role of word length (or may need to consider a different measure of word length than the number of phonemes in the word) in languages that may rely primarily on other representations during the various processes involved in speech production.

## Phonological Similarity Among Words

During spoken word recognition it is almost axiomatic that acoustic-phonetic input activates multiple phonological word forms that compete among each other, thereby influencing the speed and accuracy of lexical access (e.g. Luce & Pisoni, 1998; Marslen-Wilson & Zwitserlood, 1989; Norris et al., 2000). However, the influence of phonologically related words on the speed and accuracy of speech production is somewhat less clear. Evidence supports the hypothesis that words with similar forms compete with each other during speech production as well as the hypothesis that formally similar words facilitate retrieval during speech production. The influence that phonologically related words have on speech production is further complicated when languages other than English are considered.

Evidence for competition among phonological word forms during speech production comes from the phenomenological experience of phonologically similar words 'blocking' the retrieval of the target word during the TOT state (Schacter, 1999). Evidence from laboratory-based tasks also supports the idea that phonologically similar words compete during speech production. Using a TOT elicitation task, Jones (1989) presented definitions to participants and asked them to retrieve the word (i.e. the target) that fit the definition. Along with the definition, a prime that was semantically, phonologically or both semantically and phonologically related to the target was presented. Jones (1989; see also Jones & Langford, 1987; Maylor, 1990) found that more TOT states were elicited when a phonologically related prime was presented after hearing the definition of the target. The increase in TOT states – or the decreased ability to retrieve the target word – in the context of a phonologically related prime suggests that phonologically related words compete with each other during speech production.

An increasing amount of evidence instead suggests that phonologically similar words facilitate the activation and retrieval of lexical word forms during speech production – at least in English. For example, Meyer and Bock (1992) showed that the targets used by Jones (1989) differed across conditions in the susceptibility to TOT states. When targets with equal susceptibility to TOT states were used across conditions in a TOT elicitation task, phonological primes did not interfere with the retrieval of the target word form; rather, phonological primes facilitated the retrieval of the target word form.

The results of a TOT elicitation task also support the hypothesis that phonologically related word forms facilitate retrieval during speech production (Vitevitch & Sommers, 2003). To examine the influence of phonological similarity on speech production, Vitevitch and Sommers employed an operational definition of phonological similarity often used in experiments examining spoken word recognition, namely, *neighborhood density*. Neighborhood density refers to the number of words that are phonologically similar to a given target word (Luce & Pisoni, 1998; see also Goldrick *et al.*, 2010; Peramunage *et al.*, 2011). Two words are considered phonologically similar if a real word is created by the addition, deletion or substitution of a phoneme in the target word. For example, the word /kæt/ ('cat') has as neighbors the words /skæt/ ('scat'), /æt/ ('at'), /hæt/ ('hat'), /kʌt/ ('cut') and /kæp/ ('cap'), as well as other words. Words with many similar sounding words are said to have *dense neighborhoods*, whereas words with few similar sounding words are said to have *sparse neighborhoods*.

Vitevitch and Sommers (2005) found that more TOT states were elicited for words with sparse neighborhoods than for words with dense neighborhoods, further suggesting that similar sounding words facilitate retrieval during speech production rather than compete among each other. Evidence for facilitation by phonologically similar words during speech production in English has also been found in naturally occurring speech errors (Vitevitch, 1997), as well as in elicited speech errors and picture-naming tasks (Vitevitch, 2002). Furthermore, Gordon and Dell (2001) observed such influences in individuals with aphasia, and modeled the effect computationally. However, different results have been reported for English-speaking children who stutter (e.g. Arnold *et al.*, 2005). Additional work is needed to determine which levels of the speech production process are influenced by phonologically similar words (and *how* phonologically similar words influence processing at each level).

Additional work is also needed to determine how phonologically similar words influence processing in other languages. Work by Vitevitch and Stamer (2006, 2009) found that normal adults whose native language was Spanish produced Spanish words with dense neighborhoods more slowly than Spanish words with sparse neighborhoods, contrasting with the effects typically found in English-speaking adults (for word recognition see Vitevitch & Rodríguez, 2005). At the moment, it is unclear why neighborhood density influences production differently in Spanish than in English; however, there are several differences between the two languages that might contribute toward explaining this difference.

One major difference between English and Spanish is in the other types of relationships that exist among the phonological neighbors in the two languages. A comparative analysis of English and Spanish words by Arbesman *et al.* (2010) showed that phonologically similar words in Spanish also tended to be morphologically related, whereas phonologically similar words in English tended to be only phonologically similar. This difference in the extent to which (inflectional) morphology is used in English and Spanish may account for the differences in processing observed in English and Spanish, at least in perception.

As Arbesman *et al.* (2010) describe, the larger proportion of Spanish words that are phonologically *and morphologically* similar – sharing not just several sounds but also several semantic features – might facilitate the retrieval of the correct word form from the lexicon. Even if the wrong phonological word form is retrieved (niña instead of niño; both words refer to a small child, but differ in gender), the common semantic information in the words may enable the language processing system to recover from the acoustic-phonetic error. However, in the case of English, where words tend to be only phonologically similar, recognition of the spoken word might be more difficult, as the target word must be distinguished from neighbors with very different meanings (compare *cat* and *cap*; only one of those items fits easily on one's head).

Although the additional relationship that exists among phonological neighbors in Spanish appears to be a small difference, it may make a big difference in terms of language processing. This difference illustrates how little we know about other languages with regard to the influence of phonological similarity on production (and processing in general). Important differences in processing may be found in languages that employ lexical tone (the classic examples being Mandarin or Cantonese Chinese), or languages that employ infixation, such as the Semitic languages (Hebrew and Arabic).

## Word Frequency

One of the most robust influences observed in speech production (indeed, in many cognitive processes) is the influence of word frequency. Across multiple languages, commonly occurring words are produced with shorter latencies than less commonly occurring words (e.g. Bates *et al.*, 2003). Word frequency not only influences retrieval processes but also influences processes related to articulation. For example, Wright (1979) found that the duration of less commonly occurring words was approximately 24% longer than the duration of more commonly occurring words.

Despite the apparent ubiquity of word frequency effects, it is not entirely clear *what* word frequency is, or *how* word frequency exerts its influence on various levels of processing. For example, word frequency can be measured by subjective ratings (sometimes called *familiarity ratings*), or by objective counts of words occurring in various texts or on various websites (for concerns related to the use of internet word counts see Kilgarriff [2007]). Furthermore, word frequency is correlated with word length (i.e. Zipf's law discussed above) and with age-of-acquisition measures (e.g. Juhasz, 2005).

Also consider that Bates *et al.* (2003) found that measures of word frequency in one language predicted response latencies in other languages. One interpretation of this finding is that 'word frequency' measures something about conceptual/semantic information rather than how often a given phonological word form occurs in a language. Most models of language processing represent word frequency as thresholds for the word forms, as resting activation levels for the word forms or as a late-acting bias that affects a decision stage in lexical retrieval rather than directly influencing the activation of a word form. More recently, Besner *et al.* (2011) suggested that word frequency is represented in the connections between representations (i.e. not the resting levels of the words themselves, etc.). Although word frequency effects appear ubiquitous, it is still not clear what 'word frequency' is actually a measure of, or how it is best represented in a model of language processing. It is also not clear if research across languages or with patients with motor speech disorders can provide insight into these questions.

## Conclusion

Using English as a 'model language', researchers have greatly increased our understanding of intact and disordered language processing. If we wish to *further* advance our understanding of language-related processes, researchers will need to increasingly explore language processing in languages with characteristics that differ from English in interesting ways. The commonalities in processing observed across languages as well as the differences in processing observed across languages will ultimately increase our understanding of language processing, even though in the short run the empirical waters may only appear to be muddied by 'contradictory' findings across languages. Such 'inconsistencies' should be treated as indicators of an important linguistic characteristic that varies across languages, rather than signs of methodological shortcomings among studies or of a spurious phenomenon. After all, the other 6 billion or so people on the planet who don't speak English can't all be processing language the 'wrong' way.

## References

Abd-El-Jawad, H. and Abu-Salim, I. (1987) Slips of the tongue in Arabic and their theoretical interpretation. *Language Sciences* 9, 145–171.

Aichert, I. and Ziegler, W. (2004) Syllable frequency and syllable structure in apraxia of speech. *Brain & Language* 88, 148–159.

Altmann, G. (1980) Prolegomena to Menzerath's law. *Glottometrika* 2, 1–10.

Anderson, J.D. and Byrd, C.T. (2008) Phonotactic probability effects in children who stutter. *Journal of Speech Language Hearing Research* 51, 851–866.

Arbesman, S., Strogatz, S.H. and Vitevitch, M.S. (2010) Comparative analysis of networks of phonologically similar words in English and Spanish. *Entropy* 12, 327–337.

Arnold, H.S., Conture, E.G. and Ohde, R.N. (2005) Phonological neighborhood density in the picture naming of young children who stutter: Preliminary study. *Journal of Fluency Disorders* 30, 125–148.

Bates, E., D'Amico, S., Jacobsen, T., Szekely, A., Andonova, E., Devescovi, A., Herron, D., Lu, C.C., Pechmann, T., Pleh, C., Wicha, N., Federmeier, K., Gerdjikova, I., Guterrez, G., Hung, D., Hsu, J., Iyer, G., Kohnert, K., Mehotcheva, T., Orozco-Figueroa, A., Tzeng, A. and Tzeng, O. (2003) Timed picture naming in seven languages. *Psychonomic Bulletin & Review* 10, 344–380.

Berent, I., Lennertz, T., Jun, J., Moreno, M.A. and Smolensky, P. (2008) Language universals in human brains. *Proceedings of the National Academy of Sciences* 105, 5321–5325.

Besner, D., Moroz, S. and O'Malley, S. (2011) On the strength of connections between localist mental modules as a source of frequency-of-occurrence effects. *Psychological Science* 22, 393–398.

Bradlow, A.R., Akahane-Yamada, R., Pisoni, D.B. and Tohkura, Y. (1999) Training Japanese listeners to identify English /r/ and /l/: Long-term retention of learning in perception and production. *Perception & Psychophysics* 61, 977–985.

Brown, R. and McNeill, D. (1966) The "tip of the tongue" phenomenon. *Journal of Verbal Learning and Verbal Behavior* 5, 325–337.

Cholin, J., Dell, G.S. and Levelt, W.J.M. (2011) Planning and articulation in incremental word production: Syllable-frequency effect in English. *Journal of Experimental Psychology: Learning, Memory, & Cognition* 37, 109–122.

Cutler, A., Mehler, J., Norris, D. and Segui, J. (1986) The syllable's differing role in the segmentation of French and English. *Journal of Memory and Language* 25, 385–400.

Dell, G.S. (1986) A spreading-activation theory of retrieval in sentence production. *Psychological Review* 93, 283–321.

Fenk, A., Fenk-Oczlon, G. and Fenk, L. (2006) Syllable complexity as a function of word complexity (Menzerath's law). In V. Solovyev, V. Goldberg and V. Polyakov (eds) *The VIIIth International Conference 'Cognitive Modeling in Linguistics 2005' (Text Processing and Cognitive Technologies 11)* (pp. 324–333). Kazan: Kazan State University.

Fromkin, V.A. (1971) The non-anomalous nature of anomalous utterances. *Language* 47, 27–52.

Gathercole, S.E., Frankish, C.R., Pickering, S.J. and Peaker, S. (1999) Phonotactic influences on short-term memory. *Journal of Experimental Psychology: Learning, Memory & Cognition* 25, 85–95.

Goldrick, M., Folk, J. and Rapp, B. (2010) Mrs. Malaprop's neighborhood: Using word errors to reveal neighborhood structure. *Journal of Memory and Language* 62, 113–134.

Gordon, J.K. and Dell, G.S. (2001) Phonological neighbourhood effects: Evidence from aphasia and connectionist modeling. *Brain & Language* 79, 21–23.

Harley, T.A. and Bown, H.E. (1998) What causes a tip of the tongue state? Evidence for lexical neighbourhood effects in speech production. *British Journal of Psychology* 89, 151–174.

Johnson, C.J., Paivio, A. and Clark, J.M. (1996) Cognitive components of picture naming. *Psychological Bulletin* 120, 113–139.

Jones, G.V. (1989) Back to Woodworth: Role of interlopers in the tip of the tongue phenomenon. *Memory & Cognition* 17, 69–76.

Jones, G.V. and Langford, S. (1987) Phonological blocking in the tip of the tongue state. *Cognition* 25, 115–122.

Juhasz, B.J. (2005) Age-of-acquisition effects in word and picture identification. *Psychological Bulletin* 131, 684–712.

Kilgarriff, A. (2007) Googleology is bad science. *Computational Linguistics* 33, 147–151.

Kubozono, H. (1989) The mora and syllable structure in Japanese: Evidence from speech errors. *Language & Speech* 32, 249–278.

Kučera, H. and Francis, W.N. (1967) *Computational Analysis of Present Day American English*. Providence, RI: Brown University Press.

Laganaro, M. and Alario, F.X. (2006) On the locus of the syllable frequency effect in language production. *Journal of Memory and Language* 55, 178–196.

Lallini, N. and Miller, N. (2011) Do phonological neighbourhood density and phonotactic probability influence speech output accuracy in acquired speech impairment? *Aphasiology* 25, 176–190.

Levelt, W.J.M. and Wheeldon, L. (1994) Do speakers have access to a mental syllabary? *Cognition* 50, 239–269.

Levelt, W.J.M., Roelofs, A. and Meyer, A.S. (1999) A theory of lexical access in speech production. *Behavioral and Brain Sciences* 22, 1–75.

Luce, P.A. and Pisoni, D.B. (1998) Recognizing spoken words: The neighborhood activation model. *Ear and Hearing* 19, 1–36.

MacKain, K.W., Best, C.T. and Strange, W. (1981) Categorical perception of English /r/ and /l/ by Japanese bilinguals. *Applied Psycholinguistics* 2, 369–390.

MacKay, D.G. (1972) The structure of words and syllables: Evidence from speech errors. *Cognitive Psychology* 3, 210–227.

Marslen-Wilson, W.D. and Zwitserlood, P. (1989) Accessing spoken words: The importance of word onsets. *Journal of Experimental Psychology: Human Perception and Performance* 15, 576–585.

Maylor, E.A. (1990) Age, blocking and the tip of the tongue state. *British Journal of Psychology* 81, 123–134.

Meyer, A.S. (1992) Investigation of phonological encoding through speech error analyses: Achievements, limitations, and alternatives. *Cognition* 42, 181–211.

Mowrey, R.A. and MacKay, I.R.A. (1990) Phonological primitives: Electromyographic speech error evidence. *Journal of the Acoustical Society of America* 88, 1299–1312.

Munson, B., Swenson, C.L. and Manthei, S.C. (2005) Lexical and phonological organization in children: Evidence form repetition tasks. *Journal of Speech, Language, and Hearing Research* 14, 108–124.

Nickels, L. and Howard, D. (2004) Dissociating effects of number of phonemes, number of syllables, and syllabic complexity on word production in aphasia: It's the number of phonemes that counts. *Cognitive Neuropsychology* 21, 57–78.

Norris, D., McQueen, J.M. and Cutler, A. (2000) Merging information in speech recognition: Feedback is never necessary. *Brain and Behavioral Sciences* 23, 299–370.

O'Seaghdha, P.G., Chen, J.Y. and Chen, T.M. (2010) Proximate units in word production: Phonological encoding begins with syllables in Mandarin Chinese but with segments in English. *Cognition* 115, 282–302.

Peramunage, D., Blumstein, S.E., Myers, E., Goldrick, M. and Baese-Berk, M. (2011) Phonological neighborhood effects in spoken word production: An fMRI study. *Journal of Cognitive Neuroscience* 23, 593–603.

Pylkkänen, L., Stringfellow, A. and Marantz, A. (2002) Neuromagnetic evidence for the timing of lexical activation: An MEG component sensitive to phonotactic probability but not to neighborhood density. *Brain and Language* 81, 666–678.

Schacter, D.L. (1999) The seven sins of memory: Insights from psychology and cognitive neuroscience. *American Psychologist* 54, 182–203.

Sevald, C.A., Dell, G.S. and Cole, J.S. (1995) Syllable structure in speech production: Are syllables chunks or schemas? *Journal of Memory and Language* 34, 807–820.

Sheldon, A. and Strange, W. (1982) The acquisition of /r/ and /l/ by Japanese learners of English: Evidence that speech production can precede speech perception. *Applied Psycholinguistics* 3, 243–261.

Storkel, H.L. (2001) Learning new words: Phonotactic probability in language development. *Journal of Speech, Language, and Hearing Research* 44, 1321–1337.

Storkel, H.L. (2004) The emerging lexicon of children with phonological delays: Phonotactic constraints and probability in acquisition. *Journal of Speech, Language, and Hearing Research* 47, 1194–1212.

Storkel, H.L. and Hoover, J.R. (2010) An on-line calculator to compute phonotactic probability and neighborhood density based on child corpora of spoken American English. *Behavior Research Methods* 42, 497–506.

The Chimpanzee Sequencing and Analysis Consortium (2005) Initial sequence of the chimpanzee genome and comparison with the human genome. *Nature* 437, 69–87.

Vitevitch, M.S. (1997) The neighborhood characteristics of malapropisms. *Language and Speech* 40, 211–228.

Vitevitch, M.S. (2002) The influence of phonological similarity neighborhoods on speech production. *Journal of Experimental Psychology: Learning, Memory and Cognition* 28, 735–747.

Vitevitch, M.S. (2012) What do foreign neighbors say about the mental lexicon? *Bilingualism: Language & Cognition* 15, 167–172.

Vitevitch, M.S., Luce, P.A., Charles-Luce, J. and Kemmerer, D. (1997) Phonotactics and syllable stress: Implications for the processing of spoken nonsense words. *Language and Speech* 40, 47–62.

Vitevitch, M.S. and Luce, P.A. (1999) Probabilistic phonotactics and neighborhood activation in spoken word recognition. *Journal of Memory & Language* 40, 374–408.

Vitevitch, M.S., Pisoni, D.B., Kirk, K.I., Hay-McCutcheon, M. and Yount, S.L. (2002) Effects of phonotactic probabilities on the processing of spoken words and nonwords by postlingually deafened adults with cochlear implants. *Volta Review* 102, 283–302.

Vitevitch, M.S. and Sommers, M.S. (2003) The facilitative influence of phonological similarity and neighborhood frequency in speech production in younger and older adults. *Memory & Cognition*, 491–504.

Vitevitch, M.S., Armbruster, J. and Chu, S. (2004) Sublexical and lexical representations in speech production: Effects of phonotactic probability and onset density. *Journal of Experimental Psychology: Learning, Memory and Cognition* 30, 514–529.

Vitevitch, M.S. and Luce, P.A. (2004) A web-based interface to calculate phonotactic probability for words and nonwords in English. *Behavior Research Methods, Instruments, and Computers* 36, 481–487.

Vitevitch, M.S. and Rodríguez, E. (2005) Neighborhood density effects in spoken word recognition in Spanish. *Journal of Multilingual Communication Disorders* 3, 64–73.

Vitevitch, M.S. and Stamer, M.K. (2006) The curious case of competition in Spanish speech production. *Language and Cognitive Processes* 21, 760–770.

Vitevitch, M.S. and Stamer, M.K. (2009) The influence of neighborhood density (and neighborhood frequency) in Spanish speech production: A follow-up report. University of Kansas, *Spoken Language Laboratory Technical Report* 1, 1–6.

Wright, C.E. (1979) Duration differences between rare and common words and their implications for interpretation of word frequency effects. *Memory & Cognition* 7, 411–419.

Zamuner, T.S. (2009) Phonotactic probabilities at the onset of language development: Speech production and word position. *Journal of Speech, Language, and Hearing Research* 52, 49–60.

# 6 Cross-Language Studies in Deaf Signers

## Martha E. Tyrone

## Introduction

### Sign language structure and use

Sign languages are natural languages, which have evolved in instances where Deaf people have had the opportunity to form social and linguistic communities (the capitalised form 'Deaf' is used to refer to members of signing communities, and the lower-case form 'deaf' is used to refer to individuals with hearing loss). Sign languages have the lexical and grammatical complexity of spoken languages, but they use the hands and arms as their primary articulators, which results in formational differences between sign and speech, as outlined below. As with speech, the production of sign language can be disrupted due to a movement disorder. Traditionally, dysarthria and other acquired speech motor disorders have been viewed as specific to the speech production mechanism, so they have not been explored much in the context of sign languages. The varied effects of movement disorders on sign production are the focus of this chapter.

There are multiple sign languages worldwide. Different sign languages have distinct lexicons and distinct grammars, but some structural commonalities have been observed across languages. This chapter will focus on research from two mutually unintelligible languages, American Sign Language (ASL) and British Sign Language (BSL), because these are the sign languages that have been studied most in the context of neurogenic language and motor deficits.

First, sign languages can convey morphological, syntactic and discourse information through the placement of signs in the physical space in front of the signer (Klima & Bellugi, 1979; Sandler & Lillo-Martin, 2006; Schembri & Johnston, 2007; Sutton-Spence & Woll, 1999). For instance, certain verbs can be inflected for person and number based on the direction and number of repetitions of a sign's movement. For example, the ASL sign GIVE can be inflected to mean 'you give me', 'she gives him', or any other combination of subject and object, depending on the direction in which the hands move.

Similarly, if a sign representing an agent is placed at a given position in signing space, verbs and pronouns that refer to the same agent can move toward or away from that position to specify that reference. This type of grammatical use of the signing space has been documented in several sign languages.

Sign languages, cross-linguistically, also make use of head movement and facial expression to convey linguistic information. For example, in Greek Sign Language, a specific head movement is used to mark negation (Antzakas & Woll, 2002). Other sign languages also use head and facial actions to mark negation, topicalization and wh-questions, among other functions (Herrmann & Steinbach, 2013; Klima & Bellugi, 1979; Sutton-Spence & Woll, 1999). Researchers have debated whether these non-manual components of sign language serve primarily a syntactic or intonational role, or some combination of the two (cf. Wilbur, 2009), but there is broad agreement that the use of face and head actions in sign language is rule governed and is an integral part of sign structure.

In terms of phonology, four major phonological parameters have been identified that can differentiate signs from each other. Those parameters are: movement, handshape, location and orientation (Battison, 1978; Stokoe, 1960). Movement refers to the shape, direction and number of repetitions in the arm's movements. Handshape refers to the configuration of the hand(s). Location refers to where the hands are located on the body or in front of the body as a sign is produced. In ASL, there are 12 contrastive locations on the body, plus the space in front of the body, which is also called neutral space. For example, the ASL signs FATHER, MOTHER and FINE are contrastive because they differ in location (Figure 6.1). Finally, orientation refers to which way the palm of the hand is facing. Orientation seems to serve a less important role than the other parameters in differentiating signs. Like the grammatical uses of space and of facial expression, the major phonological

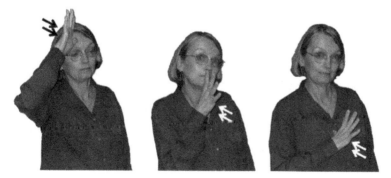

**Figure 6.1** ASL Signs FATHER, MOTHER, FINE: These signs differ only by location. For each sign, the open hand moves toward a location on the body. FATHER is located at the forehead, MOTHER at the chin, and FINE at the torso

parameters of sign language have been documented cross-linguistically (Crasborn, 2001; Johnston & Schembri, 2009).

Phonetics in the realm of sign language refers to the physical transmission of the linguistic signal through the manual-visual channel by the movement of hands and arms. A growing body of research suggests that sign languages undergo some of the same phonetic processes as spoken languages. Signs in ASL and in other sign languages can exhibit undershoot and coarticulation, so that the handshape or location of a sign becomes more like the handshape or location of the signs that surround it (Grosvald, 2009; Mauk, 2003; Mauk et al., 2008). Likewise, signs can undergo phonetic reduction, such that movement trajectories are reduced in amplitude, as an effect of rate or phonetic environment (Tyrone & Mauk, 2010). In addition, phonetic reduction in sign language can occur when sign movements originate from distal articulators (e.g. the finger rather than the wrist), as observed when a signer is close to their interlocutor (Crasborn, 2001).

Sign languages are made up primarily of lexical signs that correspond to spoken words. In addition to these lexical signs, sign languages use systems of fingerspelling to borrow words from spoken/written languages. During fingerspelling production, the fingers or hands represent the individual letters of a written word. Some languages (such as ASL) have a one-handed fingerspelling system and others (such as BSL) have a two-handed system, but for both types of systems, the movements for the individual letters are small compared to the movements used for most lexical signs. Because multiple elements have to be produced to represent a single word, and because the movements are small, fingerspelling is produced at a faster rate than signing.

Many researchers have investigated the neural basis of sign language, in part because such studies allow the examination of language independent of a specific physical production system and a set of perceptual organs (cf. Poizner et al., 1987). Based on research on clinical case studies and normative imaging data, it is apparent that the same neural structures underlie sign language as well as spoken language. Numerous studies have demonstrated the activation of traditional language areas during sign language processing and production. These areas include the inferior frontal lobe (Levanen et al., 2001; MacSweeney et al., 2002; Neville et al., 1998; Petitto et al., 2000) and the superior, posterior temporal lobe (Braun et al., 2001; MacSweeney et al., 2002; Nishimura et al., 1999). The latter finding is of interest because the superior temporal gyrus has traditionally been associated with auditory function, but in Deaf signers it seems to serve a role in perceiving visual-manual language. In addition, in terms of brain function for sign production, Corina et al. (2003) found activity in secondary motor areas of the left hemisphere during the production of ASL signs, irrespective of which hand was used to produce the sign. This suggests that the linguistic nature of the movements influenced which motor areas of the brain were recruited during sign production.

## Comparing sign and speech

Perhaps the most obvious difference between sign and speech lies in the size and configuration of the articulators used for each system. Sign language uses the hands and arms as its primary articulators, while spoken language uses the larynx and vocal tract as its primary articulators. The sign articulators are paired on opposite sides of the body, and some signs require bimanual coordination (all sign languages include both one-handed and two-handed signs). By contrast, the speech articulators are located along the midline of the body, and they produce speech sounds by means of a source-filter mechanism.

Because sign languages use large articulators and large movement trajectories, their production rate tends to be slower than the typical rate of speech production. Despite this, sign language users are able to communicate the same amount of information in the same amount of time as users of spoken languages. While producing an individual sign takes more time than producing an individual spoken word, sign language grammar employs fewer function words and it makes use of space so that sign language relies more on information presented simultaneously in the signing space and less on information that is sequential (Bellugi & Fischer, 1972; Vermeerbergen et al., 2007).

One sociocultural difference between signed and spoken language is that most sign language users do not acquire their language natively in the home. Most Deaf people are born into hearing families and do not acquire sign language until they go to school or come in contact with other Deaf children. The effect of this is that most signers are non-native users of their primary language, and unlike hearing speakers, many Deaf signers do not have full exposure to any language early in infancy. Similarly, sign languages are minority languages. They always coexist with a spoken language that is used by the majority of people in any given country or language region. As a result, almost all sign language users are bilingual, using a sign language in the Deaf community and a spoken or written language at work, with family and in other contexts.

# Sign Production Disorders: Aphasia and Apraxia

Although this chapter is focused on the motor disorders affecting sign production, it is worth discussing sign language and aphasia, in part because early research on motor deficits and sign language focused on how the characteristics of aphasia and limb motor disorders differed in the sign modality (Brentari et al., 1995; Loew et al., 1995; Poizner et al., 1987; Poizner & Kegl, 1992). Prior to that time, not much consideration had been given to linguistic as opposed to non-linguistic deficits in sign production, and a differentiation between the two could constitute evidence that sign languages are distinct from non-linguistic gesture or pantomime.

Another point to bear in mind about the study of aphasia in a sign language is that aphasia often co-occurs with limb apraxia following left hemisphere stroke. In a hearing speaker with a left hemisphere lesion, the two deficits can be differentiated based on which body part is affected. In the case of sign language users, the two deficits would affect the same articulators. Along similar lines, non-speech oral apraxia and apraxia of speech affect the same articulators as aphasia in a spoken language, but there is a more substantial literature delineating the distinctions among these disorders (Haley & Martin, 2011; Miller, 2002; Ziegler, 2002). While there has been extensive research differentiating sign aphasia from apraxia, as discussed below, there have been no documented cases of apraxia in the complete absence of aphasia in a sign language user.

Multiple studies suggest that the same types of aphasia occur in sign language as occur in spoken languages, and that those types of aphasia correspond to similarly located lesions (Corina et al., 1992; Hickok et al., 1996; Marshall et al., 2004; Poizner et al., 1987). For both language modalities, Broca's aphasia is characterised by limited and non-fluent language production, disruptions to phonology and reasonably intact language comprehension. By contrast, Wernicke's aphasia is characterised by fluent production that lacks semantic content, and more severely disrupted comprehension.

Poizner et al. (1987) were the first to examine sign aphasia and apraxia and to show that the two could differ from each other in sign language users. The study included three signers with left hemisphere lesions and aphasia. Only one of the three signers was impaired on pantomime production and imitation; and none of the signers was impaired on pantomime recognition. Thus, the signers did not have the same severity of disorder in sign and gesture. Corina et al. (1992) and Kegl and Poizner (1997) also identified dissociations between aphasia and apraxia in individual Deaf signers with left hemisphere damage. Corina et al. (1992) described a signer with a left posterior lesion who had limited sign comprehension and fluent but non-grammatical sign production. At the same time, the signer could produce and understand non-linguistic gestures, and imitate sequences of gestures, suggesting that his representation of symbolic movements was largely preserved, and his deficit was fundamentally linguistic in nature. Kegl and Poizner (1997) described a signer who had a lesion in the left parietal lobe and exhibited severe comprehension deficits and mild production deficits. Despite his signing deficits, the signer performed within the normal range on tests of ideomotor apraxia and pantomime recognition, and on kinematic measures of joint coordination. Similarly, Hickok et al. (1996) studied a group of ASL signers who had left hemisphere damage and found no correlation between their aphasia scores and their apraxia scores. Apraxia and aphasia were assessed by the Kimura gestures task (Kimura, 1993) and by an ASL translation of the Boston Diagnostic Aphasia Exam (Goodglass & Kaplan, 1975).

Findings from British Deaf signers following stroke are consistent with many of the findings from case studies in the USA. Marshall *et al.* (2004, 2005) described two sign language users who had left hemisphere damage and aphasia, and who both showed different degrees of impairment on sign and gesture tasks. Marshall *et al.* (2005) described one Deaf signer with a left anterior lesion whose aphasia was severe, with extensive comprehension deficits and no spontaneous language production. Although her performance on the Kimura box task and the Kimura gesture task suggested apraxia (Kimura, 1993), her gesture comprehension was far superior to her comprehension of BSL signs.

Marshall *et al.* (2004) described a signer who had good comprehension of single signs, but who exhibited anomia and used a large amount of non-linguistic gesture. Like the other BSL signer with aphasia, he exhibited apraxia, as assessed by the Kimura box task, but his production and comprehension of gestures were much better than his production and comprehension of BSL signs. Notably, these studies carefully controlled for the potential role of iconicity in sign comprehension and production. In particular, their tests of sign comprehension included potential visual distractors, so that if a signer was using iconic information to perceive signs, they might choose the distractor rather than the BSL sign. It is interesting that both the aphasic individuals described by Marshall and colleagues showed better performance on gesture comprehension tasks than on sign comprehension tasks, but neither signer confused BSL signs with iconic gestures representing the same objects. So even though signers could use an iconic strategy to comprehend gestures, they apparently did not use this strategy for sign comprehension.

# Sign Production Disorders: Right Hemisphere Damage

Like apraxia and aphasia, right hemisphere damage can provide an interesting contrast to other sign production disorders. Some well-documented sensory effects of right hemisphere damage are hemispatial neglect and a more general deficit in processing visuospatial information. In terms of motor deficits, individuals with right hemisphere damage often exhibit paresis or paralysis on the left side of the body, affecting voluntary hand and arm movement as well as other movements. Additionally, individuals with right hemisphere damage in some cases experience language-related deficits, such as aprosodia, pragmatic disorders and discourse processing deficits. These types of deficits have been observed in sign language as well as spoken language.

Poizner *et al.* (1987) demonstrated that language function could be preserved in signers who had right hemisphere damage, in spite of disruptions to visuospatial processing. This finding was important because sign languages use the spatial relationships between signs to mark how those signs are related grammatically or in discourse, as described above. Consequently, signers must keep track of signs' positions in order to know how they are related in the discourse. The two signers with right hemisphere damage and visuospatial processing deficits described by Poizner *et al.* (1987) were able to comprehend and produce complex sentences in ASL, in spite of the visuospatial processing demands of the task. Similarly, Marshall *et al.* (2003) compared BSL signers with left hemisphere damage and with right hemisphere damage and found that the signers with right hemisphere damage were impaired in their comprehension of spatial information but not in their general comprehension of BSL sentences or their ability to match signs to pictures.

Most studies of right hemisphere damage and sign language have focused on signers' receptive skills or on the grammaticality of their signing (Emmorey *et al.*, 1996; Loew *et al.*, 1997; Poizner *et al.*, 1987). However, a few studies have examined the phonetics of sign production in individuals with right hemisphere damage. Poizner and Kegl (1993) describe a hearing ASL signer with right hemisphere damage who exhibited a mild articulatory deficit. Specifically, she had difficulty coordinating her two arms during two-handed signs, and the authors interpreted this as motor neglect on the side of the body affected by stroke. They pointed out that the signer with right hemisphere damage showed movement lagging. When she produced two-handed signs, the initiation of movement in the left hand was delayed relative to the right hand.

One British signer with right hemisphere damage was studied in terms of his sign production (Tyrone, 2005). His signing and fingerspelling were compared to his performance on a range of non-linguistic movement tasks. In addition, both his linguistic and non-linguistic movement behaviours were compared to those of an age-matched control signer. In comparison to the control signer, the signer with right hemisphere damage exhibited lowering of high signs, laxed handshape and difficulty with fine motor control. The fine motor control deficit occurred across tasks but was more pronounced during signing. Finally, this signer showed minimal deficits with coordination, as would be expected for an individual with unilateral right hemisphere damage.

## Sign Production Disorders: Hypokinesia

### Parkinson's disease

Hypokinetic movement disorders are characterised primarily by reduced movement amplitude and speed, and by difficulty in initiating voluntary movements. The most common hypokinetic disorder is Parkinson's disease (PD), which results from the loss of dopamine neurons in the substantia nigra. The hallmark symptoms of PD are slowed movement, reduced movement size, resting tremor, muscle rigidity and postural instability (Fahn & Elton, 1987). In addition, individuals with PD often experience stooped posture, shuffling gait and dementia in the later stages of the disease. Dysarthria from PD is characterised by reduced loudness, reduced pitch range, strained and breathy voice quality and, for some speakers, occurrence of short, rapid bursts of speech. This last characteristic is of interest because it is unlike hypokinetic limb movement, which appears markedly slow.

A series of studies in the 1990s focused on sign production in ASL users with PD (Brentari & Poizner, 1994; Brentari *et al.*, 1995; Loew *et al.*, 1995; Poizner & Kegl, 1993). The goals of these studies were to characterise the effects of the disease on signing and fingerspelling and to compare the motoric deficits from PD to linguistic deficits resulting from left hemisphere damage. ASL signers with PD were compared to healthy Deaf controls and to signers with aphasia on descriptive and kinematic measures of sign production, and on kinematic measures of non-linguistic motor tasks. Results from these studies suggested that the signers with PD produced signs using mostly distal articulators, used laxed articulatory configurations, reduced the size of the signing space, showed minimal facial expression and decoupled the coordinated movements of the hand and arm. This last deficit was apparent in signs that included a handshape change as the arm was in motion, such as in the ASL sign ASK (Figure 6.2). Loew *et al.* (1995) emphasised that PD signing was spatially reduced but preserved crucial linguistic contrasts. By contrast, the errors produced by signers with aphasia consisted largely of phonological substitutions.

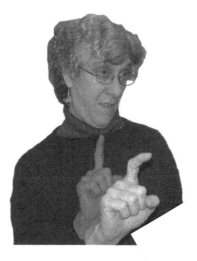

**Figure 6.2** ASL Sign ASK: The first two joints of the in. forward

Tyrone *et al.* (1999) discussed similar phenomena but examined fingerspelling rather than signing. This study suggested that signers with PD exhibited incoordination, articulatory undershoot, blending of handshapes and irregular pausing in fingerspelling. Moreover, it suggested that the rapid, sequential nature of fingerspelling made it particularly challenging for signers with PD. All of these studies emphasised that PD signing deficits were phonetic rather than phonological in nature and that incoordination was a hallmark characteristic of PD signing.

Tyrone and Woll (2008a) described a BSL signer with PD. His case was unique in that he was younger than previously documented signers with PD, 54 years old at the time of testing. Also, unlike previous signers with PD, he was a native signer, which could affect which aspects of production might be disrupted or preserved, given that he acquired the motor routines for sign production at an early age. This BSL signer was tested on individual sign production, fingerspelling and a range of non-linguistic movement tasks. In addition, because of the well-known side effects of some PD medications, he was tested both on- and off-medication for all tasks.

The signer with PD exhibited some of the same patterns reported in the literature on speech motor control and PD. The disease was not at an advanced stage when he was tested, and his sign production deficits were not severe. Moreover, this signer did not exhibit significant incoordination in signing or fingerspelling, either on- or off-medication. This is consistent with findings from past dysarthria research, suggesting that PD dysarthria does not specifically affect inter-articulator coordination. However, this finding is in contrast to the results of Brentari *et al.* (1995), which suggested that coordination specifically was impaired in PD sign production. The British signer with PD also exhibited irregular pauses and difficulty initiating movement, but less so in signing than in other movement tasks.

In various ways, the signs produced by the BSL signer with PD resembled dysarthric speech resulting from PD, while his non-linguistic limb movements resembled the limb movements of hearing speakers with PD. This suggests that the nature of the specific movement deficit depended more on the function for which the articulator was used than on the properties of the articulator itself. The BSL signer with PD often produced signs with laxed handshapes and sometimes laxed orientations. In addition, he produced slow movements both during signing and during other movement tasks. This signer did not exhibit the coordination deficits that were emphasised in the earlier research on PD and signing in the USA (Brentari *et al.*, 1995; Poizner & Kegl, 1993); nor did he lower sign locations (Kegl *et al.*, 1999). One final distinction between the BSL signer and the ASL signers with PD is that the BSL signer did not use more distal articulators in his sign production. It may be that the patterns observed [in AS]L signers with PD resulted not only from the movement disorder but [fro]m normal aging, since the BSL signer with PD was relatively young.

Unfortunately, there have been no studies of age-related changes in motor control for signing, and the studies on ASL and PD did not include age-matched controls.

## Progressive supranuclear palsy

Only one case of hypokinetic dysarthria not resulting from PD has been identified in a sign language user. The individual was a British Deaf man who developed progressive supranuclear palsy (PSP; Tyrone & Woll, 2008b). At the time of testing, he was 79 years old. He was born deaf. At seven years of age he began learning BSL, which became his primary language. Following the onset of PSP, he showed limited mobility, slow and reduced spontaneous movement, intention tremor and stooped posture. His score on the Mini-Mental State Examination (Folstein *et al.*, 1975) suggested mild dementia, but his comprehension and production of BSL were intact at the time of testing, as determined by a battery of naming, lexical recognition and sentence comprehension tasks (Atkinson *et al.*, 2005), and by observation of his spontaneous productions.

PSP is similar to PD in that it causes reduced movement amplitude and slowed movement. PSP affects the rostral portion of the brainstem and its projections to the cerebral cortex, cerebellum and basal ganglia. Unlike PD, PSP typically results in reduced eye movement and a severe form of dysarthria early in the course of the disease. PSP speech is characterised by reduced loudness, limited pitch range, articulatory undershoot and palilalia, the repetition of entire words with progressively decreasing amplitude.

The signer with PSP produced movements that were small, hypoarticulated and gradual. When the signer with PSP produced individual signs, he often used laxed handshapes and palm orientation, and sign locations were often lowered. He also exhibited incoordination in the production of two-handed signs. Unlike other signers with hypokinesia, the signer with PSP produced involuntary movements and palilalia during signing. Palilalia in spoken language is defined as the repetition of an entire word, with decreasing volume over multiple repetitions. The BSL signer with PSP also exhibited palilalia, since entire signs were repeated, and sign repetitions had decreased movement amplitude. Unlike in descriptions of spoken palilalia, individual signs were not repeated more than once.

In several ways, the signer with PSP produced signs similarly to the signers with PD who were described earlier. Like them, he produced slow, small movements with laxed articulators. Unlike signers with PD, he exhibited palilalia during signing, but he had no analogous type of movement error during fingerspelling or non-linguistic movement tasks. Like hearing speakers with PSP, his spontaneous repetition disorder was specific to the production of words. In other words, his sign production disorder was somewhat distinct from what has been reported for signers with PD, and similar to what has been reported for speakers with PSP.

## Sign Production Disorders: Ataxia

Ataxia refers to the motor deficits that result from damage to the cerebellum. These often include movement inaccuracy and incoordination (Timmann et al., 2001), intention tremor, dysdiadochokinesia (disturbance to rapidly alternating movements), dysrhythmia and dysmetria (movement undershoot or overshoot) (Bastian, 2002; Topka et al., 1998). Ataxic speech has been characterised as slow, distorted and imprecise, with a scanning rhythm, and irregular variation in pitch and loudness (Kent et al., 2000). Both clinical and experimental research suggests that ataxic dysarthria affects multiple speech articulators, instead of affecting articulators in isolation (Kent et al., 1997, 2000).

There has only been one documented case of ataxia in a sign language user, who was a Deaf BSL signer (Tyrone et al., 2009). The individual was 36 years old at the time of testing. He had developed ataxia due to extensive haemorrhaging in the cerebellum during surgery to correct an arteriovenous malformation. He was born deaf into a hearing family, and began acquiring BSL at age five when he began attending an oral school for the deaf. Following the onset of ataxia, he was tested on sign comprehension, sign production and fingerspelling tasks, over the course of multiple sessions. In addition, he was tested on a range of non-linguistic movement tasks, such as pointing, reach and grasp, and the Kimura box (Kimura, 1993).

The BSL signer with ataxia was quite different from the other signers with movement disorders. In contrast to signers with PD, who have been reported to use laxed handshapes, his handshapes during signing were hyperextended, so that his fingers extended backwards from the base knuckle of the hand. The signer with ataxia also had a tendency to use articulators that were proximal to those normally used for a given sign (for example, flexing the wrist instead of the fingers). This is the opposite of what has been reported for ASL signers with PD, who sometimes produced signs using more distal articulators. The signer with ataxia also showed intention tremor during signing and non-linguistic tasks, and he exhibited incoordination of the movements of proximal and distal articulators (such as the elbow and the fingers) and incoordination of the two hands during signing. The ataxic signer's motor symptoms more often affected aspects of sign structure that changed over the course of a sign's production (e.g. the configuration of the hand in a sign with handshape change). In some cases, he added movements to signs where they were not required.

One movement pattern that occurred across linguistic and non-linguistic tasks for the signer with ataxia was the tendency to perform one-handed tasks with two hands. In BSL and in other sign languages, some signs are produced with one hand, and others are produced with two hands. The signer with ataxia tended to spontaneously produce one-handed BSL signs using two hands and mirroring the right hand's actions on his left hand. Similarly, on the reach and grasp task, he was asked to grasp cylinders of different sizes and move them a short distance forward. On this task as well, he used both hands to accomplish the movement task.

Past research has suggested that one of the defining characteristics of cerebellar ataxia is dysmetria (Bastian, 2002; Topka *et al.*, 1998), but the signer with ataxia did not exhibit a clear pattern of dysmetria in his signing. At the same time, he exhibited more dysmetric movements during a non-linguistic pointing task, which suggests that past findings on limb movements may have been influenced by the movement task as well as by the effectors used for the tasks. The motor demands of signing are different from the demands of standard motor control tasks such as pointing, and thus signing may elicit a different pattern of movement deficits in individuals with cerebellar ataxia.

## Discussion

The studies outlined here suggest that dysarthria, as distinct from disruptions to simpler movement tasks, occurs in sign language as well as spoken language. Moreover, sign and non-sign movements may be affected differentially by the same movement disorder in the same individual, in terms of the severity of the symptoms exhibited or in terms of which specific symptoms are present. Acquired speech production deficits are often described in articulator-specific terms (Ackermann *et al.*, 1997; Yunusova *et al.*, 2008), but the fact that similar deficits occur in signed as well as spoken language suggests that the articulators may not be the only relevant variable for differentiating speech movement deficits from other types of movement deficits.

Just as dysarthria is not articulator specific, it may not necessarily be linguistic in nature. The reason that dysarthria can occur in either an oral or a manual language is because both modalities use complex, rapid, coordinated movements. Movement speed and complexity are necessary for the rapid information transfer required by a linguistic system, but this does not imply that motoric disruptions to language output are inherently linguistic. Individuals with dysarthria would probably also show impairments in any task with similar motor demands, but since few ordinary movement tasks require such speed and precision, production deficits appear predominantly in speech or sign.

The sign production deficits that have been identified so far show patterns that would be expected, based on the form that dysarthria takes in spoken language for the same movement disorders. For instance, the signer with PSP shows a distinctive production deficit, which is characterised in part by palilalia, and this is what would be predicted based on the form that dysarthria takes in hearing speakers with dysarthria. In the same way, the signer with ataxia exhibits incoordination and exaggerated sign movements, similar to the speech production deficits exhibited by hearing speakers with ataxic dysarthria. In light of findings like these, research on sign production should move beyond oppositions between motor disorders and linguistic disorders to consider more nuanced comparisons within each of those categories.

## Differences and similarities across modalities

There are a few types of production deficits that occur in both sign and speech as well as some deficits that do not, which may provide insight into the structure of signed and spoken language and into the nature of speech motor disorders. Specific deficits that occur in both sign and speech include palilalia, incoordination, reduced movement size and slowed movement. Palilalia is a particularly interesting example of a production deficit that can occur across modalities, because the movement sequences produced by the hands or by the vocal mechanism are fairly lengthy and complex – they are the combinations of movements required to repeat an entire word. With respect to reduced movement size across modalities, the size of an articulatory movement in a sign language is described only in those terms, whereas reduced movement displacements in speech can also be discussed in terms of their acoustic consequences (e.g. acoustic undershoot or reduced amplitude).

In terms of deficits that do not occur cross-modally, none of the studies so far suggests that a sign equivalent to festination occurs in PD. Hearing speakers with PD produce rapid bursts of speech (which some interpret as adaptation to altered expiratory control for speech – see below), even though their targeted limb movements tend to be slow. It does not seem that signers with PD produce rapid, brief bursts of signing. This could be related to the fact that individual signs are produced more slowly than individual spoken words to begin with (Bellugi & Fischer, 1972). The difference in production rate across modalities could create qualitative differences in the production strategies that language users employ.

There are aspects of sign and speech that cannot be easily compared, either for individuals with motor disorders or more generally. Certain differences in the articulators themselves or in their innervation make it counterproductive to search for analogues across modalities. For example, there is no obvious sign analogue to phonation, nasality or respiration. Likewise, with the exception of the vocal folds, the speech mechanism does not employ articulators that are paired across the midline of the body. The primary sign articulators are positioned on opposite sides of the body and are controlled by opposite sides of the brain, whereas the speech articulators are mostly unitary structures positioned along the midline of the body, and many of them receive bilateral innervation. For these reasons, it is best not to search for parallels between sign and speech where the comparisons are too strained.

## Methodological considerations

In addition to considering the similarities and differences in production mechanisms and deficits for sign and speech, it is also worth considering the limitations of current knowledge and procedures in the field. First, one issue in comparing groups with a disorder is the validity of the existing means of assessing that disorder. This is particularly problematic for sign language research, both because the field itself is young and because the pool of research participants is necessarily small, especially in research studies on disordered signing. Moreover, the standard assessments of language, cognition and motor function must be translated into a sign language if they are used with Deaf signers, which can threaten measurement accuracy and validity. The cross-linguistic validity of standardised assessments is an issue for all minority languages, but sign languages present a unique challenge because they employ a different language modality (cf. Atkinson et al., 2005). To illustrate this point, one need only consider established assessments of apraxia and aphasia. In administering these assessments, researchers must give instructions to participants in a sign language without using iconic signs or gestures that have the effect of demonstrating the gesture or sign that an individual is being asked to produce. Other assessments can pose similar challenges.

Along similar lines, there are no established measurements or procedures for analyzing phonetic variation in healthy signers. Current measures in sign language research are based on units identified from phonology, so there is no framework for describing aspects of production that are not linguistically contrastive. For example, one observation from research on sign production disorders has been that signers with certain disorders tend to use laxed handshapes (e.g. Loew et al., 1995; Tyrone et al., 1999). While several studies concur on this point, there are no standardised measures or normative data for laxing (or hyperextension) in typical signers. Quantitative, gradient measures of typical sign production have only begun to be developed in the last decade or so (Cheek, 2001; Mauk et al., 2008; Tyrone & Mauk, 2010), and they only exist for a few aspects of sign structure. Moreover, studies going back many decades have examined the physiological basis of speech in typical speakers (Lisker & Abramson, 1964; Stevens & House, 1955), but few studies have investigated the anatomical and physiological factors that influence sign language structure (Ann, 1996; Mandel, 1981).

Another limitation in comparisons of sign and speech production disorders is that there has been only minimal investigation of limb movement in clinical speech populations. Several studies have examined speech movements and non-linguistic limb movements in typical speakers (McNeill, 1993; Meister *et al.*, 2009; Rochet-Capellan *et al.*, 2008) and in speakers who stutter (Max *et al.*, 2003; Olander *et al.*, 2010), but limb movement in individuals with dysarthria has received comparatively little attention. Studies such as the one by Ackermann *et al.* (1997) have discussed speech motor deficits in dysarthria in light of central motor functions underlying both speech and limb movement, but the researchers did not directly compare the two types of movement in the same subjects. It may be informative to analyze both limb movements in isolation and gestures that accompany speech in hearing speakers with dysarthria. Similar patterns may arise in gesture and in speech, particularly since co-speech gestures are timed to coordinate with speech production in typical speakers. Deficits that appear in both speech and speech-accompanying gesture could suggest new avenues for diagnosis and therapy.

## Directions for Future Research

One challenge for the study of production deficits in sign language is that the numbers of cases of the different disorders are very small, so it is difficult to obtain instrumented measures of impaired production. More problematically, there is an insufficient amount of normative sign production data available for comparison. A few studies have collected motion capture data for signers with neurogenic motor deficits (Brentari *et al.*, 1995; Poizner *et al.*, 1987), but there is still not a sizable body of normative motion capture data available for comparison. Moreover, the normative data that do exist were collected mostly from young adult signers and not from signers who would be more closely age matched to signing individuals with acquired motor disorders. For this reason and others, there is a clear need for more normative signing data, collected from a broader range of the Deaf community.

Research in this area would be greatly enhanced by predictive models that could characterise typical and disordered sign production. Some studies are beginning to explore the explanatory value of articulatory phonology for sign language in healthy signers (Tyrone *et al.*, 2010). It would be informative to pursue other models in the same way, and to attempt to apply them to disordered sign production. Testable models could then be compared against individual case studies as they are identified by investigators.

As outlined above, most sign language users are bilingual and have extensive experience with the dominant spoken language as well as with their sign language. This being the case, future studies of acquired production disorders could focus more on comparing sign and speech skills in the same individuals, particularly now that the wide availability of videotaping can assist with premorbid assessments of both signing and speech. Marshall *et al.* (2005) studied a Deaf signer with aphasia, who had strong bilingual skills, so the researchers compared her skills in BSL and in English. With respect to motor disorders, Kegl *et al.* (1999) compared findings on speech production and signing in PD, but they were not comparing the same individuals, so they could not control for individual variation.

Finally, one goal of further research into sign language and speech motor disorders should be to develop better therapies for individuals with sign production deficits. Research in the UK suggests that speech and language services for Deaf signers are extremely lacking (Atkinson *et al.*, 2002; Marshall *et al.*, 2003). This issue has received scant attention in other countries, but the situation elsewhere is likely to be the same. It is hoped that better insight into the sign production mechanism will help to inform future diagnosis and treatment for individuals with motor disorders in general and for sign language users in particular.

## References

Ackermann, H., Hertrich, I., Daum, I., Scharf, G. and Spieker, S. (1997) Kinematic analysis of articulatory movements in central motor disorders. *Movement Disorders* 12, 1019–1027.

Ann, J. (1996) On the relation between the difficulty and the frequency of occurrence of handshapes in two sign languages. *Lingua* 98, 19–41.

Antzakas, K. and Woll, B. (2002) Head movements and negation in Greek Sign Language. In I. Wachsmuth and T. Sowa (eds) *Gesture and Sign Language in Human-Computer Interaction* (pp. 193–196). Berlin: Springer-Verlag.

Atkinson, J., Marshall, J., Thacker, A. and Woll, B. (2002) When sign language breaks down: Deaf people's access to language therapy in the UK. *Deaf Worlds* 18, 9–21.

Atkinson, J.R., Marshall, J., Woll, B. and Thacker, A. (2005) Testing comprehension abilities in users of British Sign Language following CVA. *Brain and Language* 94, 233–248.

Bastian, A.J. (2002) Cerebellar limb ataxia: Abnormal control of self-generated and external forces. *Annals of the New York Academy of Sciences* 978, 16–27.

Battison, R. (1978) *Lexical Borrowing in American Sign Language*. Silver Spring, MD: Linstok.

Bellugi, U. and Fischer, S. (1972) A comparison of sign language and spoken language. *Cognition* 1, 173–200.

Brentari, D. and Poizner, H. (1994) A phonological analysis of a Deaf Parkinsonian signer. *Language and Cognitive Processes* 9, 69–99.

Brentari, D., Poizner, H. and Kegl, J. (1995) Aphasic and Parkinsonian signing: Differences in phonological disruption. *Brain and Language* 48, 69–105.

Corina, D.P., Poizner, H., Bellugi, U., Feinberg, T. and O'Grady-Batch, L. (1992) Dissociation between linguistic and nonlinguistic gestural systems: A case for compositionality. *Brain and Language* 43, 414–447.

Corina, D.P., San Jose-Robertson, L., Guillemin, A., High, J. and Braun, A.R. (2003) Language lateralization in a bimanual language. *Journal of Cognitive Neuroscience* 15, 718–730.

Cormier, K.A. (2002) Grammaticization of indexic signs: How American Sign Language expresses numerosity. PhD dissertation, University of Texas at Austin.

Crasborn, O. (2001) Phonetic Implementation of Phonological Categories in Sign Language of the Netherlands. PhD dissertation, Leiden University. Utrecht: Landelijke Onderzoekschool Taalwetenschap.

Emmorey, K., Hickok, G. and Klima, E.S. (1996) The neural organization for sign language: Insights from right hemisphere damaged signers. *Brain and Cognition* 32, 212–215.

Fahn, S. and Elton, R.L. (1987) Unified Parkinson's disease rating scale. In S. Fahn, C.D. Marsden, D.B. Calne and M. Golstein (eds) *Recent Developments in Parkinson's Disease* (Vol. 2; pp. 153–163). Florham Park, NJ: MacMillan Healthcare Information.

Folstein, M.F., Folstein, S.E. and McHugh, P.R. (1975) Mini-mental state: A practical method for grading the state of patients for the clinician. *Journal of Psychiatric Research* 12, 189–198.

Goodglass, H. and Kaplan, E. (1975) *The Assessment of Aphasia and Related Disorders.* Philadelphia, PA: Lea & Febiger.

Grosvald, M.A. (2009) Long-distance coarticulation: A production and perception study of English and American Sign Language. PhD thesis, University of California at Davis.

Haley, K.L. and Martin, G. (2011) Production variability and single word intelligibility in aphasia and apraxia of speech. *Journal of Communication Disorders* 44, 103–115.

Herrmann, A. and Steinbach, M. (eds) (2013) *Nonmanuals in Sign Languages.* Philadelphia, PA: John Benjamins.

Hickok, G., Bellugi, U and Klima, E.S. (1996) The neurobiology of sign language and its implications for the neural basis of language. *Nature* 381, 699–702.

Johnston, T. and Schembri, A. (2007) *Australian Sign Language (Auslan): An Introduction to Sign Language Linguistics.* Cambridge: Cambridge University Press.

Kegl, J. and Poizner, H. (1997) Crosslinguistic/crossmodal syntactic consequences of left-hemisphere damage: Evidence from an aphasic signer and his identical twin. *Aphasiology* 11, 1–37.

Kegl, J., Cohen, H. and Poizner, H. (1999) Articulatory consequences of Parkinson's disease: Perspectives from two modalities. *Brain and Cognition* 40, 355–386.

Kent, R.D., Kent, J.F., Rosenbek, J.C., Vorperian, H.K. and Weismer, G. (1997) A speaking task analysis of the dysarthria in cerebellar disease. *Folia Phoniatrica* 49, 63–82.

Kent, R.D., Kent, J.F., Duffy, J.R., Thomas, J.E., Weismer, G. and Stuntebeck, S. (2000) Ataxic dysarthria. *Journal of Speech, Language, and Hearing Research* 43, 1275–1289.

Kimura, D. (1993) *Neuromotor Mechanisms in Human Communication.* Oxford: Oxford University Press.

Klima, E.S. and Bellugi, U. (1979) *The Signs of Language.* Cambridge, MA: Harvard University Press.

Levanen, S., Uutela, K., Salenius, S. and Hari, R. (2001) Cortical representation of sign language: Comparison of Deaf signers and hearing non-signers. *Cerebral Cortex* 11, 506–512.

Lisker, L. and Abramson, A.S. (1964) A cross-language study of voicing in initial stops: Acoustical measurements. *Word* 20, 384–422.

Loew, R.C., Kegl, J.A. and Poizner, H. (1995) Flattening of distinctions in a Parkinsonian signer. *Aphasiology* 9, 381–396.

MacSweeney, M., Woll, B., Campbell, R., McGuire, P.K., David, A.S., Williams, S.C.R., Suckling, J., Calvert, G.A. and Brammer, M.J. (2002) Neural systems underlying British Sign Language and audiovisual English processing in native users. *Brain* 125, 1583–1593.

Mandel, M.A. (1981) Phonotactics and morphophonology in ASL. PhD dissertation, University of California–Berkeley.

Marshall, J., Atkinson, J., Thacker, A. and Woll, B. (2003) Is speech and language therapy meeting the needs of language minorities? The case of Deaf people with neurological impairments. *International Journal of Language and Communication Disorders* 38, 85–94.

Marshall, J., Atkinson, J., Smulovitch, E., Thacker, A. and Woll, B. (2004) Aphasia in a user of British Sign Language: Dissociation between sign and gesture. *Cognitive Neuropsychology* 21, 537–554.

Marshall, J., Atkinson, J.R., Woll, B. and Thacker, A. (2005) Aphasia in a bilingual user of British Sign Language and English: Effects of cross-linguistic cues. *Cognitive Neuropsychology* 22, 719–736.

Mauk, C.E. (2003) Undershoot in two modalities: Evidence from fast speech and fast signing. PhD dissertation, University of Texas at Austin.

Mauk, C.E., Lindblom, B. and Meier, R.P. (2008) Undershoot of ASL locations in fast signing. In J. Quer (ed.) *Signs of the Time: Selected Papers from TISLR 2004* (pp. 3–24). Seedorf: Signum.

Max, L., Caruso, A.J. and Gracco, V.L. (2003) Kinematic analyses of speech, orofacial nonspeech, and finger movements in stuttering and nonstuttering adults. *Journal of Speech, Language, and Hearing Research* 46, 215–232.

McNeill, D. (1992) *Hand and Mind: What Gestures Reveal about Thought.* Chicago, IL: University of Chicago Press.

Meister, I.G., Buelte, D., Staedtgen, M., Boroojerdi, B. and Sparing, R. (2009) The dorsal premotor cortex orchestrates concurrent speech and fingertapping movements. *European Journal of Neuroscience* 29, 2074–2082.

Miller, N. (2002) The neurological bases of apraxia of speech. *Seminars in Speech and Language* 23, 223–230.

Neville, H., Bavelier, D., Corina, D., Rauschecker, J., Karni, A., Lalwani, A., Braun, A., Clark, V., Jezzard, P. and Turner, R. (1998) Cerebral organization for language in deaf and hearing subjects: Biological constraints and effects of experience. *Proceedings of the National Academy of Sciences* 95, 922–929.

Nishimura, H., Hashikawa, K., Doi, K., Iwaki, T., Watanabe, Y., Kusuoka, H., Nishimura, T. and Kubo, T. (1999) Sign language 'heard' in the auditory cortex. *Nature* 397, 116.

Olander, L., Smith, A. and Zelaznik, H.N. (2010) Evidence that a motor timing deficit is a factor in the development of stuttering. *Journal of Speech, Language, and Hearing Research* 53, 876–886.

Petitto, L.A., Zatorre, R.J., Gauna, K., Nikelski, E.J., Dostie, D. and Evans, A.C. (2000) Speech-like cerebral activity in profoundly deaf people processing signed languages: Implications for the neural basis of human language. *Proceedings of the National Academy of Sciences* 97, 13961–13966.

Poizner, H., Klima, E. and Bellugi, U. (1987) *What the Hands Reveal About the Brain.* Cambridge, MA: MIT Press.

Poizner, H. and Kegl, J. (1992) Neural basis of language and motor behaviour: Perspectives from American Sign Language. *Aphasiology* 6, 219–256.

Poizner, H. and Kegl, J. (1993) Neural disorders of the linguistic use of space and movement. In P. Tallal, A. Galaburda, R. Llinas and C. von Euler (eds) *Annals of the New York Academy of Science, Temporal Information Processing in the Nervous System* (Vol. 682; pp. 192–213). New York: New York Academy of Sciences Press.

Rochet-Capellan, A., Laboissiere, R., Galvan, A. and Schwartz, J.L. (2008) The speech focus position effect on jaw-finger coordination in a pointing task. *Journal of Speech, Language, and Hearing Research* 51, 1507–1521.

Sandler, W. and Lillo-Martin, D. (2006) *Sign Language and Linguistic Universals.* Cambridge: Cambridge University Press.

Stevens, K.N. and House, A.S. (1955) Development of a quantitative description of vowel articulation. *Journal of the Acoustical Society of America* 27, 484–493.

Stokoe, W.C. (1960) *Sign Language Structure: An Outline of the Visual Communication Systems of the American Deaf.* Silver Spring, MD: Linstok Press.

Sutton-Spence, R. and Woll, B. (1999) *The Linguistics of British Sign Language*. London: Cambridge University Press.

Timmann, D., Citron, R., Watts, S. and Hore, J. (2001) Increased variability in finger position occurs throughout overarm throws made by cerebellar and unskilled subjects. *Journal of Neurophysiology* 86, 2690–2702.

Topka, H., Konczak, J., Schneider, K., Boose, A. and Dichgans, J. (1998) Multijoint arm movements in cerebellar ataxia: Abnormal control of movement dynamics. *Experimental Brain Research* 119, 493–503.

Tyrone, M.E. (2005) Sign and speech articulation: Right and left. Paper at the Winter Meeting of the Linguistic Society of America. Oakland, CA.

Tyrone, M.E., Kegl, J. and Poizner, H. (1999) Interarticulator co-ordination in Deaf signers with Parkinson's disease. *Neuropsychologia* 37, 1271–1283.

Tyrone, M.E. and Woll, B. (2008a) Sign phonetics and the motor system: Implications from Parkinson's disease. In J. Quer (ed.) *Signs of the Time: Selected Papers from TISLR 2004* (pp. 43–68). Seedorf: Signum.

Tyrone, M.E. and Woll, B. (2008b) Palilalia in sign language. *Neurology* 70, 155–156.

Tyrone, M.E., Atkinson, J.R., Marshall, J. and Woll, B. (2009) The effects of cerebellar ataxia on sign language production: A case study. *Neurocase* 15, 419–426.

Tyrone, M.E. and Mauk, C.E. (2010) Sign lowering and phonetic reduction in American Sign Language. *Journal of Phonetics* 38, 317–328.

Tyrone, M.E., Nam, H., Saltzman, E., Mathur, G. and Goldstein, L. (2010) Prosody and movement in American Sign Language: A task-dynamics approach. *Speech Prosody 2010* 100957:1–4. See www.speechprosody2010.illinois.edu/papers/100957.pdf (accessed 20 June 2011).

Vermeerbergen, M., Leeson, L. and Crasborn, O. (2007) *Simultaneity in Signed Languages: Form and Function*. Amsterdam: John Benjamins.

Wilbur, R.B. (2009) Effects of varying rate of signing on ASL manual signs and nonmanual markers. *Language and Speech* 52, 245–285.

Yunusova, Y., Weismer, G., Westbury, J.R. and Lindstrom, M.J. (2008) Articulatory movements during vowels in speakers with dysarthria and healthy controls. *Journal of Speech, Language, and Hearing Research* 51, 596–611.

Ziegler, W. (2002) Task-related factors in oral motor control: Speech and oral diadochokinesis in dysarthria and apraxia of speech. *Brain and Language* 80, 556–575.

# 7 Apraxia of Speech in Bilingual Speakers as a Window into the Study of Bilingual Speech Motor Control

Marina Laganaro and
Mary Overton Venet

## Introduction

Understanding the nature of motor speech disorders and their assessment and treatment is a difficult task even in monolinguals, as the definition and classification between diagnostic categories (phonological, phonetic, motor disorder) represent a challenge for both clinicians and researchers. When it comes to bilingual speakers, the issue is even more complicated, especially regarding the characterisation of impairments in their second language (L2). Indeed, it is often difficult to disentangle speech characteristics that are due to premorbid L2 mastery from those that are due to impaired speech planning and control processes. In addition, models of speech processing in bilinguals are underspecified and interpreting bilingual impairments in the light of monolingual speech production models is often inadequate. This situation becomes particularly complicated in the clinical context, as the ideal scenario, i.e. the clinician mastering the same languages as the patient, is rarely found or feasible.

In the present chapter, we focus on impairments at the level of speech planning. First, we present an overview of psycholinguistic models of speech production in bilingual speakers; then we address the clinical implications for the assessment of speech planning disorders and we suggest how the investigation of apraxia of speech (AoS) in a bilingual population can inform models of speech production. Finally, we briefly describe a clinical-experimental assessment of a bilingual speaker presenting with AoS following a stroke.

# Theory (Models) of Speech Planning in Monolingual and Bilingual Speakers

Speech planning refers to the encoding of the phonetic form of an utterance before its articulation. Current psycholinguistic models of speech production postulate that an abstract linguistic phonological make-up is planned before a more specified motor plan is encoded (Levelt, 1989; Levelt *et al.*, 1999). Although the representations and processes attributed to the proposed encoding levels vary according to their different theoretical positions, in most accounts phonological encoding includes the retrieval of suprasegmental and segmental representations. At this encoding level, the segmental representation is totally underspecified in some proposals (Béland *et al.*, 1990); in other theoretical proposals, phonological features are partially specified along with segmental representations (Levelt *et al.*, 1999). Phonetic encoding processes specify an articulation plan that will be used as motor commands. These (monolingual) theories of speech production suggest the independent organisation of phonological and phonetic encoding processes. In this case, motor planning can proceed as an independent process once the linguistic properties of the message have been encoded. Alternative proposals claim that lexical representations are associated with detailed phonetic representations rather than with abstract phonological codes (Browman & Goldstein, 1989; Pierrehumbert, 2002); however, some recent accounts suggest an interaction between phonological and phonetic levels of encoding. The main arguments for this proposition lie in the observation that lexical-phonological properties (e.g. phonological neighborhood, lexical frequency) affect the phonetic properties of the produced words (Baese-Berk & Goldrick, 2009; McMillan & Corley, 2010; McMillan *et al.*, 2009). To account for these effects, interaction in the sense of cascading from phonological to phonetic levels of encoding was postulated (see Goldrick & Blumstein, 2006), decreasing the independence between these two encoding processes. Interaction between phonological and phonetic processing has consequences on the classical definition of patterns of impairment in AoS (see Laganaro, 2012), which are based on serial and independent phonological encoding processes and motor planning. In sum, the question of a clear distinction between symbolic abstract phonological codes and phonetic plans is still debated and theoretical positions vary even in monolingual models of speech production. A related question concerns the size of stored phonological/phonetic linguistic units and their specification. Here, we focus on syllables as they seem good candidates for coding phonetic plans. The representation of syllabic units has been suggested in prominent models of monolingual language production; in addition, investigation has recently focused on syllabic representation in bilingual speakers.

## Syllables as Units of Phonetic Encoding

The specification of articulatory gestures on the basis of an abstract phonological representation is thought to involve the retrieval of syllable-sized representations. In this view, the syllabary (Crompton, 1982) is a store containing a chunked representation for each syllable of the language, specifying its articulatory plan. The theoretical account of stored phonetic syllables has been validated empirically with data from both psycholinguistic experimental studies and patient accuracy data. In particular, it has been shown that the frequency of use of syllabic plans affects production speed in terms of response latency in non-brain-damaged speakers (Cholin et al., 2006, 2011; Laganaro & Alario, 2006; Levelt & Wheeldon, 1994) and errors in brain-damaged speakers presenting with impaired phonological/phonetic encoding (Aichert & Ziegler, 2004; Laganaro, 2008; Staiger & Ziegler, 2008). The convergence between psycholinguistic and neurolinguistic data on the representation of syllabic units involved during speech planning was confirmed in a recent, fully parallel neurolinguistic and psycholinguistic investigation (Perret et al., 2012). Production accuracy was investigated in 14 brain-damaged speakers producing phonological and/or phonetic errors (patients deemed to have conduction aphasia and patients classified as having AoS) and production latencies in 24 non-brain-damaged speakers: an effect of the frequency of use of syllables was observed in both populations (on production accuracy and production latency, respectively) independently of other sub-lexical variables. Thus, syllabic units seem to play a central role in speech planning and this theoretical account has been particularly investigated in (monolingual) AoS. A central question then is how units coding speech plans are represented and processed in bilingual speakers.

## Phonetic Encoding in Bilingual Speakers

Lexical and phonological organisation in two languages has been widely investigated in the literature on bilingual speech production, but much less attention has been paid to the processes involved in motor speech planning. The study of bilingual language processing has addressed the following core questions: (i) whether linguistic representations are shared or language specific; (ii) whether both languages are activated while processing one language; and (iii) whether the type of bilingualism has an impact on the organisation of two languages in the bilingual brain.

Current modes of bilingual speech production claim that both languages are activated at lexical and phonological levels when a bilingual speaker plans an utterance in one of his/her languages (Costa et al., 2000, 2005; Green, 1998). In addition, some authors hold that the phonological representations of two languages are not separate and that common phonological representations are shared across languages (Roelofs, 2003;

Roelofs & Verhoef, 2006). In the framework of models assuming abstract phonological representations, the authors claim that (abstract) phonemic segments that are common across the two languages of bilingual speakers (such as /m/ or /t/ in French and English) are represented only once. By contrast, language-specific phonological units (such as English /θ/ or French /ã/) and rules (e.g. lexical stress which differs across French and English, or liaison, which is specific to French) are bound to be separated. The same holds for phonetic programs: they are thought to be separate because of language-specific rules and realisations (Flege, 2002; Roelofs, 2003, 2006).

Models of bilingual speech processing also suggest that the effective degree of parallel activation and of shared representations is modulated by the type of bilingualism. In particular, age of L2 acquisition and proficiency modulate the organisation of two languages in the brain (Grosjean, 2008). For instance, while proficient early bilinguals tend to produce the same phoneme with distinct acoustic properties across languages (Caramazza et al., 1973; Fowler et al., 2008; Flege et al., 2003), this is not always the case for less-proficient bilinguals (Flege, 1981, 2002). For the latter but not for the former, speech motor plans may be shared between the two languages because phonetic encoding in the L2 may rely on motor programs acquired in the first language (L1).

The question of common vs separate phonetic representations across languages has been addressed empirically with French–Spanish bilinguals (Alario et al., 2010). This study was aimed at investigating whether syllables which are phonologically identical across the two languages of bilingual speakers (such as /ka/ or /pi/ for Spanish and French) have a single representation for both languages or if two separate representations are stored, one for each language. To analyze this question, the authors took advantage of the syllable frequency effect. As phonologically similar syllables may have different frequency counts across languages, analyzing whether language-specific frequency counts or cumulative frequency across languages affects production speed would inform about common or separate representations for identical syllables. It appeared that early proficient bilinguals were affected by language-specific frequency counts, while late bilinguals were only affected by frequency counts in the other language. Alario et al. (2010) concluded that two different phonetic representations were stored for phonologically identical syllables across languages in early proficient bilinguals, while a single syllabic motor plan was used in late (less-proficient) speakers, which corresponded to the phonetic plan of their first language.

In summary, during language production lexical and phonological activation spreads across the two languages and those phonological units and rules that are common between the two languages seem to be shared. By contrast, phonetic implementation seems to be much more language specific and stored motor plans are shared between languages only in less-proficient (late) bilinguals, i.e. on those who rely on their L1 motor plans to produce their L2.

## Phonetic Encoding Impairments in Bilingual Brain-Damaged Speakers (Aphasia and Apraxia of Speech)

Any impairment at the level of planning of speech gestures (phonetic encoding in psycholinguistic models of speech processing) is usually clinically labeled as AoS. Impairment in accessing or generating phonetic programs results in a series of changes including phonetic and phonemic errors, groping and effortful speech initiation, changes in inter- and intra-syllabic transitions, increased syllabic duration and decreased speech rate (Code, 1998; Darley *et al.*, 1975; McNeil *et al.*, 2004).

A crucial question regarding AoS in bilingual speakers is whether a breakdown in motor speech planning will necessarily affect both languages in the same way. When linguistic levels of speech encoding are damaged in bilingual speakers (bilingual aphasia), such damage generally affects both languages but with variability in the relative impairments of the two languages (Paradis, 2001). As a consequence, one may assume that AoS also affects both languages, with some variations across the two languages. According to the framework presented above, phonological representations and rules common to the two languages should be shared, whereas phonetic implementation is mainly language specific except in cases of late low-proficient bilinguals. Therefore, one may expect a similar breakdown across languages when these languages have many similar phonological features and rules (e.g. Spanish and Italian) and in late low-proficient bilinguals. By contrast, dissociated patterns may arise in patients with AoS across two very different languages (e.g. English vs Japanese), in particular in early highly proficient speakers. So, the severity of the impairment in bilingual AoS may vary across languages as a function of L1–L2 similarity, of L2 proficiency and age of acquisition. To the best of our knowledge, there are very few reports of bilingual patients presenting with AoS. Two studies have been carried out on Afrikaans–English bilinguals by Van der Merwe and Tesner (2000) and by Theron *et al.* (2009). The authors compared impairment in L1 and L2 on the basis of the hypothesis that L2 should be more impaired because of the higher demand on the control of motor planning in a less practiced language. A single case study (Van der Merwe & Tesner, 2000) confirmed more severe patterns of AoS in L2 than in L1. In the second preliminary study on three bilingual patients with AoS, the authors analyzed the adaptation to increased speech rate demands in L1 and L2. Durational analyses were carried out on speech elicited with material described as 'phonetically similar' across the two languages. In contrast with the control subjects (but similarly to three speakers with phonological impairment), the three patients had less durational adjustments (in terms of vowel and sentence duration) in their L2 than in their L1 under conditions of increased speech rate.

It seems thus that these first reports of AoS in bilingual stroke patients confirm a parallel impairment with increased consequences for the less familiar/less practiced language. This issue needs to be further investigated. In particular, most late bilingual speakers face increased difficulty in planning and articulating specific 'unfamiliar' speech sequences in their L2 (when these sequences are not shared with their L1). This means that even in premorbid speech production, one might find features in the L2 that are similar to those observed in AoS, such as slowed speech rate, increased transition duration and off-target articulations. It is therefore very difficult to tease apart which characteristics of speech are due to impaired phonetic encoding and which are linked to low proficiency in the L2. The comparison with premorbid L2 speech samples would be the best way to apprehend the apraxic features in low-proficiency L2. Alternatively, as phonologically common syllables seem to be shared in late bilingual speakers (Alario *et al.*, 2010, see previous section), the analysis of common syllables compared to language-specific syllables may be a promising approach to assess parallel/ divergent impairment across languages. In the following section, we will illustrate a clinical application of these propositions.

## Clinical-Experimental Case Study and Implications for Assessment and Treatment

Here, we will present an approach to the clinical management of bilingual AoS and discuss how in turn bilingual AoS can inform models of bilingual speech planning. In particular, we will illustrate by means of a single case, how the question of shared vs independent syllabic motor plans can be addressed in bilingual AoS.

Let us first address some general problems regarding the assessment of bilingual aphasia in general, and bilingual AoS in particular. There is a recognised paucity of standardised tools for bilingual populations. The most commonly used composite bilingual aphasia evaluation instrument is the Bilingual Aphasia Test (BAT; Paradis & Libben, 1987; http://www.mcgill.ca/linguistics/research/bat). Here, AoS is not specifically addressed, but we can use the subtests that provide oral output to inform us about the patient's phonological and/or phonetic encoding abilities: the spontaneous speech sample, word and sentence repetition tasks, the series and naming tasks and finally the sentence construction tasks. We still have to be inventive, however, to find a way around the major practical difficulty posed here: accessing speech production in languages not shared between patient and therapist. For this, therapists may find it useful to recruit a native speaker to administer the evaluation (mindful of the issues surrounding employing untrained volunteers to deliver clinical assessments).

Another important challenge is the accurate estimation of the patient's premorbid L2 competency. The BAT questionnaire goes some way to providing descriptive biographical data, including information about age of acquisition. However, assessing premorbid L2 proficiency remains a real challenge, as it is not always correlated with age of acquisition (Grosjean, 1998). In particular, self-report cannot provide a reliable indication of phonological-phonetic L2 mastery. We would therefore recommend obtaining, among other things and where possible, a sample of the patient's premorbid speech production in their L2.

Another essential point is that of the linguistic properties of the two languages. How can we estimate the commonality of phonological features and phonological rules between the languages in question? The identification of parallel linguistic properties and rules is the crucial point. In the absence of standard materials, we need to construct them in a relevant patient-driven manner.

These three points will be illustrated in the following: we outline a possible procedure for the  assessment of bilingual AoS. Our proposals for evaluation involve two complementary aspects: (i) collecting and comparing the patient's speech production in their L1 and L2, while also taking into account their premorbid L2 competencies; and (ii) assessing production on material composed of shared and language-specific syllables.

The patient, a 76-year-old, native Swedish engineer, living in Geneva and using French (L2) in the home environment for over 50 years, presented with residual moderate AoS in both languages following a stroke a year earlier. He was a fluent and competent communicator in French, with a mild foreign accent. In order to estimate his premorbid L2 skills and specific changes after his stroke, we were provided with a premorbid speech sample (extracted from a family video). We extracted 50 short and clearly audible sentences from the premorbid French audio-track and asked the patient to repeat each sentence.

A composite assessment of his aphasic impairments was carried out in both languages with the BAT. As the therapist (second author) had no mastery of the patient's L1 (Swedish), a native speaker of Swedish administered the relevant subtests in the patient's L1.

In addition, we aimed to assess speech production with material composed of French–Swedish common and French-specific syllables. French sub-lexical units and frequency counts are available in the Lexique database (New et al., 2004; www.lexique.org). We conducted an internet search on the structure and characteristics of the Swedish language and contacted a psycholinguist who could provide us with information about its phonology and syllable frequency counts. As computerised databases seem not to be available for Swedish, he proposed estimations of sub-lexical frequency counts on the basis of a small sample. We were also provided with an account of the phonotactic and prosodic properties of Swedish.

French and Swedish have very different phonological properties, but also some common phonemic and phonotactic characteristics. We therefore took advantage of their common features to create pseudoword stimuli composed of shared phonological material (common syllables), following the criteria described in Alario *et al.* (2010). We selected 192 phonologically shared syllables that were present in both Swedish and French (e.g. /fu/, /pin/) to create 96 bisyllabic pseudowords, in which we manipulated syllable frequency (high vs low) in each language (L1 and L2) with a 2 × 2 factorial design. In addition, we created 48 bisyllabic pseudowords with French-specific syllables of high or low syllabic frequency. Syllabic structure and inter-syllabic transitions were controlled across the experimental conditions. We administered these 144 pseudowords in a pseudorandom order during two separate sessions in two modalities: oral reading and repetition in a French mode setting. Two Swedish–French bilinguals with an L2 mastery similar to our patient underwent the same tasks as the control subjects.

Below, we will summarise some preliminary results on the pseudoword production task (Overton Venet & Laganaro, 2013). Two hypotheses could be contrasted with this experimental design: (i) the production of French–Swedish common phonological syllables is underpinned by a unique (shared) motor plan; and (ii) a language-specific motor plan is used to output a common syllable. The first hypothesis predicts an effect of syllabic frequency counts in the L1 when producing the L2 or of summed frequency counts from the two languages. The second hypothesis predicts that only frequency counts of the tested language will affect the behavior.

Production accuracy was higher on pseudowords composed of syllables of high frequency in both languages relative to pseudowords containing syllables which were of low frequency in one language (whether French or Swedish) and the highest error rate was observed on pseudowords composed of low-frequency syllables in both languages. Accuracy was comparable across frequency categories in two bilingual matched controls. The observation that frequency of use summed across languages influences production accuracy in this patient suggests shared syllabic motor plans (a unique representation used in L1 and L2), which is consistent with the hypothesis of common gestural scores in late bilingual speakers presented above.

## Implications for Treatment

The principles that we have developed above regarding the assessment of bilingual AoS can also drive the development of therapy materials. To the best of our knowledge, no published studies on bilingual AoS treatment are available. We therefore have no input concerning issues of generalisation of treatment benefits from the treated language to the other language. Some insights can be derived from the few published studies on the bilingual treatment of lexical-phonological impairment after a stroke. It has been shown that treatment in one language generalises to the other language only when common representations or processes are targeted in treatment (Detry *et al.*, 2005; Junqué *et al.*, 1995; Kohnert, 2004; Laganaro & Overton Venet, 2001). This would imply that those impaired motor plans that are shared between the two languages, as seems to be the case for instance for common French–Swedish syllables in the late bilingual patient presented above, should benefit from transfer. By contrast, features that are language specific may not improve unless targeted specifically in treatment. This hypothesis needs to be tested in experimental treatment studies on bilingual AoS, although any attempt at generalisation is likely to be limited by the marked heterogeneity of L2 mastery in this population.

## Conclusion

As we have seen, there is a lack of published reports regarding theoretical accounts as well as assessment and treatment in cases of bilingual AoS. In spite of this state of affairs, in this chapter we presented a number of theoretical aspects and clinical proposals contributing to the management of AoS in bilingual populations. We also illustrated how the experimental investigation of production accuracy in bilingual AoS patients may allow us to tease apart the role played by language-specific vs shared motor plans. According to current theoretical positions reviewed in this chapter, specific dissociations and associations should be observed in AoS. For instance, if motor plans are shared in languages with similar phonological features and rules or in low-proficient bilinguals, we expect largely parallel impairments and the transfer of treatment effects in those cases. By contrast, dissociations would be expected in early proficient bilinguals for whom separate motor plans are hypothesised between their L1 and L2.

### Acknowledgments

The authors are very grateful to Joost van de Weijer from the University of Lund for his generous help with providing Swedish phonological properties and syllable data, and wish to thank Jessica Marillat for her collaboration with the ongoing study. The first author is supported by the Swiss National Science Foundation (SNF) grant N. PP001-118969.

## References

Aichert, I. and Ziegler, W. (2004) Syllable frequency and syllable structure in apraxia of speech. *Brain and Language* 88, 148–159.

Alajouanine, Th., Ombredane, A. and Durand, M. (1939) *Le syndrome de désintégration phonétique dans l'aphasie*. Paris: Masson.

Alario, F.X., Goslin, J., Michel, V. and Laganaro, M. (2010) The functional origin of foreign accent: Evidence from the syllable frequency effect in bilingual speakers. *Psychological Science* 21, 15–20.

Baese-Berk, M. and Goldrick, M. (2009) Mechanisms of interaction in speech production. *Language and Cognitive Processes* 24, 527–554.

Béland, R., Caplan, D. and Nespoulous, J.L. (1990) The role of abstract phonological representations in word production. Evidence from phonemic paraphasias. *Journal of Neurolinguistics* 5, 125–164.

Browman, C.P. and Goldstein, L. (1989) Articulatory gestures as phonological units. *Phonology* 6, 201–251.

Caramazza, A., Yeni-Komshian, G., Zurif, E. and Carbone, E. (1973) The acquisition of a new phonological contrast: The case of stop consonants in French-English bilinguals. *Journal Acoustical Society of America* 54, 421–428.

Cholin, J., Levelt, W.J.M. and Schiller, N.O. (2006) Effects of syllable frequency in speech production. *Cognition* 99, 205–235.

Cholin, J., Dell, G.S. and Levelt, W.J.M. (2011) Planning and articulation in incremental word production: Syllable-frequency effects in English. *Journal of Experimental Psychology: Learning, Memory, and Cognition* 37, 109–122.

Code, C. (1998) Major review: Models, theories and heuristics in apraxia of speech. *Clinical Linguistics and Phonetics* 12, 47–65.

Costa, A., Caramazza, A. and Sebastián-Gallés, N. (2000) The cognate facilitation effect: Implications for models of lexical access. *Journal of Experimental Psychology: Learning, Memory, and Cognition* 26, 1283–1296.

Costa, A., Santesteban, M. and Caño, À. (2005) On the facilitating effects of cognate words in bilingual speech production. *Brain and Language* 94, 94–103.

Crompton, A. (1981) Syllables and segments in speech production. *Linguistics* 19, 663–716.

Darley, F., Aronson, A. and Brown, J. (1975) *Motor Speech Disorders*. Philadelphia, PA: Saunders.

Detry, C., Pillon, A. and de Partz, M. (2005) A direct processing route to translate words from the first to the second language: Evidence from a case of a bilingual aphasic. *Brain and Language* 95, 40–41.

Duffy, J.R. (2006) Apraxia of speech in degenerative neurologic disease. *Aphasiology* 20, 511–527.

Flege, J.E. (1981) Age of learning affects the authenticity of voice-onset time (VOT) in stop consonants produced in a second language. *Journal Acoustical Society of America* 89, 395–441.

Flege, J.E. (2002) Interactions between the native and second-language phonetic systems. In P. Burmeister, T. Piske and A. Rohde (eds) *An Integrated View of Language Development: Papers in Honor of Henning Wode* (pp. 217–244). Trier: Wissenschaftlicher Verlag.

Flege, J.E., Schirru, C. and MacKay, I.R. (2003) Interaction between the native and second language phonetic subsystems. *Speech Communication* 40, 467–491.

Fowler, C.A., Sramko, V., Ostry, D.J., Rowland, S. and Halle, P. (2008) Cross-language phonetic influences on the speech of French-English bilinguals. *Journal of Phonetics* 36, 649–663.

Goldrick, M. and Blumstein, S.E. (2006) Cascading activation from phonological planning to articulatory processes: Evidence from tongue twisters. *Language and Cognitive Processes* 21, 649–683.

Green, D.W. (1998) Mental control of the bilingual lexicosemantic system. *Bilingualism: Language and Cognition* 1, 67–81.

Grosjean, F. (1998) Studying bilinguals: Methodological and conceptual issues. *Bilingualism: Language and Cognition* 1, 131–149.

Grosjean, F. (2004) Studying bilinguals: Methodological and conceptual issues. In T.K. Bhatia and W.C. Ritchie (eds) *The Handbook of Bilingualism* (2nd edn: pp. 32–63). Oxford: Blackwell Publishing.

Grosjean, F. (2008) *Studying Bilinguals*. New York: Oxford University Press.

Josephs, K.A., Duffy, J.R., Strand, E.A., Whitwell, J.L., Layton, K.F., Parisi, J.E., Hauser, M.F., Witte, R.J., Boeve, B.F., Knopman, D.S., Dickson, D.W., Jack Jr, C.R. and Petersen, R.C. (2006) Clinicopathological and imaging correlates of progressive aphasia and apraxia of speech. *Brain* 129, 1385–1398.

Junqué, C., Vendrell, J. and Vendrell, P. (1995) Differential impairments and specific phenomena in 50 Catalan-Spanish bilingual aphasic patients. In M. Paradis (ed.) *Aspects of Bilingual Aphasia* (pp. 177–209). New York: Pergamon Press.

Kohnert, K. (2004) Cognitive and cognate-based treatments for bilingual aphasia: A case study, *Brain and Language* 91, 294–302.

Laganaro, M. (2008) Is there a syllable frequency effect in aphasia or in apraxia of speech or both? *Aphasiology* 22, 1191–1200.

Laganaro, M. (2012) Patterns of impairments in AoS and mechanisms of interaction between phonological and phonetic encoding. *Journal of Speech Language and Hearing Research* 55, S1535–1543.

Laganaro, M. and Overton Venet, M. (2001) Acquired alexia in multilingual aphasia and computer-assisted remediation in both languages: Issues of generalisation and transfer. *Folia Phoniatrica* 53, 135–144.

Laganaro, M. and Alario, F.X. (2006) On the locus of syllable frequency effect. *Journal of Memory and Language* 55, 178–196.

Levelt, W. (1989) *Speaking: From Intention to Articulation*. Cambridge, MA: MIT Press.

Levelt, W. and Wheeldon, L.R. (1994) Do speakers have access to a mental syllabary? *Cognition* 50, 239–269.

Levelt, W.J.M., Roelofs, A. and Meyer, A.S. (1999) A theory of lexical access in speech production. *Behavioral and Brain Sciences* 22, 1–75.

McMillan, C.T., Corley, M. and Lickley, R.J. (2009) Articulatory evidence for feedback and competition in speech production. *Language and Cognitive Processes* 24, 44–66.

McMillan, C.T. and Corley, M. (2010) Cascading influences on the production of speech: Evidence from articulation. *Cognition* 117, 243–260.

McNeil, M.R., Pratt, S.R. and Fossett, T.R.D. (2004) The differential diagnosis of apraxia of speech. In B. Maassen (ed.) *Speech Motor Control in Normal and Disordered Speech* (pp. 389–413). New York: Oxford University Press.

Overton Venet, M. and Laganaro, M. (2013) Production of L1-L2 common syllables in apraxia of speech: A study if bilingual production in a late Swedish-French bilingual. Poster presented at the 29th IALP World Congress, Torino (Italy), August 2013.

Paradis, M. (2001) Bilingual and polyglot aphasia. In R.S. Berndt (ed.) *Language and Aphasia* (pp. 69–91). Amsterdam: Elsevier Science.

Paradis, M. and Libben, G. (1987) *The Assessment of Bilingual Aphasia*. Hillsdale, NJ: LEA Inc.

Perret, C., Schneider, L., Dayer, G. and Laganaro, M. (2012) Convergences and divergences between neurolinguistic and psycholinguistic data in the study of phonological and phonetic encoding: A parallel investigation of syllable frequency effects in brain-damaged and healthy speakers. *Language and Cognitive Processes* 1–20.

Pierrehumbert, J. (2002) Word-specific phonetics. In C. Gussenhoven and N. Warner (eds) *Laboratory Phonology VII* (pp. 101–139). Berlin: Mouton de Gruyter.

Roelofs, A. (2003) Shared phonological encoding processes and representations of languages in bilingual speakers. *Language and Cognitive Processes* 18, 175–204.

Roelofs, A. and Verhoef, K. (2006) Modeling the control of phonological encoding in bilingual speakers. *Bilingualism: Language and Cognition* 9, 167–176.

Staiger, A. and Ziegler, W. (2008) Syllable frequency and syllable structure in the spontaneous speech production of patients with apraxia of speech. *Aphasiology* 20, 1201–1215.

Theron, K., Van der Merwe, A., Robin, D.R. and Groenewald, E. (2009) Temporal parameters of speech production in bilingual speakers with apraxic or phonemic paraphasic errors. *Aphasiology* 23, 557–583.

Van der Merwe, A. and Tesner, H. (2000) Apraxia of speech in a bilingual speaker: Perceptual characteristics and generalisation of non-language specific treatment. *South African Journal of Communication Disorders*. Special edition: *Communication Disorders in Multilingual Populations* 47, 79–89.

Ziegler, W. (2008) Apraxia of speech. In G. Goldenberg and B. Miller (eds) *Neuropsychology and Behavioral Neurology* (3rd edn; pp. 269–286). Edinburgh: Elsevier.

# 8 Phonological and Speech Output in Adult Non-Literate Groups

Dora Colaço, Ana Mineiro
and Alexandre Castro-Caldas

## Introduction

Many assessments and treatment approaches for speech output and speech perception involve the manipulation of sounds, syllables and words, so-called metaphonological tasks, e.g. sound and word segmentation, order judgements. A number of these tasks have been incorporated into assessment batteries and employed to differentially diagnose between different underlying disorders. However, it remains far from clear to what extent or in what ways sound processing is dependent on or exploits these manipulations, whether or not they constitute simply a set of linguistic exercises or whether they reflect actual psycholinguistic processes involved in speech. Answers to these questions have implications for models of speech perception and output as well as direct implications for clinical and educational practice.

Cross-language studies of fundamentally differing sound structures and sound-grapheme correspondences can assist in addressing these questions. One approach that has been taken in this line of investigation is an examination of sound manipulation tasks in speakers of languages with and without an orthographic system or in individuals with and without schooling that has involved training in some form of phonics. The aim of this chapter is to present an overview of key issues and studies surrounding literacy levels and performance on metaphonological and similar tasks. Additionally, we will take a detour into some of these questions in relation to bilingual speakers to provide further interesting points in relation to metaphonological awareness.

## Literacy

The effects of literacy, defined as the ability to read and write, have been a focus of interest since the days of the ancient Greek philosophers.

In more recent studies, despite some differences across the literature in terms of methodology and results which give rise to some apparent discrepancies, the idea that literacy is associated with differences in language processing and brain activation is accepted by the majority of the researchers who work in this field.

Literacy has been defined as knowledge of a written code. Underlying the learning of alphabetised reading and writing skills is an abstract knowledge concerning the conversion of graphemes to phonemes and phonemes to graphemes, that is, an operation of linking auditory-verbal information in a time sequence with visual-verbal units in a spatial sequence. Through this, a new strategy is created in language processing, one which is concerned with giving a phonological correspondence to units that are smaller than words, i.e. letters. This visual-graphic correspondence is independent from semantics. In this way, besides the ability to implicitly perceive and articulate phonemes, explicit perception is developed, allowing the lexicon to be orthographically represented. This skill is usually learned at school and is related to other skills that are shaped and developed in the same space.

## The Impact of School Attendance: What Happens in School?

When studying literacy, it can be difficult to isolate the variable 'school attendance', which can be confused with the effects of schooling. Likewise, literate and illiterate individuals can be confused with schooled and unschooled individuals. In addition, there are several other variables that can critically interfere when examining literacy, such as economic and cultural status or the differences between rural and urban environments. However, among these variables, schooling has been considered to be the most relevant issue (Ardila *et al.*, 2000; Coppens *et al.*, 1998).

If they have never attended school, illiterate individuals have never learned topics and skills in subjects such as geography, mathematics, sciences, drawing, etc. They have not been educated in a system which organises knowledge and they have not acquired study skills.

A number of works have shown that some of the illiterate subjects' difficulties come from a lack of experience with visual analysis tasks, and with the analytic operations that these tasks require (Morais, 1997). This is not directly connected to the fact that they are illiterate but instead to them being unschooled individuals. In order to assess this effect, several authors have tested individuals who learned to read when adults and who can read in a rudimentary way.

Most authors agree on the importance of schooling and on how much this variable can affect cognitive processing. Some key categories identified concerning the main differences between schooled and unschooled individuals are: concrete vs abstract thinking skills; visuospatial and visuomotor skills; phonologic awareness; and working memory. For instance, the fact that unschooled subjects present a more concrete level of cognitive processing might have consequences on their visuospatial skills, such as bidimensional representations (Coppens *et al.*, 1998).

Schooling also appears to influence formal operational thinking and seems to reinforce certain skills (verbal memory and phonological awareness), making it easier to learn new knowledge. Ostrosky-Solís *et al.* (2003) conducted a study where they trained these cognitive competences in illiterate adults. They demonstrated that their participants improved on their performance in neuropsychological tests and progressed on their reading learning process.

Schooling, besides presenting students with knowledge opportunities, also broadens their linguistic knowledge, because it is through reading that one has the possibility of attaining vocabulary enrichment and learning more complex syntactic structures. It also appears that reading provides the ability to reflect on phonologic knowledge (the sounds of speech) and its relations to an abstract code system – writing. Recent functional magnetic resonance imaging (fMRI) findings demonstrated that the auditory cortex is reliably activated when individuals read (Campbell *et al.*, 1999; Cohen *et al.*, 2000; Dehaene & Cohen, 2011). Literacy enhances brain responses in distinct ways; for example, Dehaene *et al.* (2010: 1359) demonstrated that literacy 'enhanced phonological activation to speech in the planum temporale and afforded a top-down activation of orthography from spoken inputs'.

## The Role of School in Metaphonological Knowledge

Metalinguistics has been defined as implicit knowledge of a language's structural components. Metalinguistic abilities involve knowledge of a language's forms regardless of their meaning, and the ability to reflect on such knowledge. Therefore, metaphonology can be defined as the consciousness of a language's sound system. It has to do with the ability to reflect on structural components of words such as syllables and phonological segments.

The tasks used to test this type of knowledge typically include the following:

- Rhyme awareness
- Syllable segmentation
- Syllable manipulation
- Word length awareness
- Phonological recall

- Phonemic segmentation
- Phonemic manipulation
- Pseudowords repetition

From early on, studies of phonological awareness presented data that suggested that literacy assists metalinguistic development. Liberman *et al.* (1974) compared illiterate to literate children on their performance in several phonological awareness tasks, entailing manipulating syllables and phonemes. The alphabetised children obtained better results than the non-alphabetised children in every task, which suggested that orthographic knowledge helped them to do better at these tasks.

Gathercole (2006) also argued that non-word repetition and word learning both rely on phonological storage, based on results of simple tasks in children and adults and in individuals with language impairment. She concluded that learning mediated by temporary phonological storage is a primitive learning mechanism that is important in the early stages of acquiring a language.

Hatcher *et al.* (1994) conducted a study with seven-year-old children with reading difficulties. Four groups were formed – a control group that followed the stipulated reading learning plan, and three experimental groups where children attended work sessions: (1) in the 'phonology' group, children did phonology exercises (rhymes, syllable and phoneme manipulation); (2) in the 'phonology + reading' group, children underwent less intensive training but applied phonologic strategies to reading and writing; and (3) in the 'reading' group, children practised reading and writing exercises, with no reference whatsoever to phonology. The results showed that, when compared to the control group, only the 'phonology + reading' group progressed more in reading tasks, whether on isolated words, words in context and pseudowords or in comprehension of texts.

We can thus reflect on the importance of phonological knowledge in the process of learning the alphabetic code and recognise that there is a need to relate phonemic learning to reading. But when we refer to phonemic skills, we are only focusing on the phoneme level. It has been demonstrated that in the case of preliterate children and illiterate adults, the discovery of the phoneme is made in the process of learning the alphabetic code. Phonemic consciousness seems never to precede acquisition of the alphabetic code. These two types of knowledge appear together. Neither is the origin of the other but still, they influence each other mutually and continue reinforcing each other reciprocally.

It has also been established that illiterate adults have more difficulties when carrying out tasks which require more explicit language perception, that is, a certain level of phonological awareness (Morais, 1993). This suggests that there are differences in phonological processing between literate and illiterate individuals, a finding which has subsequently been demonstrated by other researchers (e.g. Ardila *et al.*, 2000, Kosmidis, 2006).

In a study of phonemic awareness with illiterate and ex-illiterate adults (learned how to read after 15 years of age), Morais *et al.* (1979) used a test where participants had to remove the first phoneme in words and pseudowords. The group of illiterate subjects obtained significantly lower results in this segmental analysis, especially in the case of pseudowords. In another test in the same study, which consisted of recalling words starting with a given phoneme, illiterate adults had yet again the worst results.

Still on the subject of phoneme-level manipulation, Morais (1997) employed pseudoword segmentation tasks using visual stimuli with illiterate poets in an attempt to test these individuals' phonemic awareness. In a task using coins (establishing a coin/phoneme correspondence), he verified that even with highly developed metaphonological skills at syllable level and rhyme level, these individuals were not able to segment small words into phonemes. Nevertheless, this also illustrates that being literate is not an obligatory prerequisite for assessing rhyme. Phonemic awareness does not emerge spontaneously, even when there are other forms of phonological awareness, such as 'rhyme awareness'.

Bertelson and de Gelder (1989) also demonstrated that children in a preliterate age (as well as illiterate subjects) were able to judge the quality of rhymes while at the same time being unable to manipulate phonemes. This is in keeping with later studies (e.g. Morais *et al.*, 1979, 1986) with illiterate adults who obtained weak results in phoneme manipulation tasks, whether subjects were required to add or omit phonemes in words, whereas most illiterate subjects succeeded in rhyme tasks.

Concerning awareness of word length, Kolinsky *et al.* (1987) concluded that this competence was actually related to different levels of literacy and not to age and its corresponding cognitive maturation stages. Nevertheless, illiterate adults do have a certain level of awareness of word length, even if they perform worse than literate adults. Such data prove that these individuals can focus their attention on the word's phonologic form, being able to calculate the word's length without there being any interference of the object's actual size. For instance, subjects manage to understand that the word 'borboleta' (butterfly) is larger than the word 'gato' (cat) without there being any interference of their knowledge on the real size of these two animals. This seems to imply a certain degree of abstract knowledge in illiterate individuals.

Together, the findings above suggest the possibility of the existence of different levels of phonological awareness. In respect of this hypothesis, Morais *et al.* (1986) compared a sample of Portuguese illiterate adults to a sample of literate adults with the same social status, on different metaphonological tasks. Their results agreed with Liberman *et al.* (1974).

Literate adults had superior results in metaphonological tasks compared to illiterate subjects. However, illiterate subjects obtained better results in rhyme tasks than in phoneme manipulation tasks. Tasks involving rhyme judgement seem to call for little metaphonological reflection, being more associated with speech than with metaphonological knowledge. This ability of rhyme judgement could be associated with nursery rhyme experiences; however, most illiterate people learn these traditional poems and songs in the family context and not at school.

Gombert (1992) and others authors who will be mentioned in this chapter, have proposed that there is a progression in the degree of metaphonological awareness. We can include sounds and syllables in the definition of metaphonological awareness. Metaphonological development needs to be studied as a continuum, starting from implicit language knowledge that gradually develops into a sort of explicit knowledge, one that is connected to a learning process.

If we admit that there is a progression in the levels of metalinguistic knowledge, from more implicit levels to more explicit levels, it is necessary to recognise literacy as a cause of this gradual change.

## Studies in Patients with Aphasia

Within the field of research on illiterate individuals, studies involving illiterate people with aphasia have afforded a unique opportunity to gain insights into error patterns and through these to make inferences concerning the nature of lexical access and phonological knowledge.

In a study by Colaço *et al.* (2010), groups were matched according to their type of aphasia, and in the case of the literate subjects according to their schooling level. There were two groups both of aphasic literate participants (six with fluent aphasia and nine with non-fluent aphasia) and aphasic illiterate participants (six with fluent aphasia and four with non-fluent aphasia). Object-naming tasks were conducted, including high frequency and morphological simple words (HFMSW), low frequency and morphological simple words (LFMSW) and low frequency and morphological complex words (LFMCW) – compounded and derivated items. Repetition tasks included morphological simple and complex words – compounded and derivated items. The group of literate people with aphasia produced more (but not statistically significant) morphophonological errors than the illiterate speakers, suggesting differences in lexical access organised by phonological programming strategies, as hypothesized by Castro-Caldas (2002).

These data reveal that illiterate people with aphasia do not seem to easily accomplish word segmentation, presumably since they have not established a grapheme-phoneme association. Their morphological errors can be argued to be caused by a deficit in lexical-phonological access, as stated in the study of Colaço *et al.* (2010). This type of error reflects the usual speech of illiterate people who do not have access to orthographic forms of the word. They produce phonetic simplifications. Illiterate people have greater difficulty in phonological decoding and create simplification rules, producing errors that correspond to the phonetically easier words. In the case of literate aphasic speakers, morphophonological errors seem to arise from their difficulty in phonetic planning, as illustrated in the following example: /alpi'neti/ instead of /alfi'neti/ (*'alfinete'* is *'pin'* in English), although we cannot define this as a systematic difference with only this sample of participants. In the same way, in the language acquisition process, unschooled children make more errors related to lexical-phonological processes than errors related to phonetic planning. Such a dichotomy between phonological access errors and planning errors is described in the literature by Kohn and Smith (1994) related to adults with aphasia.

Again in the study by Colaço *et al.* (2010), data from the literate and illiterate participants with fluent aphasia on a repetition task showed that illiterate speakers with aphasia produced a smaller number (but not statistically significant) of lexical-semantic errors than their literate pairs, and also incurred a smaller number of other errors. This fact can be interpreted again as a lexical selection strategy supported in semantic relations and more 'diffuse' activations (such as circumlocutions) than the morphophonological approaches produced by literate aphasic speakers. This difference relates to literacy and is not simply a matter of different aphasic profiles among speakers because these groups were matched for aphasia type – Wernicke's, conduction, Broca's and transcortical motor aphasia.[1]

Fonseca *et al.* (2002), contrary to other studies such as Lecours *et al.* (1987) and Rosselli *et al.* (1990), did not find any significant differences between groups of paired illiterate and literate speakers, either in object-naming and identification tasks or in sentence comprehension tasks. Differences were found only in word repetition, where illiterate subjects produced inferior results, suggesting once more that differences lie at the level of phonological knowledge in these individuals.

## Repetition and Phonological Awareness

It is claimed that word repetition can be performed through three routes: the semantic route, the lexical route and the phonological route (Chialant *et al.*, 2002; Levelt *et al.*, 1999).

Through the semantic route, after having heard a certain word, the individual analyses the auditory signal and through phonological-lexical input gains access to that word's lexical-semantical representations, decoding its meaning. This is the semantic route for word repetition, through which one accesses the meaning of a heard word and only after that produces the word.

The fact that we can repeat pseudowords for which there is no semantic representation leads us to believe that repetition can also be processed from phonological decoding (input) followed by phonological coding (output). This is the hypothesized phonological route for word repetition.

Nevertheless, there are cases where access to semantics as well as to pseudoword repetition is impaired. Here, only the repetition of known words is retained, which proves that neither the semantic route nor the phonological route is being used for word repetition. In these cases, repetition happens through a lexical route. Lexical effects appear because the words are in some way easier to access than pseudowords. Figure 8.1 illustrates how these three routes are activated in word repetition.

Since illiterate speakers seem to be more supported by information processing strategies sustained by reference to semantics, these individuals are left with a smaller range of choices concerning word repetition processing mechanisms if we assume that other routes are uniquely dependent on phonological processes.

Studies such as those of Adrián (1993) and Rosselli *et al.* (1989, 1990) demonstrated that there are differences in the ability to repeat pseudowords between literate and illiterate subjects, again suggesting illiterate speakers are poorer at segmental analysis, with a stronger tendency to process a word's meaning rather than its form.

The weaker ability to repeat words can be interpreted as follows: people who use language in its written form have their auditory-phonological decoding more trained, which facilitates access to a wider spectrum of

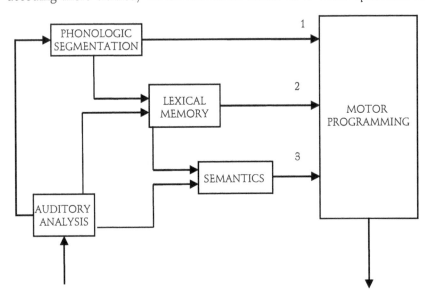

**Figure 8.1** Phonological route; 2 – Lexical route; 3 – Semantic route

information, and this favourably influences the production of errors (Castro-Caldas *et al.*, 1995). On the other hand, illiterate subjects rely on semantic clues as a cognitive strategy, ensuring a better performance in word repetition tasks than in pseudoword repetition tasks – so long as their semantic access is intact.

Castro-Caldas *et al.* (1994) demonstrated that word repetition was more altered in illiterate subjects than in literate individuals with Wernicke's aphasia. In another study (Castro-Caldas *et al.*, 1998), the group of illiterate subjects presented results that were slightly inferior in word repetition, and results considerably inferior in pseudoword repetition, indicating once again that there are different competences in certain aspects of language phonological processing. Previously, Castro Caldas *et al.* (1997) had observed a close connection between the results of auditory word comprehension tasks and those of oral word repetition tasks in the illiterate population, which was not present in the group of literate aphasics. These studies suggest that illiterate individuals need to understand the semantic content in order to make a decision, in this case word repetition.

Therefore, we can conclude that the use of a direct morphophonological route is particularly limited due to the absence of visual-graphic effects in the auditory units of spoken language. The strong conclusion of the results presented in these studies appears to be that illiterate speakers are more limited to processing the content of the information. That is, conceptual organisation in illiterate speakers is more based on lexical-semantic associations than on associations related to the words' phonological attributes. Further, if phonological coding is ineffective, it can mean that the phonological route is not sufficiently developed for lexical access.

These differences in accessing lexicon and cognitive processing in illiterate individuals raise important questions on cerebral organisation for these competences and also the importance of their underdevelopment.

# The Neurobiology of Literacy

Through the use of neuroimaging techniques, Castro-Caldas *et al.* (1998) observed that the acquisition of a phonological-orthographic system can influence the auditory-verbal processing of spoken language. This study used *positron emission tomography* (PET) and statistical parametric mapping within a brain activation study. The authors compared tasks of word and pseudoword repetition in literate and illiterate subjects. In the task of repetition of real words, the two groups activated similar areas of the brain. However, the illiterate subjects had more difficulty repeating pseudowords correctly and did not activate the same neural structures as the literate subjects. These results were taken to demonstrate that learning the written form of language (orthography) interacts with the functional organisation of the oral form of language.

These differences raise the question of how these competences are organised in the brain. Claims exist that literacy is a factor responsible for typical cortical language representation, and it enhances cerebral dominance for speech (Cameron *et al.*, 1971; Damásio *et al.*, 1979).

In a study by Petersson *et al.* (2007), evidence was presented that illiterate speakers were consistently more lateralized to the right than the literate subjects evaluated. These results suggest that a cultural factor, such as literacy, may influence the inter-hemispheric functional balance in reading tasks and in verbal working memory.

Apparently, illiterate subjects activate more participation of the right hemisphere, that is, 'mechanisms not directly related to linguistic processing' (Castro-Caldas *et al.*, 1995). Clinical follow-up of aphasic patients has led researchers to suggest that the severity of aphasia in illiterate people tends to be less, what comes against some studies that suggested that the right hemisphere is involved in language processing in illiterate subjects (Connor *et al.*, 2001; Lecours *et al.*, 1988; Parente & Lecours, 1998; Reis & Petersson, 2003).

Using the dichotic listening technique, Tzavaras *et al.* (1981) used pairs of digits and found that illiterate participants showed a larger right ear advantage than educated control subjects, which would suggest a left hemisphere preference. The authors claimed that 'the acquisition of reading and writing skills results in an ambi-hemispheric representation of strategies (mechanisms) for the solution of some language problems'.

Other studies have contributed to the idea that biofunctional organisation in the brain is altered by schooling, namely its anatomy (Carreiras *et al.*, 2009; Castro-Caldas *et al.*, 1999) and the areas activated (Petersson *et al.*, 1999, 2007). Neuroimaging studies have verified that the activation of a specific region of the brain, located in the left temporal-occipital cortex, called the 'visual word form area' (VWFA), appears to be associated with learning how to read (Dehaene *et al.*, 2010; Maurer *et al.*, 2006; Shaywitz *et al.*, 2002).

Castro-Caldas *et al.* (1998) demonstrated that on a repetition task, the illiterate participants performed significantly worse than the literate participants. Neuroimaging results showed that: (1) during real-word repetition, the left inferior parietal gyrus was more active in the literate group; and (2) during pseudoword repetition, the right frontal operculum/anterior insula, left anterior cingulate, left putamen/pallidum, anterior thalamus/hypothalamus, pons and medial cerebellum were more active in the literate group.

The question then is as follows: is it that the low performance in the illiterate group results from the weak activation of these areas or is the former the cause of the latter?

It is possible to establish a parallel with the neurobiology of bilingualism, since early acquisition, use and linguistic proficiency in two or more languages result in a more economic, neuronal 'activation' in coextensive areas in the respective languages.

One of the questions that might contribute to the understanding of the neurobiology of language in literate and illiterate subjects is how the neurobiology of bilingual speakers is organised. Is it that the brain regions utilised are identical for both languages? In which circumstances does one language overlap the other? Is it that late acquisition provokes a wider involvement of the right hemisphere, similarly to what happens to illiterate subjects when they learn how to read later in life?

## Neurobiology of Bilingualism

In neurobiological terms, scientific evidence leads us to suppose that bilingual speakers may engage different regions of the brain for both languages (Yetkin et al., 1996) as a result of the potential role of a number of environmental variables such as proficiency, language exposure and age of second language (L2) acquisition. All these variables seem to play an important role in the shaping of language representations in the bilingual brain (Abutalebi et al., 2005). There is consensus that language acquisition and its processing are associated with a specific part of the brain: the perisylvian region of the left hemisphere.

Recent studies in brain imagery investigating language production and comprehension suggest that the L2 learned later in life activates a non-overlapping area of the brain that of the L2 acquired early (Dehaene et al., 1997; Kim et al., 1997).

Research conducted by Kim et al. (1997) on early and late bilingual acquisition revealed a different physical location for L2, in the regions of Broca and Wernicke, in the case of late bilinguals. In the case of early bilingual acquisition, the regions for the two languages are identical. Dehaene et al. (1997) in a study on English–French bilingual speakers, all of whom acquired their L2 after the age of seven, showed common areas of cerebral activation in the left temporal lobe for all participants when they were using their first language (L1), and variable areas of activation when they were using their L2. Wartenburger et al. (2003) tested three groups of bilinguals: (i) 11 participants with early acquired L2, during childhood; (ii) 12 participants who acquired their L2 in adulthood, but who attained a high level of proficiency; and (iii) 9 subjects who acquired their L2 later in life and attained limited proficiency. The results demonstrated that, although acquisition age is a determinant as to grammar processing *loci*, the same does not happen with regard to semantic processing. Only if the L2 is acquired at a very early age do neuronal regions activated for L1 and L2 overlap.

In the case of late bilinguals, proficiency is vital in the brain organisation of both grammar and semantics. Regarding phonology, the study by Yetkin *et al.* (1996) showed that people who were not yet fluent in the language activated the frontal lobe when doing tasks involving with voxels. The native speakers and fluent L2 speakers produced equivalent activation. These findings are consistent with the critical period hypothesis (Lenneberg, 1964) in language acquisition, suggesting that grammatical processing is dependent on age of acquisition and is based on a neurological competence that should be 'wired in'.

Functional organisation of languages in the bilingual speaker's brain can exhibit substantial differences. Perani *et al.* (2003) in their study using fMRI concluded that a wider brain area is activated in the case of subjects who are less exposed to their L2, even if they exhibit great proficiency in that language. These results are consistent with those of Illes *et al.* (1999) who did not find any differences in brain activity concerning L1 and L2 speakers during semantic tasks, and also with the research of Chee *et al.* (2001) who found a similar pattern of brain activity for early and late bilinguals. The crucial factor in brain organisation in this case seems to be, therefore, late bilinguals' high proficiency.

In this discussion, still, we need to bear in mind the proposal of Paradis (2004) who anchors the notion of bilingualism in the distinction between implicit and explicit language knowledge. Implicit knowledge implies non-conscious processing and this is depleted in adults for processing that is not established or automatised at an early stage. In order to compensate for this deficit, late bilinguals utilise their declarative memory, that is, their 'explicit knowledge'. This neurolinguistic theory on bilingualism would explain, on the one hand, the different activation *loci* in early and late bilinguals because process memory and declarative memory might not be located in coextensive regions. On the other hand, it would also explain the reason for which semantic knowledge acquisition – declarative and non-procedural knowledge – remains unchanged beyond the critical period for language acquisition. For Paradis (2004), the fact that metalinguistic knowledge never becomes implicit competence does not mean that it is useless for the acquisition of an L2. Metalinguistic awareness helps in learning a new language, but it helps one to acquire it only indirectly, in a non-automatised fashion. Practice itself leads to the internalisation of implicit procedures that allow the individual to understand and produce well-formed sentences in an automatic way. Metalinguistic competence serves for checking the well-formedness of the automatic output of the implicit system.

Transferring these notions of age of acquisition and automaticity, explicit-implicit processing to literacy one might speculate that illiterate people show greater difficulties in producing grammatical judgements concerning speech output, because their metalinguistic knowledge is not as developed as that of literate people and they are unable to resort to wider strategies to solve task demands.

The difference in 'implicit' and 'explicit' language knowledge can be compared in these two groups of individuals – illiterate and bilingual. We know that illiteracy conditions metaphonologic knowledge during verbal production and in linguistic judgements. Late bilinguals will eventually resort to this metalinguistic knowledge, which is more explicit, when using both languages, contrary to early bilinguals, in the case of which knowledge is implicitly presented. This reinforces the idea of a critical period concerning language acquisition and particularly the acquisition of an L2.

Studies in the neurobiology of literacy and studies in bilingualism allow us to understand that activation areas do not seem to be the same, both in the case of people who learned to read and write *vs* illiterate people, and in the case of bilinguals *vs* non-bilinguals. There are indications that metaphonological knowledge is developed through learning reading and writing skills; however, it is not yet possible to explain precisely the extent to which these skills influence cerebral organisation.

Behavioural studies lead us to understand that metaphonological knowledge is an ability that is defined as 'absent' or 'present'. We would argue that this knowledge should be interpreted as a continuum of skills, given that there are differences in the ability to analyse words through smaller phonological units, either phonemes or syllables.

## Conclusion

The importance of school attendance as a variable in studying phonological processes has been broached and we argue should be taken into account in any metaphonological study, since it appears that literacy, i.e. learning how to perform grapheme-phoneme conversions and vice versa, is not the only variable that modifies knowledge in a language.

Speech output has been widely explored in different languages, but metaphonological knowledge, because it is so difficult to define and limit, is a linguistic domain that requires more research, and, most of all, more systematic comparisons between different types of languages, with different metaphonological codes, different patterns of phoneme-grapheme correspondence and different writing systems

## Note

(1)  All the subjects were evaluated through a formal evaluation using the Lisbon Evaluation Battery of Aphasia (Bateria de Avaliação de Afasias de Lisboa – BAAL), proving the aphasic diagnostic and respective type.

# References

Abutalebi, J., Cappa, S. and Perani, D. (2005) What can functional neuroimaging tell us about the bilingual brain? In J. Kroll and A.M.B. de Groot (eds) *Handbook of Bilingualism: Psycholinguistic Perspectives* (pp. 497–515). Oxford: Oxford University Press.

Adrián, J. (1993) Habilidade metafonologica en sujetos analfabetos y malos lectores. *Boletim de Psicologia* 39, 7–19.

Albert, M.L. and Obler, L.K. (1975) Mixed polyglot aphasia. Paper presented at the Academy of Aphasia, Victoria, BC.

Ardila, A., Ostrosky, F. and Mendoza, V. (2000) Learning to read is much more than learning to read: A neuropsychologically-based learning to read method. *Journal of the International Neuropsychological Society* 6, 789–801.

Bertelson, P. and de Gelder, B. (1989) Learning about reading from illiterates. In A.M. Galaburda (ed.) *From Reading to Neurons: Issues in the Biology of Language and Cognition* (pp. 1–25). Cambridge, MA: MIT Press.

Bloom, L. (1974) Talking, understanding and thinking. In R.L. Schiefelbusch and L.L. Lloyd (eds) *Language Perspectives – Acquisition, Retardation and Intervention* (pp. 285–311). Baltimore, MD: University Park Press.

Briellmann, R.S., Saling, M.M., Connel, A.B., Waites, A.B., Abbott, D.F. and Jackson, G.D. (2004) A high-field functional MRI study of quadrilingual subjects, *Brain and Language* 89, 531–542.

Cameron, R.F., Currier, R. and Haerer, A.F. (1971) Aphasia and literacy. *Journal of Language & Communication Disorders* 6, 161–163.

Campbell, R., Calvert, G., Brammer, M., MacSweeney, M., Surguladze, S., McGuire, P., Woll, B., Williams, S., Amaro, E. and David, A.S. (1999) Activation in auditory cortex by speechreading in hearing people: fMRI studies. Auditory-Visual Speech Processing Conference (AVSP'99), 7–10 August, Santa Cruz, CA.

Carreiras, M., Seghier, M., Baquero, S., Estévez, A., Lozano, A., Devlin, J.T. and Price, C.J. (2009) An anatomical signature for literacy. *Nature* 461, 983–U245.

Castro-Caldas, A. (2000) *A herança de Franz Joseph Gall*. Lisbon: McGraw-Hill.

Castro-Caldas, A. (2002) *O cérebro analfabeto: A influência do conhecimento das regras da leitura e da escrita na função cerebral*. Lisbon: Bial.

Castro-Caldas, A., Reis, A. and Parreira, E. (1994) Word repetition by illiterate aphasics: The importance of phonological awareness. Poster presented at the Research Group Meeting on Aphasia & Cognitive Disorders, Budapest, 17–18 June, Hungary.

Castro-Caldas, A., Ferro, J., Guerreiro, M., Mariano, G. and Farrajota, L. (1995) Influence of literacy (vs illiteracy) on the characteristics of acquired aphasia in adults. In C. Leong and R. Joshi (eds) *Developmental and Acquired Dyslexia* (pp. 79–81). Dordrecht: Kluwer Academic.

Castro-Caldas, A., Reis, A. and Guerreiro, M. (1997) Neuropsychological aspects of illiteracy. *Neuropsychological Rehabilitation* 7, 327–338.

Castro-Caldas, A., Petersson, K.M., Reis, A., Stone-Elander, S. and Ingvar, M. (1998) The illiterate brain: Learning to read and write during childhood influences the functional organization of adult brain. *Brain* 121, 1053–1063.

Castro-Caldas, A., Miranda, P., Carmo, I., Reis, A., Leote, F., Ribeiro, C. and Ducla-Soares, E. (1999) Influence of learning to read and write on the morphology of the corpus callosum. *European Journal of Neurology* 6, 23–28.

Chee, M.W.L., Caplan, D., Soon, C.S., Sriram, N., Tan, E.W.L., Thiel, T. and Weekes, B. (1999) Processing of visually presented sentences in Mandarin and English studied with fMRI. *Neuron* 23, 127–137.

Chialant, D., Costa, A. and Caramazza, A. (2002) Models of naming. In A.E. Hillis (ed.) *The Handbook of Adult Language Disorders: Integrating Cognitive Neuropsychology, Neurology and Rehabilitation* (pp. 123–163). New York: Psychology Press.

Cohen, L., Dehaene, S., Naccache, L., Lehéricy, S., Dehaene-Lambertz, G., Hénaff, M.A. and Michel, F. (2000) Visual word form area: Spatial and temporal characterization of an initial stage of reading in normal subjects and posterior split-brain patients. *Brain* 123, 291–307.

Colaço, D., Mineiro, A., Leal, G. and Castro-Caldas, A. (2010) Revisiting 'The influence of literacy in paraphasias of aphasic speakers'. *Clinical Linguistics Phonetics* 24, 890–905.

Connor, L.T., Obler, L.K., Tocco, M., Fitzpatrick, P.M. and Albert, M.L. (2001) Effect of socio-economic status on aphasia severity and recovery. *Brain and Language* 78, 254–257.

Coppens, P., Parente, M.A. and Lecours, A.R. (1998) Aphasia in illiterate individuals. In P. Coppens, Y. Lebrun and A. Basso (eds) *Aphasia in Atypical Populations* (pp. 175–202). Mahwah, NJ: Lawrence Erlbaum Associates.

Curtiss, S. (1977) *Genie: A Psycholinguistic Study of a Modern-Day "Wild Child"*. New York: Academic Press.

Damásio, H., Damásio, A.R., Castro Caldas, A. and Hamsher, K. (1979) Reversal of ear advantage for phonetically similar words in illiterates. *Journal Clinical Neuropsychology* 1, 331–338.

De Groot, A.M.B. and Kroll, J.F. (eds) (1997) *Tutorials in Bilingualism: Psycholinguistic Perspectives*. Mahwah, NJ: Erlbaum.

Dehaene, S., Dupoux, E., Mehler, J., Cohen, L. and Perani, P. (1997) Anatomical variability in the cortical representation of the first and second language. *NeuroReport* 8, 3809–3815.

Dehaene, S., Pegado, F., Braga, L.W., Ventura, P., Nunes Filho, G., Jobert, A., Dehaene-Lambertz, G., Kolinsky, R., Morais, J. and Cohen, L. (2010) How learning to read changes the cortical networks for vision and language. *Science* 330, 1359–1364.

Dehaene, S. and Cohen, L. (2011) The unique role of the visual word form area in reading. *Trends in Cognitive Sciences* 15, 254–262.

Fonseca, J., Guerreiro, M. and Castro-Caldas, A. (2002) Analfabetismo e recuperação da afasia. *Sinapse* 2, 39–50.

Gathercole, S.E. (2006) Nonword repetition and word learning: The nature of the relationship. *Applied Psycholinguistics* 27, 513–543.

Gombert, J. (1992) *Metalinguistic Development*. Hemel Hempstead: Harvester Wheatsheaf.

Hatcher, P., Hulme, C. and Elli, A.W. (1994) Ameliorating early reading failure by integrating the teaching of reading and phonology skills: The phonological linkage hypothesis. *Child Development* 65, 41–57.

Illes, J., Francis, W.S., Desmond, J.E., Gabrieli, J.D.E., Glover, G.H., Poldrack, R., Lee, C.J. and Wagner, A.D. (1999) Convergent cortical representation of semantic processing in bilinguals. *Brain and Language* 70, 347–363.

Kim, K.H., Hirsch, J., Relkin, N., De Laz Paz, R. and Lee, K.M. (1997) Distinct cortical areas associated with native and second languages. *Nature* 388, 171–174.

Kohn, S.E. and Smith, K.L. (1994) Distinctions between two phonological output deficits. *Applied Psycholinguistics* 15, 75–95.

Kolinsky, R., Cary, L. and Morais, J. (1987) Awareness of words as phonological entities. The role of literacy. *Applied Psycholinguistics* 8, 223–232.

Kosmidis, M.H., Tsapkini, K. and Folia, V. (2006) Lexical processing in illiteracy: Effect of literacy or education? *Cortex* 42, 1021–1027.

Lecours, A.R., Mehler, J., Parente, M.A., Caldeira, A., Cary, L., Castro, M.J., Dehaut, F.P., Delgado, R., Gurd, J., Karmann, D.F., Jakubovitz, R., Osorio, Z., Cabral, L.S.

and Junqueira, A.M.S. (1987) Illiteracy and brain damage: 1. Aphasia testing in culturally contrasted populations. *Neuropsychologia* 25, 231–245.

Lecours, A.R., Mehler, J. and Parente, M.A.M.P. (1988) Illiteracy in brain damage: A contribution to the study of speech and language disorders in illiterates with brain damage. *Neuropsychologia* 104, 98–108.

Lenneberg, E. (1964) *New Directions in the Study of Language.* Cambridge: MIT Press.

Levelt, W.J.M., Roelofs, A. and Meyer, A.S. (1999) A theory of lexical access in speech production. *Behavioral and Brain Sciences* 22, 1–75.

Liberman, I.Y., Shankweiler, D., Fischer, F.W. and Carter, B. (1974) Explicit syllable and phoneme segmentation in the young child. *Journal of Experimental Child Psychology* 18, 201–212.

Maurer, U., Brem, S., Kranz, F., Bucher, K., Benz, R., Halder, P., Steinhausen, H.C. and Brandeis, D. (2006) Coarse neural tuning for print peaks when children learn to read. *Neuroimage* 33, 749–758.

Morais, J. (1993) Phonemic awareness language and literacy. In R.M. Joshi and C.K. Leong (eds) *Reading Disabilities: Diagnosis and Component Processes* (pp. 175–184). Dordrecht: Kluwer Academic.

Morais, J. (1997) *A arte de ler: Psicologia cognitiva da leitura.* Lisbon: Edições Cosmo.

Morais J., Cary, L., Alegria, J. and Bertelson, P. (1979) Does awareness of speech as a sequence of phones arise spontaneously? *Cognition* 7, 323–331.

Morais, J., Bertelson, P., Cary, L. and Alegria, J. (1986) Literacy training and speech segmentation. *Cognition* 24, 45–64.

Newport, E. (1991) Contrasting concepts of the critical period for language. In S. Carey and R. Gelman (eds) *The Epigenesis of Mind: Essays on Biology and Cognition* (pp. 111–130). Hillsdale, NJ: Lawrence Erlbaum Associates.

Ostrosky-Solís, F., Lozano, A., Ramírez, M., Picasso, H., Gomez, E. and Velez, A. (2003) Estudio neuropsicologico de poblacion mexicana en proceso de alfabetizacion. *Revista Mexicana de Psicologia* 20, 5–17.

Paradis, M. (1977) Bilingualism and aphasia. In H. Witaker and H.A. Witaker (eds) *Studies in Neurolinguistics* (pp. 65–121). New York: Academic Press.

Paradis, M. (1985) On the representation of two languages in one brain. *Languages Sciences* 7, 1–39.

Paradis, M. (2004) *A Neurolinguistic Theory of Bilingualism.* Amsterdam: John Benjamins.

Parente, M. and Lecours, A.R. (1998) Participação do hemisfério direito na recuperação das afasias de analfabetos. *Neuropsychologia Latina* 4, 73–78.

Perani, D., Abutalebi, J., Paulesu, E., Brambati, S., Scifo, P., Cappa, S.F. and Fazio, F. (2003) The role of age acquisition and language usage in early, high-proficient bilinguals: A fMRI study during verbal fluency. *Human Brain Mapping* 19, 170–182.

Petersson, K.M., Reis, A., Castro-Caldas, A. and Ingvar, M. (1999) Effective auditory-verbal encoding activates the left prefrontal and the medial temporal lobes: A generalization to illiterate subjects. *NeuroImage* 10, 45–54.

Petersson, K., Reis, A., Askelof, S., Castro-Caldas, A. and Ingvar, M. (2000) Language processing modulated by literacy: A network analysis of verbal repetition in literate and illiterate subjects. *Journal of Cognitive Neuroscience* 12, 364–382.

Petersson, K., Silva, C., Castro Caldas, A., Ingvar, M. and Reis, A. (2007) Literacy: A cultural influence on functional left-right differences in the inferior parietal cortex. *European Journal of Neuroscience* 26, 791–799.

Reis, A., Guerreiro, M. and Castro Caldas, A. (1994) Influence of educational level of non brain-damaged subjects on visual naming capacities. *Journal of Clinical and Experimental Neuropsychology* 16, 939–942.

Reis, A. and Petersson, K. (2003) Education level, socioeconomic status and aphasia research: A comment on Connor et al. (2001) – effect socioeconomic status on aphasia severity and recovery. *Brain and Language* 87, 449–452.

Rosselli, M., Ardila, A. and Rosas, P. (1989) Neuropsychological assessment in illiterates: Visuospatial and memory abilities. *Brain and Cognition* 11, 147–166.

Rosselli, M., Ardila, A. and Rosas, P. (1990) Neuropsychological assessment in illiterates: Language and praxic abilities. *Brain and Cognition* 12, 281–296.

Shaywitz, B.A., Shaywitz, S.E., Pugh, K.R., Mencel, E., Fulbright, R., Skudlarski, P., Constable, T., Marcxhione, K., Fletcher, J.M., Lyon, G.R. and Gore, J. (2002) Disruption of posterior brain systems for reading in children with developmental dyslexia. *Biological Psychiatry* 52, 101–110.

Tzavaras, A., Kaprinis, G. and Gatzoyas, A. (1981). Literacy and hemispheric specialization for language: Digit dichotic listening in illiterates. *Neuropsychologia* 19, 565–570.

Wartenburger, I., Heekeren, H.R., Abutalebi, J., Cappa, S.F., Villringer, A. and Perani, D. (2003) Early setting of grammatical processing in the bilingual brain. *Neuron* 37, 1–20.

Yetkin, O., Yetkin, F.Z., Haughton, V.M. and Cox, R.W. (1996) Use of functional MR to map language in multilingual volunteers. *American Journal of Neuroradiology* 17, 473–476.

# Part 2

# Language Specific Profiles and Practices

# 9 Dysarthria and Apraxia of Speech in Selected African Languages: Zulu and Tswana

Anita van der Merwe
and Mia Le Roux

## Introduction

South Africa has 11 official languages. Two of these are English and Afrikaans and the other nine are African languages belonging to the Bantu language family. Zulu is spoken as first language (L1) by almost 24% of the population of approximately 50 million people. As L1, Tswana is spoken by 8.2%, English by 8.2% and Afrikaans by 13.35% of the population (Lewis, 2009). However, the language of communication is English. Most speakers in South Africa are bilingual or multilingual. Zulu and Tswana will be the focus of this chapter as these are two of the most prevalent languages spoken in South Africa.

Approximately 2000 speech-language pathologists are registered with the South African Speech-Language-Hearing Association. Of these, a small percentage (around 10%) is L1 Bantu language speakers. It is a young profession and the rendering of services to all language groups remains a daunting challenge. Some of the major difficulties in devising materials are the prevalence of dialectal variation in the Bantu languages and the multilingual nature of communities where different languages impact on each other. Pure forms of these languages are spoken only in remote rural areas (Jacobson & Traill, 1986). A need exists to adapt many criteria characterising English materials and there is an argument that published English tests need to be adapted to English as spoken in the local contexts. A survey done by Mphahlele (2006) revealed that the first clinical assessment tool developed for a local language was the Afrikaans articulation test by Lotter in 1974. Since the first assessment tool for a local language was developed, numerous assessment protocols for different speech, language and hearing disorders have been developed in different official languages, but most of these are not standardised or adequately verified and remain informal clinical instruments.

In the field of neuromotor speech disorders, the manifestation of these disorders in the speech of L1 and second language (L2) English and Afrikaans speakers has been studied extensively (Erasmus *et al.*, 1993; Gillmer & Van der Merwe, 1983; Klopper *et al.*, 1984; Theron *et al.*, 2009; Van der Merwe, 2007; Van der Merwe & Grimbeek, 1990; Van der Merwe & Tesner, 2000; Van der Merwe *et al.*, 1987, 1988, 1989). However, *neuromotor* speech disorders in speakers of southern Bantu languages have only been addressed in four recent studies (Coetzee *et al.*, 2011; Dogil & Mayer, 1998; Fouché & Van der Merwe, 1999; Mahwayi *et al.*, 2011). Some of these results are reported in this chapter.

## Bantu Language Groups

Bantu languages belong to one fairly homogeneous family of languages. Early linguists noted the linguistic homogeneity of this family of languages. The name that was attributed to this family of languages in 1862 has been credited to the father of Bantu linguistics, Wilhelm Bleek (Ziervogel, 1967: 7). Between 300 and 600 Bantu languages are geographically spread across the sub-Saharan African continent. These languages can be classified into different language groups. Language groups that are found in the south-eastern zone of Africa include the language groups of South Africa, namely Nguni, Sotho, Venda and Tsonga. Each of these language groups is subdivided

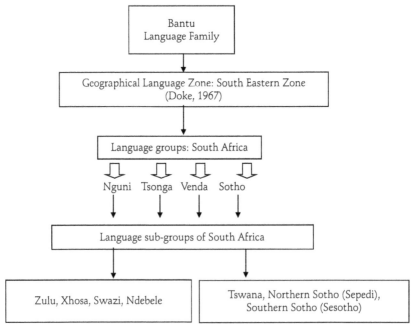

**Figure 9.1** Subdivisions within the Bantu language groups found in the south-eastern zone of Africa with special reference to the Nguni and Sotho sub-groups in South Africa

to form dialect clusters (Cole, 1992; Doke, 1967; Jacobson & Traill, 1986; Poulos & Bosch, 1997). Figure 9.1 provides an overview of the language groups found in South Africa. In this chapter, the focus is on Tswana which belongs to the Sotho group and on Zulu which belongs to the Nguni group. In the text, reference will be made to African languages as this is the more popular term, but the intention is to refer to Bantu languages.

## The Sound Systems of Tswana and Zulu

English contains 24 consonants and 14 vowels. Tswana has 29 consonants and seven basic vowel phonemes (Cole, 1992). Zulu contains 59 consonants and five basic vowels (Ziervogel, 1967). The consonant systems of Bantu languages, and Zulu in particular, are thus more varied than that of the English language.

Information in the following sections was compiled from several sources. Various phoneticians have worked in this field (e.g. Cole, 1992; Cope, 1983; Doke, 1967; Poulos & Bosch, 1997; Poulos & Msimang, 1998; Taljaard & Snyman, 1993; Westerman & Ward, 1990; Ziervogel, 1967). Aspects of the phonetics of Bantu languages are still debated and some of these points of debate will be mentioned in the following sections.

### The vowels

Traditional vowel charts for Tswana and Zulu, based on a perceptual comparison with the cardinal vowels are presented in Figure 9.2 (Tswana) and Figure 9.3 (Zulu).

The seven Tswana vowel phonemes are differentiated into 11 vowel phones. Four *raised* allophones of the mid-high and mid-low vowels are distinguished (Cole, 1992). Vowel raising is the process whereby vowels

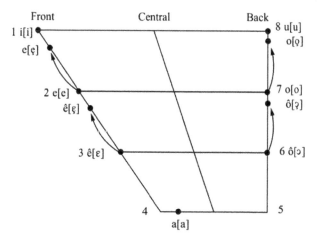

**Figure 9.2** Vowel chart of Tswana

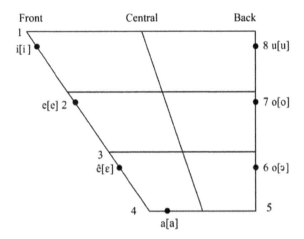

**Figure 9.3** Vowel chart of Zulu

with a higher tongue position influence those pronounced with the tongue in a lower position when they appear in succeeding syllables (Snyman, 1989). The positioning of vowels on the vowel chart of Tswana is still debated. Based on perceptual analysis, their positions are traditionally portrayed as equidistant from one another. An acoustic investigation indicates that the vowels are not evenly spaced along the outer limits of the vowel chart and also that the issue of vowel raising is not as simplistic as suggested by traditional vowel charts and descriptions (Le Roux & Le Roux, 2008).

Zulu has five basic vowels and two variants of the basic vowels /o/ and /e/. Vowel raising does not take place, but vowel assimilation does (Ziervogel, 1967: 82, 166). When the mid-low front vowel /ɛ/ and mid-low back vowel /ɔ/ are succeeded by high vowels /i/ and /u/, the /ɛ/ will become the mid-high front vowel /e/ and the /ɔ/ will become the mid-high back vowel /o/. Example: [–ɓɔna] (to see) > [–ɓonisa] (to show).

## The consonants

The consonants of Tswana are summarised in Table 9.1 and that of Zulu in Table 9.2. The information in the tables was adapted from Snyman (1989) and Taljaard and Snyman (1993).

## Manner of articulation of consonants

### Manner of airstream release

The following sounds occur in Tswana and Zulu: plosives, implosives (present in Zulu), ejectives, affricates, trills, fricatives, approximants, nasals and clicks. Clicks are characteristic of Nguni languages. The different click positions are dental, palatal and alveo-lateral.

Clicks are perceptually sharp and distinct as a class, but to the untrained ear there is much confusion within the class. From a universal perspective, clicks are highly marked consonants, but there is virtually no existing discussion of the question of markedness *within* the class (Herbert, 1990). Three issues are regarded as unresolved with regard to the description of click sounds. These are the different phonetic transcription systems for clicks, a controversy regarding the places of articulation and the phonetic content of so-called affricated clicks (Roux, 2007).

Prenasalisation or partial nasalisation of sounds are features of Zulu. In Zulu, affricates, plosives and clicks can be prenasalised or partially nasalised (Cope, 1983; Ladefoged & Maddieson, 1996: 119; Naidoo *et al.*, 2005). Example of a prenasalised stop in Zulu: *i.mbu.zi* (goat) > /i.mbu.zi/. Although multiple articulatory gestures form the 'mb' (also 'nd' and 'ng'), these are generally regarded as single phonemes. However, phonetically they are noted as [mb], [nd] and [ŋg] (Ladefoged & Maddieson, 1996: 119). Prenasalised stops are also referred to as nasal compounds.

Affricates occur frequently in Bantu languages. The affricates such as [kxʰ] or the aspirated [tʃʰ] are regarded as one consonant phoneme, but orthographically multiple symbols are implemented (Cole, 1992: 52; Ziervogel, 1967: 11). Example: Tswana: *kgɔ.mo.ga.di* (cow) > [kxʰo.mo.xa.di]; Zulu dialect: *-tshe.tsha* (hurry) > [tʃʰɛ.tʃʰa].

## Nature of airstream

Tswana and Zulu speech sounds can be voiced, voiceless, aspirated or, in Zulu, breathy voiced. The mechanism of production of aspiration is similar to aspiration in English. However, in Tswana and Zulu, aspiration of sounds changes the *meaning* of a word (Van Rooy & Grijzenhout, 2000). In African languages, aspiration is written phonetically as a superscript /ʰ/ after the aspirated consonant. In the majority of words, aspiration is also indicated in normal orthography by an 'h'. Examples: Tswana: *tha.ba* (mountain) > /tʰa.ba/; *ta.ba* (case, such as legal case) > /ta.ba/; Zulu: *-pha.na* (give to one another) > /-pʰa.na/; *-pa.na* (to knee-halter/hobble) > /-pa.na/.

Zulu sounds can also be breathy or partially voiced. Breathy voice, which Ladefoged and Maddieson (1996: 48) equal to murmur, differs from aspiration in that during the production of breathy voice, vocal fold vibration does occur but without appreciable contact. Breathy voice can be implemented as a paralinguistic feature, but in Zulu breathy voice is phonemic and differentiates lexical meaning. A distinction is made between delayed breathy-voiced and fully breathy-voiced sounds. Zulu sounds such as /b/, /d/ and /g/ are described as delayed breathy-voiced sounds. When

**Table 9.1** The consonants of Tswana

| | Manner of articulation | | | Place of articulation | | | | | | | | | | | | | | | | | | | | | |
|---|---|---|---|---|---|---|---|---|---|---|---|---|---|---|---|---|---|---|---|---|---|---|---|---|---|
| Manner of airstream release | Nature of airstream | Airstream mechanism | Channel of airstream release | Bilabial | Labio-dental | Labio-prepalatal | Labio-palatal | Labio-velar | Apico-labio-alveolar | Apico-dental | Apico-alveolar | Apico-alveolabiodental | Apico-postalveolar | Apico-palatalalveolar | Lamino-dental | Lamino-postalveolar | Lamino-palatoalveolar | Dorsopalatal | Dorso-postpalatal | Dorsopalato-lateral | Dorsovelar | Uvular | Glottal | Practical orthography |
| **Plosive** | VL | | M | p | | | | | | | t | | | | | | | | | | k | | | p, t, k |
| | A | P | M | ph | | | | | | | th | | | | | | | | | | kh | | | ph, th, kh |
| | VL | | L | | | | | | | | tl | | | | | | | | | | | | | tl |
| | A | | L | | | | | | | | tlh | | | | | | | | | | | | | tlh |
| | V | | M | b | | | | | | | d | | | | | | | | | | | | | b, d |
| **Implosive** | | | | | | | | | | | | | | | | | | | | | | | | |
| **Affricate** | VL | | M | | | | | | | | ts | | | | | ʧ | | | | | | | | ts, tš |
| | A | P | M | | | | | | | | tsh | | | | | ʧh | | | | | kxh | | | tsh, tšh, kg |
| | V | | M | | | | | | | | | | | | | ʤ | | | | | | | | j |
| **Click** | VL | Li | M | | | | | | | | | | ǃ | | ǀ | | | | | | | | | q, c |
| | V | P+Li | N+M | | | | | | | | | | | | ŋǀ | | | | | | | | | nc |
| | VL | Li | L | | | | | | | | ǁ | | | | | | | | | | | | | x |
| | V | P+Li | N+L | | | | | | | | ŋǁ | | | | | | | | | | | | | nx |

CONTINUANT

| | | | | f | s | ʃ | x | h | |
|---|---|---|---|---|---|---|---|---|---|
| Fricative | VL | P | M | f | s | ʃ | x | h | f, s, š, g, h |
| Trill* | V | P | M | | r | | | | r |
| Approximant* | V | P | M | w | | | j | | w, y |
| | V | P | L | | l | | | | l |
| Nasal* | V | P | N | m | n | | ɲ | ŋ | m, n, ny, ng |

*Indicates Resonant

| | | |
|---|---|---|
| D = Delayed Breathy Voice | P = Pulmonic | M = Medial |
| F = Full Breathy Voice | L = Laryngeal | L = Lateral |
| A = Aspirated | Li = Lingual (velaric) | R = Retroflex |
| V = Voiced | | N = Nasal |
| VL = Voiceless | | |

**Table 9.2** The consonants of Zulu

| Manner of articulation | | | | Place of articulation | | | | | | | | | | | | | | | | | | | | Practical orthography |
|---|---|---|---|---|---|---|---|---|---|---|---|---|---|---|---|---|---|---|---|---|---|---|---|---|
| Manner of airstream release | Nature of airstream | Airstream mechanism | Channel of airstream release | Bilabial | Labio-dental | Labio-prepalatal | Labio-palatal | Labio-velar | Apico-labio-alveolar | Apico-dental | Apico-alveolar | Apico-alveolabiodental | Apico-postalveolar | Apico-palatalalveolar | Lamino-dental | Lamino-postalveolar | Lamino-palatoalveolar | Dorsopalatal | Dorso-postpalatal | Dorsopalato-lateral | Dorsovelar | Uvular | Glottal | |
| Plosive | VL | L | M | pʼ | | | | | | | tʼ | | | | | | | | | | kʼ | | | p, t, k |
| | A | P | M | pʰ | | | | | | | tʰ | | | | | | | | | | kʰ | | | ph, th, kh |
| | D | P | M | ɓ̥ | | | | | | | d̥ | | | | | | | | | | g | | | bh, d, g |
| | F | P | M | b̤ː | | | | | | | d̤ː | | | | | | | | | | ɡ̈ː | | | (m)b, (n)d, (n)g |
| | PF | P | M | | | | | | | | | | | | | | | | | | k̚ | | | k |
| Implosive | V | P + L | M | ɓ | | | | | | | | | | | | | | | | | | | | b |
| | VL | L | M | | | | | | | | | | | | | tʃʼ | | | | | | | | tsh |
| Affricate | F | P | L | | | | | | | | dɮ̥ | | | | | | | | | | | | | (n)dl |
| | F | P | M | | ɸv | | | | | | dz̤ː | | | | | ɮ̤ | | | | | | | | (m)v, (n)z, (n)j |
| | D | P | M | | pɸ | | | | | | tsʼ | | | | | dʒ | | | | | | | | (m)f, ts |
| | VL | L | L | | | | | | | | tɬʼ | | | | | | | | | | kɬʼ | | | (n)hl, kl |

Phonetic chart (rotated landscape table)

| Manner | Voice | Airstream | Position | | | | Orthography |
|---|---|---|---|---|---|---|---|
| Click | VL | Li | M | | ǃ | ǀ | q, c |
| | A | Li+P | M | | ǃh | ǀh | qh, ch |
| | D | Li+P | M | | ǃg° | ǀg° | gq, gc |
| | F | Li+P | M | | ǃg | ǀg | (n)gq, (n)gc |
| | ♥ | P+Li | N+M | | ŋǃ̃ | ŋǀ̃ | nq, nc |
| | V | P+Li | N+M | | ŋǃ | ŋǀ | (n)kq, (n)kc |
| | VL | Li | L | ǁ | | | x |
| | A | Li+P | L | ǁh | | | xh |
| | L | Li+P | L | ǁg° | | | gx |
| | F | Li+P | L | ǁg | | | (n)gx |
| | V | P+Li | L | ŋǁ̃ | | | (n)x |
| | V+VL | P+Li | L | ŋǁ | | | (n)kx |
| C O N T I N U A N T — Fricative | VL | P | M | s | ʃ | x | h f, s, sh, h, h |
| | F | P | M | z̤ | | | ɦ v, z, hh |
| | VL | P | L | ɬ | | | hl |
| | F | P | L | ɮ | | | dl |
| Trill* | F | P | M | r̩ | | | r |
| Approximant* | V | P | L | l | | | l |
| | F | P | L | l̩ | | | l |
| | V | P | M | w | j | w, y | w, y |
| Nasal* | V | P | N | n | ɲ | ŋ | m,(m)v, n, ny, (n)g |
| | F | P | N | n̥ | | | m, n |

*Indicates Resonant

| | | |
|---|---|---|
| D = Delayed Breathy Voice | P = Pulmonic | M = Medial |
| F = Full Breathy Voice | L = Laryngeal | L = Lateral |
| A = Aspirated | Li = Lingual | R = Retroflex |
| V = Voiced | (velaric) | N = Nasal |
| VL = Voiceless | | |
| PV = Partially Voiced | | |

they occur in nasal compounds these sounds become fully breathy-voiced sounds. Tswana does not contain breathy-voiced sounds.

### Airstream mechanism

The airstream utilised during the articulation of the sounds of Tswana and Zulu is pulmonic, glottalic egressive, glottalic ingressive or velaric (lingual). The latter is used to produce clicks. When nasalised clicks are articulated, both the pulmonic and velaric airstream mechanisms are employed: the pulmonic airstream mechanism for the articulation of the nasal segment and the velaric airstream mechanism for the articulation of the click component (Cole, 1992; Zerbian, 2009; Ziervogel, 1967). Example: [ŋǁ] in –*nxu.ma* (to cut off) > [-ŋǁu.ma].

## Syllable structure of Tswana and Zulu

In Bantu languages, syllables are characteristically open-ended or consist of syllabic phonemes. The syllable structure is either V (vowel), C (consonant) or CV. Words in Bantu languages are fundamentally disyllabic, i.e. the majority of *word stems* with all prefixes and suffixes removed have two syllables (Cole, 1992:52).

Due to the agglutinating nature of the Bantu languages and especially of the Nguni languages such as Zulu, words may contain several syllables. The most prominent feature of agglutinating languages is that prefixes and suffixes are conjunctively written with roots and word stems to form words. In agglutinative languages, each *affix* represents one unit of meaning such as a noun class prefix, diminutive, female gender, past tense, passive form of the verb, locative adverbs and plural. Zulu makes use of an even more conjunctive orthography than Tswana. Examples: Tswana: *Monnamogolo* > mo.n.na.mo.go.lo (an old man). Zulu: *Izihlabamkhosi* > I. zi.hla.ba.m.kho.si (a piercing noise).

Vowels and consonants can function as syllables. In Zulu, all noun class prefixes start with vowels. Example: Zulu: *u.ma.ma* (mother). The consonants 'r, l, m, ny, ng' > [r, l, m, ɲ, ŋ] function as syllables. Examples: Tswana: *m.ma.la* (colour). The nasal /ŋ/ is always syllabic when it occurs at the end of a word. Example: *le.sa.kê.ng* (at the kraal) > /le.sa.kɛ.ŋ/. The nasals /m/ and /n/ are syllabic when occurring immediately before consonants other than nasals. Example: *mpa* (stomach) > /m.pa/; *le.bê.n.kê. lê* (shop) > /le.bɛ.ŋ.kɛ.lɛ/. Zulu: When the objectival concord of the third person (singular) is added to the verb stem, the vowel /u/ of the objectival concord /mu-/ is elided and the remaining nasal functions as a syllabic consonant. Example: *ngi.ya.m.tha.nda* (I love him) > [ŋgi.ja.m.tʰa.nda].

When loanwords are adopted into Tswana and Zulu, the syllable structure of the words is modified to fit the open structure. Examples:

Tswana: *ga.la.se* from glass, *pê.nê* from pen; Zulu: *i.pi.pi* from pipe, *i.ka.ti* from cat.

## Tone

Tswana and Zulu, like all Bantu languages, are tone languages in which word-level pitch variations convey lexical and grammatical meaning (Cole, 1992; Zerbian & Barnard, 2008). Tone is apparent on *vowels and syllabic consonants* and may distinguish meaning between two otherwise identical words. Examples: Tswana: *bó.nà* (to see) and - *bò.ná* (they). Zulu: *í.nyá.ngá* (moon) and *í.nyà.ngà* (doctor). Tonal information is not indicated in the orthography of most Bantu languages. Most southern Bantu languages have two *phonological* tones, high (H>') and low (L>`). These tones sometimes cluster to form a high-low tone (H-L>'`) (Khumalo, 1990: Preface). Doke (1967) identifies two types of tones, namely *level* and *gliding* tones. The latter is broken down into rising, falling and rising-falling tones. Coarticulation and assimilation caused by the *phonetic* environment determine gliding phonetic tone (Khumalo, 1990: Preface). Cole (1992) regards these as non-significant varieties of the two phonological tonal values. Although most southern Bantu languages only have two level tones, a systematic account is complicated by the agglutinative morphology, the significant influence of grammar and the occurrence of tone sandhi within and across words (Zerbian & Barnard, 2008).

## Length and stress

Lengthening of syllables is a prosodic feature of African languages. Length is perceptible on the second last syllable of words. Examples: Tswana: *mo.n:.na* (man); *mo.sa:.di* (woman). Zulu: *u.ma:.ma* (mother). Increased length also occurs on the final syllable of the final word of sentences and phrases. The presence/absence and function of stress in Bantu languages is still being debated (Cole, 1992).

# Dysarthria and Apraxia of Speech in Speakers of Tswana and Zulu

## Clinical and research materials

Development of clinical and research assessment material in African languages is restricted, among other things, by the absence of a Dewey-type index of relative phoneme and syllable frequency, sound transitional probabilities, an index of word frequency for languages other than southern Sotho and the absence of standardised passages or other comparable word lists for reading or other elicitation of speech (Jacobson & Traill, 1986).

Further restricting factors are, for example, the difference between the vocabulary of rural and urban speakers in South Africa, the influence of different languages on each other in multilingual communities, some illiterate clients and the scarcity of professionals who are proficient in African languages.

Jacobson and Traill (1986) developed intelligibility word lists for five Bantu languages with the aim of assessing intelligibility in speakers with glossectomy. To our knowledge, these have not been used further for the purpose of research. Fouche and Van der Merwe (1999) developed an Intelligibility Test for Sepedi (which belongs to the Sotho language family and is similar to Tswana). The test contains four word lists, each consisting of 27 words, and a set of 12 multiple-choice items for each word. All the vowels of the language occur in controlled phonetic environments in combination with plosives, fricatives, continuants and trills. Language-appropriate aspirated bilabial, alveolar and velar sounds are included. The syllable structure of words is CVCV. The multiple-choice items represent typical phonetic errors that may result from dysarthric speech. The speaker produces the word and the listener selects the word from the multiple-choice list. The test also contains four sentence lists, each with sentences and words of increasing length. Both authors had some knowledge of the language, but a lack of in-depth knowledge of the sound system prohibited development of stimuli that are representative of all the sounds of the language and which consider tone differences between words that are phonemically similar.

It also became clear that only speakers of African languages with a background in speech pathology/phonetics are suitable as listeners. Other listeners do not perceive tone errors and other subtle phonetic errors such as de-aspiration – though even if they cannot label the change, at some level of consciousness they do perceive an alteration (see below). The lack of literacy of some of the participants was also found to be a problem. Development of a test consisting only of pictures as stimuli holds its own challenges in an African context consisting of a rural as well as a multilingual urban population (Fouche & Van der Merwe, 1999).

Research and assessment material should be developed for Tswana and Zulu and for other Bantu languages. To make comparison of error types across different populations possible, the frequency of occurrence of, for example, the different vowels, consonants, aspirated consonants, clicks and tone differentiations should be controlled within a set of stimuli. For the studies by Coetzee et al. (2011) and Mahwayi et al. (2011), material was developed, but strict phonetic criteria were not applied. In future, such material should be developed further and then utilised across studies to achieve some form of standardised research material.

# Studies in Dysarthria and Apraxia of Speech (AOS) in Speakers of Tswana and Zulu

## Studies in dysarthria

The validity of the Sepedi Intelligibility Test (Fouche & Van der Merwe, 1999) was verified by application to four L1 Sepedi speakers. Two participants presented with unilateral upper motor neuron (UMN) dysarthria, one with spastic dysarthria due to bilateral UMN lesions and one with ataxic dysarthria due to cerebellar dysfunction. One L1 Sepedi-speaking and three Afrikaans-speaking individuals acted as listeners. All were fourth-year speech-language pathology students. Speech signs typical of dysarthria (Duffy, 2005: 418) occurred in the Sepedi-speaking individuals. Wrong identification by the listeners of the target words from the multiple-choice sets revealed errors such as a plosive sound perceived as a fricative, voiced as voiceless and a low vowel as a high vowel. Spasticity, flaccidness, incoordination and involuntary movements of speech structures may induce distortion of place and manner of articulation. Such errors may cause the listener to perceive a target word as another word with related phonetic features. A generic example from this study (from the participant with spastic dysarthria) is the target word /pêpa/ that was confused with /fêpa/ probably due to inadequate lip closure and plosive release. A generic example which may cause lexical confusion in a Bantu language is the aspirated target *'phapa'* confused with *'papa'* probably due to an inability to achieve the greater rate of airflow through the vocal folds or other poor coordination between the larynx and articulators (Ladefoged & Maddieson, 1996).

In another study, dysarthria speech characteristics of two Zulu-speaking individuals were studied (Mahwayi *et al.*, 2011). One participant presented with a severe mixed dysarthria (including spasticity) and the other with unilateral UMN dysarthria after a stroke. The latter participant had spastic paresis of the lower quarter of the face and half of the tongue on the left side and no apparent aphasia or acquired AOS. Both were non-literate and could only produce the stimuli on imitation of a multilingual African language speaker (first author). A two-syllable word list containing 30 words and a list of 28 sentences with words of increasing length was developed. Some of the words required tone differentiation. An African language speaker and two bilingual English and Afrikaans speakers (the authors) performed narrow phonetic transcriptions and perceptual analysis of errors by consensus. The participant with mixed dysarthria was severely impaired and presented with a consistently strained voice, excess loudness variation, nasality, slow speech, general distortion, telescoping of syllables and articulatory breakdown towards the end of long words or sentences. Signs that were language specific were weakening/distortion or deletion of all six clicks in the stimuli and omission of syllabic tone variation.

The other participant with less severe dysarthria served as a better model to demonstrate Zulu-specific signs, as he was more intelligible. The generic signs he displayed were de-aspiration of consonants and telescoping, simplification (example: [ŋgi-] > [ŋ] a syllabic consonant) or deletion of syllables in multisyllabic words. Duffy (2005) mentions telescoping as a sign of ataxic dysarthria only. The occurrence of syllabic telescoping, simplification and deletion is therefore unexpected and may indicate its Zulu-specific nature. Language-specific signs were omission of syllabic tone variation and weakening/distortion of all click sounds in the stimuli (examples: the palatal [!] and dental clicks [|] > distorted [k]). In Zulu, these errors all change the meaning of a word or change it to a non-word, rendering the message highly unintelligible. In this way, the consequences of such changes are probably more pronounced than the effects of a unilateral UMN dysarthria in speakers of languages such as English or Afrikaans. Traditionally, this type of dysarthria is regarded as just a slight impediment, but this is based on judgements of English and closely related languages.

## Studies in apraxia of speech

An exploratory study by Coetzee et al. (2011) examined AOS signs across four languages in an L1 Tswana speaker. The participant was a 48-year-old male who suffered a traumatic localised brain injury 10 years prior to the research. He reported to be multilingual, able to speak English, Afrikaans and Zulu. After the injury, he was unable to produce speech for many months. He was then treated with the speech motor learning approach (Van der Merwe, 2011) that implements non-words and is not language specific. Treatment was not applied under controlled conditions. He regained his ability to speak Tswana and English to the extent that he could take on an occupation where verbal communication was necessary.

Word lists containing 30 single- to multiple-syllable words, and three sets of sentences of increasing length were developed for each of the four languages. The words included different sound types and tone requirements. Included in the sentence set for English were for example: I sit; I sit on a chair; I sit on a chair without cushions. Although the participant was literate, an African language speaker modelled three words or sentences at a time and then the participant was requested to read the words or sentences. Production, therefore, was produced in self-initiated mode. An African language speaker (a fourth-year speech-language pathology student) and the three researchers performed narrow phonetic transcriptions and perceptual analyses by consensus.

The presenting speech signs were those typical of AOS (McNeil et al., 2009). Language-independent, but also African language-specific errors were observed. The typical presenting signs as described in English language studies were consonant distortions, vowel production errors (noted as errors as it was not always clear whether it was a distortion or substitution), start-restart behaviour, syllable segregation, distorted consonant substitutions, cluster reduction, distorted cluster reduction and self-corrections of phoneme substitutions, omissions and trans-positioning. Additional errors specific to the sound systems of the two African languages were click distortion, click deletion, de-aspiration and omission of syllabic tone variation. The Zulu material included four clicks and all four were impaired. Syllable deletion and addition also occurred, particularly in the multisyllabic Zulu words and in Zulu sentences. These errors changed the meaning of words or changed real words to non-words.

In English 16 errors (7% of total errors) occurred, in Afrikaans 50 (20%), in Tswana 54 (22%) and in Zulu 127 (51%). The higher frequency of errors in Tswana than in English and Afrikaans may be due to the high frequency of use of the latter two in the workplace. Another explanation is that subtle changes such as de-aspiration and omission of tone variation in Tswana have a linguistic impact and are therefore noted as errors, while this is not the case in English and Afrikaans. The higher frequency of errors in the two African languages may also indicate that speech production in these languages is motorically more complex than speech production of English and Afrikaans. The high number of errors in Zulu may have been due to less proficiency in this language or due to the sound structure of the language.

Dogil and Mayer (1998) performed a case study on an L1 Xhosa-speaking individual with reported AOS. Production of 64 Xhosa words by imitation in three test sessions revealed only 17 errors. No errors on click sounds occurred. The authors found the results surprising. They mention the important fact that imitated speech is less impaired than self-initiated speech and that this variable may have influenced the results. The authors do not report if analyses implemented broad or narrow transcription and who performed the analyses. Perceptual analysis of disordered speech is a highly specialised task and this variable may have contributed to the unexpected results.

The occurrence of tone production deficits in both dysarthric and apraxic speakers in the reported studies confirms the results of Kadyamusuma et al. (2011). These authors found lexical tone disruption and an inability to manipulate pitch in left hemisphere damaged and in right hemisphere damaged Shona-speaking participants. They do not report on the presence of neuromotor speech disorders. Two types of tone errors are identified: substitutions and non-words. Tone errors found in the reported studies would probably belong to the latter type.

# The Nature of Neuromotor Speech Disorders in Tswana and Zulu

The speech signs of AOS and dysarthria as found in the studies involving speakers of Tswana and Zulu, confirm views of breakdown derived from English language studies. Language-independent speech signs such as sound distortion are evident, but African language-specific signs such as omission or distortion of tone variation and click weakening/distortion also occur. Though language specific, these signs are in accord with the underlying disorders in speech motor planning and execution (McNeil *et al.*, 2009; Van der Merwe, 2009).

Effects of motor complexity on output are common to AOS and dysarthria (albeit for quite different reasons). Demands like click production, controlled nasalisation, tone variation and alternation between different airstream mechanisms within a single word may increase motor complexity and may impact speech motor planning *and* execution. These simultaneous demands may particularly affect multisyllabic words. Click production involves coordinated movements among the articulators and complex articulatory adjustments when coarticulated with other sounds (Bernhardt & Stemberger, 1998; Vilakati & Kimberley, 2010). Naidoo *et al.* (2005) found that nasals, plosives, approximants and fricatives develop earlier in the speech of Zulu-speaking children than affricates, clicks and prenasalised consonants. This finding suggests higher motor complexity of the latter sound classes. Tone production requires fine control of vocal fold length for pitch variation. The sound features together with the multisyllabic nature of particularly Zulu words appear to increase motor planning and execution load.

These preliminary studies in Tswana and Zulu provide evidence that this field of research needs to be explored in much greater depth. The sound systems of African languages provide a rich opportunity to gain further insight into the intricacies of speech motor planning and execution, and its disorders.

## References

Ball, M.J. and Rahilly, J. (1999) *Phonetics: The Science of Speech*. London: Arnold.

Bernhardt, B.H. and Stemberger, J.P. (1998) *Handbook of Phonological Development from the Perspective of Constraint-based Nonlinear Phonology*. San Diego, CA: Academic Press.

Coetzee, M., De Jager, L. and Van der Merwe, A. (2011) Apraxia of speech in a multilingual individual: Speech signs across languages. Research project, University of Pretoria.

Cole, D.T. (1992) *An Introduction to Tswana Grammar*. Johannesburg: Longman Penguin SA.

Cope, A.T. (1983) *A Comprehensive Course in the Zulu Language* (revised edition). Department of African Studies Textbook. Durban: University of Natal.

Dogil, G. and Mayer, J. (1998) Selective phonological impairment: A case of apraxia of speech. *Phonology* 15, 143–188.

Doke, C.M. (1967) *The Southern Bantu Languages*. London: Dawsons.

Duffy, J.R. (2005) *Motor Speech Disorders: Substrates, Differential Diagnosis and Management*. St Louis, MO: Elsevier Mosby.

Erasmus, I., Van der Merwe, A. and Groenewald, E. (1993) Speech sound distortion in neuromotor speech disorders: A comparison between cerebellar dysarthria and apraxia of speech (title translated). *South African Journal of Communication Disorders* 40, 85–96.

Fouche, S. and Van der Merwe, A. (1999) Sepedi test for speech intelligibility (title translated). *South African Journal of Communication Disorders* 46, 25–35.

Gillmer, E. and Van der Merwe, A. (1983) Voice onset time of apraxic and dysarthric speakers (title translated). *South African Journal of Communication Disorders* 30, 34–39.

Herbert, R.K. (1990) The relative markedness of click sounds: Evidence from language change, acquisition, and avoidance. *Anthropological Linguistics* 32, 120–138.

Jacobson, M.C. and Traill, A. (1986) Assessment of speech intelligibility in five South-Eastern Bantu languages: Critical considerations. *South African Journal of Communication Disorders* 33, 15–27.

Kadyamusuma, M.R., De Bleser, R. and Mayer, J. (2011) Lexical tone disruption in Shona after brain damage. *Aphasiology* 25, 1239–1260.

Khumalo, J.S.M. (1990) *English-Zulu-Zulu-English Dictionary*. Johannesburg: Witwatersrand University Press.

Klopper, K., Willemse, A., Van der Merwe, A. and Tesner, H. (1984) *An Afrikaans Intelligibility Test* (title translated). Research project, University of Pretoria.

Ladefoged, P. and Maddieson, I. (1996) *The Sounds of the World's Languages*. Oxford: Blackwell Publishers.

Le Roux, M. and Le Roux, J. (2008) An acoustic assessment of Setswana vowels. *South African Journal of African Languages* 2, 156–171.

Lewis, M.P. (2009) *Ethnologue: Languages of the World* (16th edn). Dallas, TX: SIL International. See http://www.ethnologue.com/ (accessed June 2011).

Lotter, E.C. (1974) The development of articulation in Afrikaans-speaking children and the development of an appropriate articulation test. Master's degree dissertation, University of Pretoria.

Mahwayi, L., Uys, W. and Van der Merwe, A. (2011) Dysarthria speech characteristics of African language speakers. Research project, University of Pretoria.

McNeil, M.R., Robin, D.A. and Schmidt, R.A. (2009) Apraxia of speech. In M.R. McNeil (ed.) *Clinical Management of Sensorimotor Speech Disorders* (2nd edn; pp. 249–268). New York: Thieme.

Mphalele, C. (2006) Inventory of linguistically and culturally sensitive material for speech and language assessment in South Africa. Research report, University of Pretoria.

Naidoo, Y., Van der Merwe, A., Groenewald, E. and Naude, E. (2005) Development of speech sounds and syllable structure of words in Zulu-speaking children. *Southern African Linguistics and Applied Language Studies* 23, 59–79.

Poulos, G. and Bosch, S.E. (1997) *Zulu*. Munich: Lincom-Europa.

Poulos, G. and Msimang, C.T. (1998) *A Linguistic Analysis of Zulu*. Cape Town: Via Africa.

Roux, J. (2007) Unresolved issues in the representation and phonetic description of click articulation in Xhosa and Zulu. *Language Matters* 38, 8–25.

Snyman, J.W. (1989) *An Introduction to Tswana Phonetics*. Houtbaai: Marius Lubbe.

Taljaard, P.C. and Snyman, J.W. (1993) *An Introduction to Zulu Phonetics*. Cape Town: Marius Lubbe.

Theron, K., Van der Merwe, A., Robin, D.R. and Groenewald, E. (2009) Temporal parameters of speech production in bilingual speakers with apraxic or phonemic paraphasic errors. *Aphasiology* 23, 557–583.

Van der Merwe, A. (2007) Self-correction in apraxia of speech: The effect of treatment. *Aphasiology* 21, 658–669.

Van der Merwe, A. (2009) A theoretical framework for the characterization of pathological speech sensorimotor control. In M.R. McNeil (ed.) *Clinical Management of Sensorimotor Speech Disorders* (2nd edn; pp. 3–18). New York: Thieme.

Van der Merwe, A. (2011) A speech motor learning approach to treating apraxia of speech: Rationale and effects of intervention with an adult with acquired apraxia of speech. *Aphasiology* 25, 1174–1206.

Van der Merwe, A., Uys, I.C., Loots, J.M. and Grimbeek, R.J. (1987) The influence of certain contextual factors on the perceptual symptoms of apraxia of speech (title translated). *South African Journal of Communication Disorders* 34, 10–22.

Van der Merwe, A., Uys, I.C., Loots, J.M. and Grimbeek, R.J. (1988) Perceptual symptoms of apraxia of speech: Indications of the nature of the disorder (title translated). *South African Journal of Communication Disorders* 35, 45–54.

Van der Merwe, A., Uys, I.C., Loots, J.M., Grimbeek, R.J. and Jansen, L.P.C. (1989) The influence of certain contextual factors on voice onset time, vowel duration and utterance duration in apraxia of speech (title translated). *South African J Communication Disorders* 36, 29–41.

Van der Merwe, A. and Grimbeek, R.J. (1990) A comparison of the influence of certain contextual factors on the symptoms of acquired apraxia of speech and developmental apraxia of speech (title translated). *South African Journal of Communication Disorders* 37, 27–34.

Van der Merwe, A. and Tesner, H. (2000) Apraxia of speech in a bilingual speaker: Perceptual characteristics and generalization of non-language specific treatment. *The South African Journal of Communication Disorders* 47, 79–89.

Van Rooy, B. and Grijzenhout, J. (2000) Voicing phenomena in Zulu-English. Unpublished paper. International Conference on Linguistics in Southern Africa, Cape Town.

Vilakati, T. and Kimberley, D. (2010) *Coproduction and Coarticulation in isiZulu Clicks.* Berkeley, CA: University of California Press.

Westerman, D. and Ward, I.C. (1990) *Practical Phonetics for Students of African Languages.* London: Kegan Paul International.

Zerbian, S. (2009) Phonology and phonetics of tone in Northern Sotho, a Southern Bantu language. In P.K. Austin, O. Bond, M. Charette, D. Nathan and P. Sells (eds) *Proceedings of Conference on Language Documentation and Linguistic Theory 2* (pp. 313–321). London: SOAS.

Zerbian, S. and Barnard, E. (2008) Phonetics of intonation in South African Bantu languages. *Southern African Linguistics and Applied Language Studies* 26 (2), 235–254.

Ziervogel, D. (1967) *Handboek vir die Spraakklanke en Klankveranderinge in die Bantoetale van Suid-Afrika (Textbook on the Speech Sounds and Sound Changes in the Bantu Languages of South Africa).* Pretoria: University of South Africa Press.

# 10 Motor Speech Disorders in Chinese

## Tara L. Whitehill[1] and Joan K-Y. Ma

Chinese, spoken by approximately 20% of the world's population, is the most commonly spoken language in the world (Fung, 1990). There is some debate regarding whether varieties of spoken Chinese should be considered dialects or separate languages. Here, we regard them as separate languages. The various languages of Chinese are considered united by a common written system, although this characterisation is problematic for Cantonese, which has many colloquial expressions with no written form (Bauer & Benedict, 1997). In this chapter, we focus on two of the most common Chinese languages, Cantonese and Mandarin (Putonghua). Cantonese is spoken in Hong Kong, southern China and many overseas Chinese communities. Mandarin, also known as standard Chinese, is the official national language of China and Taiwan, and is one of the four official languages of Singapore.

## Cantonese

Detailed descriptions of Cantonese phonology can be found in Bauer and Benedict (1997), Cheung (1986) and Zee (1991). There have been active debates about several aspects of Cantonese phonology, including (a) the treatment of final glides/diphthongs, (b) the nature of the consonants /kw/ and /kwʰ/ and (c) the number of lexical tones. In this chapter, we have generally adopted the positions of Bauer and Benedict (1997).

### Syllable structure

Traditionally, Chinese syllables have been described using an onset, a rime (comprising an obligatory vowel and an optional coda) and a tone. We adopt here an alternate model of the syllable structure (Bauer & Benedict, 1997), which takes account of the two permissible syllabic nasals, /m/ and /ŋ/. The structure is: (C1) V1 or Cn (C2 or V2), where C1 = initial consonant, V1 = vowel, Cn = syllabic nasal consonant, C2 = final consonant and V2 = ending vowel (second portion of diphthong); portions in parentheses are optional. Over 98% of Cantonese syllables are CV or CVC in structure

(Wang, 1941, cited in Lau & So, 1988). Tone, which is carried on the vowel portion of the syllable, is obligatory.

## Phonology

Cantonese has 19 initial consonants: /p, pʰ, t, tʰ, k, kʰ, ts, tsʰ, f, s, h, m, n, ŋ, l, w, j, kw, kwʰ/. The initial nasal /ŋ/ is optionally deleted in contemporary Cantonese, and there is a free variation between initial /n/ and /l/. There is some debate about the segments /kw/ and /kwʰ/, which are considered either as coarticulated unitary phonemes or as clusters. The six final consonants are /p, t, k, m, n, ŋ/. The final plosives are unreleased. There are eight primary vowels, /i, y, u, ɛ, œ, ɔ, a, ɐ/, each of which has allophonic variations. The short vowel, /ɐ/, only appears with a final consonant, whereas the other vowels can form a rime component independently. In addition, Cantonese has 10 diphthongs: /ai, ui, ɐi, ɔi, ɛi, au, ɔu, ɐu, iu, œy/. Cantonese is a lexical tonal language, where variations in fundamental frequency are used to differentiate minimal word pairs that are not distinctive by segmental information. There are six contrastive tones in contemporary Cantonese: high level (55), high rising (25), mid level (33), low falling (21), low rising (23) and low level (22). There are several methods to describe Cantonese tones; here, we have combined traditional verbal descriptors with the numeric system developed by Chao (1947), with a modification to the tone value of the high-rising tone from 35 to 25, which has been found to be a better description of the fundamental frequency contour (Ma *et al.*, 2006).

## Stress and rhythm

In contrast to English, which is stress timed, Cantonese is syllable timed. Stress is not phonemic in Cantonese.

## Syntax/morphology considerations

A thorough description of Cantonese syntax and morphology can be found in Mathews and Yip (1994) and a shorter summary in Fung (2009). To our knowledge, possible interactions between syntax/morphology and phonology have not received any attention in the literature on Chinese motor speech disorders.

## Features of particular interest

As most of the literature about motor speech disorders has focused on English speakers, here we note the features of Cantonese which are most in contrast with English. These are the features most likely to be of interest in investigating possible language-specific aspects of motor speech (as well as other speech) disorders. First is the tonal nature of Cantonese. Second is the relatively simple syllable structure (i.e. with /kw/ and /kwʰ/ being the only clusters or, in some cases, considered as unitary phonemes, and 98% of syllables either CV or CVC). Third, the relatively small fricative system (only three fricatives, only one of which is produced intra-orally). Fourth, the fact that Cantonese has an aspirated vs unaspirated contrast for plosives, as opposed to the voiced–voiceless contrast in English (both contrasts involve differences in voice onset time [VOT]; see Clumeck et al., 1981). Fifth, that Cantonese is not stress timed. Finally, the logographic vs alphabetic nature of the written language (which raises issues for treatment, in particular).

# Mandarin

Detailed descriptions of Mandarin phonology can be found in Ladefoged and Maddieson (1996), Hashimoto (1970), Lee and Zee (2003) and Hua (2002). Controversies regarding Mandarin phonology have included (a) the characterisation of /ɹ/ (sometimes described as /r/) and /x/ (sometimes described as /χ/); (b) the surface value of certain vowels, given their allophonic variations; and (c) whether the vowels /i/ and /u/ should be considered as semivowels when occurring in diphthongs or tripthongs (Hua, 2002: 42).

## Syllable structure

The syllable structure of Mandarin is (C) V (N). That is, the initial consonant is optional, the vowel is obligatory, and the final consonant, which can only be a nasal consonant, is optional. As with Cantonese, tone is obligatory and is carried on the vowel portion of the syllable.

## Phonology

Mandarin has 22 initial consonants: / p, pʰ, t, tʰ, k, kʰ, m, n, ŋ, ts, tsʰ, tʂ, tʂʰ, tɕ, tɕʰ, f, s, ʂ, ɕ, x, ɹ, l /. There are only two final consonants, /n, ŋ/. There are nine simple vowels, /i, y, ɛ, ə, ɚ, a, ɤ, u, o/; 9 diphthongs, /ae, ɑo, ei, oʊ, ia, iɛ, ua, uo, yɛ/; and 4 triphthongs, /iɑo, ioʊ, uae, uei/. Mandarin has four tones, described as high level (55), rising (35), falling-rising (214) and high falling (51); the numbers again refer to the numeric system of Chao (1930).

## Stress and rhythm

Unlike Cantonese (but as in English), Mandarin is a stress-timed language. Weak stress (also termed weak syllable or neutral tone) is a particular characteristic of Mandarin, and it has attracted considerable debate in terms of the relationship between weak syllable and tone, and relevant phonological and morphological rules (Hua, 2002).

## Syntax/morphology considerations

A detailed description of Mandarin grammar can be found in Chao (1968); a more succinct and recent description is provided by Fung (2009). As with Cantonese, we are not aware of any reports of interactions between syntax/morphology and phonology in the literature on motor speech disorders in Mandarin speakers.

## Features of particular interest

Some of the same features mentioned above for Cantonese are also of interest when contrasting Mandarin with English. Namely, the tonal nature of Mandarin, the relatively simple syllable structure, the aspiration contrast for plosives and the logographic nature of the written language. Several additional features are of interest when contrasting Mandarin phonology with both English and Cantonese. First is the relatively restricted final consonant system and the fact that the only permissible finals are two nasals. Second, the fricative/affricate system is relatively rich in comparison to Cantonese, with retroflex fricative/affricate, alveolo-palatal fricative/affricate and velar fricative. Third, the place of articulation involves both retroflex and alveolar-palatal, which does not exist in Cantonese. Again, these are features that should be of particular interest when investigating possible language-specific influences on motor speech disorders.

# Studies of Motor Speech Disorder in Chinese

Whitehill (2010) provided a recent review of studies of motor speech disorder in Chinese, which focused on adults with Parkinson's disease (PD), and teenagers or young adults with cerebral palsy. Here, we focus primarily on acquired disorders. This chapter also takes a more applied focus, reviewing the available clinical materials as well as treatment studies.

## Characterisation of motor speech disorders

There are limited studies focusing on the general characterisation of motor speech disorders in Chinese. Using the classic Mayo Clinic approach (Darley et al., 1969a, 1969b, 1975), Whitehill et al. (2003) investigated the perceptual characteristics of hypokinetic dysarthria in Cantonese speakers. The findings were largely similar to those found for English (e.g. Darley et al., 1975) and Japanese (Fukusake et al., 1983). Interestingly, lexical tone production was found to be relatively robust in this group of speakers, particularly in comparison with the dimension of 'monotone'. To our knowledge, no similar studies have been done for other types of dysarthria in Cantonese or Mandarin.

Kwan (1998) investigated the acoustic variables of speech in one Cantonese speaker with apraxia and three speakers with ataxic dysarthria. The acoustic measures included variables associated with vowels and diphthongs, temporal organisation, pause duration and the intensity of syllable-initial consonants and vowels. The findings were generally consistent with those of previous studies of English speakers with similar motor speech disorders. The fundamental frequency (F0) contours of tones were deviant for all four speakers, compared with those of non-impaired speakers.

## Assessment and treatment materials

There are few published tests or materials for the assessment of motor speech disorders in Chinese speakers. The National Institutes of Health Stroke Scale (NIHSS) is a well-known 15-item scale to evaluate patients following a stroke (Brott et al., 1989). The scale contains one item on facial palsy (rated on a four-point scale), and one item on dysarthria, which involves the patient reading or repeating a list of words, and is rated using a three-point scale. The NIHSS has been translated and validated for Cantonese (Cheung et al., 2010) and Mandarin (Cheung et al., 2010; Sun et al., 2006).

Whitehill and colleagues developed a series of materials to be used in evaluating Cantonese speakers with dysarthria. These materials include a single-word list for evaluating phonology (Whitehill, 1994); a contrastive single-word Intelligibility Test (Whitehill, 1995; Whitehill & Ciocca, 2000a) that is based on the test developed by Kent et al. (1989); and a Cantonese sentence intelligibility battery (Whitehill, 2003; Whitehill et al., 2004), based on the sentence portion of the Assessment of Intelligibility of Dysarthric Speech (AIDS) (Yorkston & Beukelman, 1981). These materials have been primarily used in research studies but have not been published. Most clinicians working in Hong Kong evaluate dysarthria based on the principles and procedures outlined by Duffy (2005). Apraxia is generally evaluated using an informal translation of the *Apraxia Battery for Adults* (Dabul, 2000). The non-standardised adaptation of the speech materials, such as in the increasing word length task, was relatively straightforward given the syllabic nature of Cantonese. Yiu (1992) developed a Chinese (Cantonese) version of the Western Aphasia Battery (WAB) (Kertesz, 1982), which includes a 15-item section for the evaluation of apraxia.

A single-word Intelligibility Test was developed in Taiwan for Mandarin speakers with dysarthria (Liu et al., 2000). The test was partly based on that developed by Kent et al. (1989). Liu et al. (2000) describe the use of the test with young men with cerebral palsy but the test should be suitable for use with other groups of Mandarin speakers with dysarthria. Currently, the test appears to be primarily a research tool and we are not aware if it is being used clinically.

There are few published treatment materials available for Chinese speakers with motor speech disorders. The only material currently publicly available is on the website for Lee Silverman Voice Treatment (LSVT®), which lists the availability of a Cantonese version of the DVD for treatment materials.

## Treatment studies

Reports of treatment studies with Chinese speakers with dysarthria are, unfortunately, sparse. A recent study by Whitehill and colleagues described the use of LSVT with a group of Cantonese patients with PD (Whitehill et al., 2011). The primary focus of the study was to investigate the effect of LSVT on lexical tone errors. The speakers made significant improvement on a number of measures already well-documented to improve following LSVT treatment in English speakers, such as loudness (Ramig et al., 2001) and vowel articulation (Sapir et al., 2007). However, there was no significant improvement in lexical tone. This confirmed the findings of an earlier pilot study with a smaller group of Cantonese speakers with PD, using treatment based on the principles of LSVT (Whitehill & Wong, 2007). The authors discussed the relatively intact nature of tone pretreatment as well as a possible dissociation between tone and intonation. A more detailed discussion on the interaction between intonation and tone in speakers with dysarthria is included in the following section.

The effects of surgical treatment (bilateral subthalamic nucleus deep brain stimulation [STN-DBS]) on speech in a group of Mandarin-speaking patients with PD were investigated by a team of researchers in Beijing (Xie et al., 2011). The results confirmed those of several previous studies of DBS surgery for this population. That is, while the procedure improved motor abilities, there was effectively no improvement in speech performance. The study did not focus on language-specific aspects of performance, pre- or post-surgery.

# Language-Specific Studies

## Tone

One of the main characteristics of Chinese languages (Cantonese and Mandarin) is that they are tonal languages. In tone languages, F0 variation at the syllabic level is used to mark semantic meaning, while F0 changes at the sentential level are used to mark intonation. The production of lexical tone in Cantonese speakers with dysarthria has been the focus of investigation in two etiological groups, PD and cerebral palsy, for different reasons. Speakers with PD are characterised by monotonous speech and reduced pitch variation within sentences due to rigidity, while speakers with cerebral palsy tend to display extreme variability related to reduced control of the laryngeal mechanism (Darley *et al.*, 1969b; Jacques *et al.*, 1985). As a result of these different characteristics, both groups are susceptible to errors in tone production.

Wong and Diehl (1999) investigated the production and perception of Cantonese tones produced by a PD speaker and a non-impaired speaker. They reported that the PD speaker had a more restricted tonal space, as defined by the pitch range of all tones, when compared with the healthy control speaker. Additionally, the tones produced by the PD speaker were less accurately identified than those of the non-PD speaker. However, they provided little detail about their methodology. Also, their study used only one PD speaker. As speech produced by individuals with dysarthria is known to be highly heterogeneous (Lowit-Leuschel & Docherty, 2001), it is questionable whether the pattern reported in Wong and Diehl (1999) was representative of PD speakers. Using perceptual analysis, Whitehill *et al.* (2003) established a perceptual profile of the speech characteristics of Cantonese PD speakers. The dimension of 'tone distortion' was included specifically for the linguistic property of Cantonese. They found that tone production was relatively unaffected in Cantonese PD speakers. Ma (2009) investigated the acoustic pattern of the Cantonese lexical tones produced by five speakers with PD, with the target tones embedded at three different positions (initial, medial and final) of a five-syllable question or statement. The results showed that speakers with PD contrasted the six lexical tones in a similar manner compared with control speakers across positions and intonations, except at the final position of questions. Significantly lower fundamental frequency (F0) values were found towards the end of the syllable at the final position of questions for the speakers with PD than for the control speakers. This showed a different pattern of interaction between intonation and tone for the speakers with PD and the control speakers. In investigating the effect of medication on speech in Mandarin speakers with PD, Tseng (2000) included tonal contrast as one of the measures. Using perceptual analysis, the results showed that the lexical tones produced by 10 PD speakers were very similar to those of the control speakers.

A series of studies were conducted to investigate lexical tone production by Cantonese speakers with cerebral palsy and perception of tone production by non-dysarthric speakers (Ciocca *et al.*, 2000, 2002, 2004). The F0 patterns of the monosyllabic tone targets were analysed acoustically and the results showed excessive variability in the F0 patterns by speakers with cerebral palsy. The six tones showed a much larger degree of overlap than in non-dysarthric speakers. Abnormal patterns in both tone level and tone contour were observed. The F0 level of the high-level tone was found to be lower than for non-dysarthric speakers. Additionally, falling F0 patterns were found for both level tones and rising tones, while rising F0 patterns were observed in some falling tone production. These errors patterns had a significant impact on perception, with level tones being perceived as rising or falling, and errors perceived in the perception of tone level. Jeng *et al.* (2006) conducted a similar investigation of tone production and its perception in Mandarin speakers with cerebral palsy. They found that the high-rising and low falling-rising tones were produced less accurately than the high-level and the high falling tones but commented that, in general, the F0 contours of the four tones were to a large extent retained by the speakers. Instead, the acoustic analysis showed that the most significant problem in lexical tone production in this group of speakers was related to the precision of the F0 contour.

## Voice onset time

Another specific feature of Chinese languages is that, instead of contrastive voicing, plosives and affricates are contrasted by aspiration. This applies to both Cantonese and Mandarin. VOT serves as an acoustic correlate and perceptual cue of the aspiration contrast, as for the voicing contrast in English. One study has examined the VOT of plosives in Mandarin speakers with dysarthria (Tseng, 2000). Ten speakers with PD were asked to produce a series of words contrasting in both tone and aspiration. The results of the acoustic analysis indicated that speakers with PD showed a larger number of VOT overlaps than control speakers, reducing the contrast between aspirated and unaspirated consonants. Tseng (2000) hypothesized that the VOT overlap was related to reduced coordination of the speech mechanism in speakers with PD. Interestingly, some speakers in the same study showing no VOT overlap before L-dopa medication were found to have VOT overlap after L-dopa. Another study investigating the effect of various acoustic parameters on intelligibility in 20 Mandarin speakers with cerebral palsy showed longer VOT for unaspirated stops than in control speakers (Liu *et al.*, 2000).

## Consonant cluster

Reduction of consonant clusters /kw/ and /kwʰ/ was found to be one of the most common errors in the manner of articulation among Cantonese individuals with cerebral palsy (Whitehill & Ciocca, 2000b). The consonants /kw/ and /kwʰ/ were realised as either [k] or [kʰ], which are considered acceptable variations in Cantonese (in some contexts), or as [w], which is regarded as an error. The simplification of the manner of articulation in these consonant clusters reflected the nature of the dysarthrias associated with cerebral palsy, whereby individuals lack skills in precise articulatory movement rather than an inability to contrast phonemic prominence (Platt et al., 1980). The findings also have implications for the controversy on the consonant cluster vs unitary phoneme nature of the /kw/ and /kw$^h$/ phonemes in Cantonese, as the error patterns showed cluster reduction rather than simplification of a unitary phoneme.

## Theoretical Implications

Speech prosody has been found to be one of the main impairments in Chinese speakers with dysarthria (e.g. Ciocca et al., 2001; Whitehill et al., 2003), as in other languages. As F0 is used to mark both intonation (at sentential level) and lexical tone (at syllabic level), it was traditionally believed that an impairment in intonation marking in speakers with dysarthria would unavoidably be generalised to the production of lexical tones. Vance (1976) hypothesized that there might be separate control mechanisms for lexical tone and intonation, but did not provide any evidence to support the claim. Ma et al. (2006, 2011) provided evidence to suggest that the production of tone and intonation in Cantonese are independent of each other. That is, an impairment in the production of either lexical tone or intonation might not necessarily lead to the other.

However, the interpretation of tone and intonation production is complicated by the fact that there is a bidirectional interaction between them; for example, the final intonation contour might affect the F0 contour of a tone, and the tone contour of the final syllable might have an impact on intonation identification (Ma et al., 2006, 2011).

As for other languages, monotone speech is one of the key perceptual characteristics of Cantonese speakers with PD (Whitehill et al., 2003). In studying the question–statement contrast in Cantonese, it has been shown that speakers with PD marked the intonation of questions in a similar manner to control speakers, but were less efficient in exploiting some of the cues (e.g. final F0 rise and increase in F0 level) (Ma & Whitehill, 2008; Ma et al., 2010). That is, the speakers with PD retained the phonological distinction in marking questions and statements, but the physiological constraints of PD led to a reduction in the F0 excursions at the phonetic level for some speakers. The reduction in intonation marking caused perceptual confusion among native listeners (Ma et al., 2010). On the other hand, Cantonese speakers with PD were reported to have relatively intact lexical tone production (Ma, 2009; Whitehill et al., 2003). Although the reduction in the F0 range of speakers with PD resulted in a smaller tonal space than control speakers, speakers with PD preserved similar F0 contours and tonal contrast to control speakers (Ma, 2009). It is also interesting to note that the largest difference in lexical tone production between speakers with and without hypokinetic dysarthria occurs at the final position of questions (Ma, 2009). In non-dysarthric speakers, the canonical form of lexical tone at the final position of questions was modified to a rising contour as a result of F0 final-rise in questions. However, the magnitude of this interaction between intonation and tone was reduced in speakers with PD (Ma, 2009).

In summary, although both intonation and tone have F0 as the primary acoustic cue, findings from Cantonese speakers with PD showed that it is possible to have different degrees of impairment in tone and intonation production. This serves as an example to researchers and clinicians to exercise caution when generalising the findings from one language to another without consideration of the specific features of each language.

## Conclusion

In this chapter, we reviewed studies of the assessment, treatment and characterisation of motor speech disorders in Cantonese and Mandarin. We focused on publications in English with the addition of a few easily accessible publications in Chinese. Overall, the review highlighted that the characteristics of motor speech disorders in Chinese are similar to those reported in English-speaking individuals. This reflects the fact that motor speech disorders such as dysarthria are brought about by a neurophysiological impairment, which impedes individuals similarly regardless of language. However, there is also some level of interactions between the neurophysiological impairment and the linguistic features of Chinese, such as tones. Studies have shown that tone is severely impaired in some speakers with dysarthria (e.g. with dysarthrias associated with cerebral palsy) but remains relatively intact in some other speakers (e.g. speakers with hypokinetic dysarthria associated with PD). Research in motor speech disorders in Chinese is still limited in many areas, especially in the areas of standardised assessment tools and treatment studies. In addition, the diversity of languages in Chinese-speaking regions provides an additional challenge to the study of motor speech disorders in Chinese.

## Note

(1) This chapter is dedicated to the memory of Professor Tara L. Whitehill, who passed away in August 2013. Professor Whitehill was wholeheartedly committed to the professional development of speech-language therapy in Hong Kong. She focused her research on motor speech disorders and cleft lip and palate, and made an exceptional contribution to our understanding of the manifestation of motor speech disorders in Chinese. Professor Whitehill was also instrumental in the development of several research and clinical tools in motor speech disorders in Cantonese. Professor Whitehill's memory is cherished by all of us who were fortunate enough to have known her intelligence, eloquence, thoughtfulness and compassion. A teacher, mentor, colleague and friend who is greatly missed.

# References

Bauer, R.S. and Benedict, P.K. (1997) *Modern Cantonese Phonology*. Berlin: Mouton de Gruyter.

Brott, T., Adams Jr, H.P., Olinger, C.P., Marler, J.R., Barsan, W.G., Biller, J., Spilker, J., Holleran, R., Eberle, R., Hertzberg, R., Rorick, M., Moomaw, C.J. and Walker, M. (1989) Measurements of acute cerebral infarction: A clinical examination scale. *Stroke* 20, 864–870.

Chao, Y.R. (1930) A system of tone-letters. *Le Maître Phonétique* 45, 24–27.

Chao, Y.R. (1947) *Cantonese Primer*. Cambridge: Cambridge University Press.

Chao, Y.R. (1968) *A Grammar of Spoken Chinese*. Berkeley, CA: University of California Press.

Cheung, K.L. (1986) The phonology of present day Cantonese. PhD thesis, University College London.

Cheung, R.T.F., Lyden, P.D., Tsoi, T.H., Huang, Y., Liu, M., Hong, S.F.K., Raman, R. and Liu, L. (2010) Production and validation of Putonghua- and Cantonese-Chinese language National Institutes of Health Stroke Scale training and certification videos. *International Journal of Stroke* 5, 74–79.

Ciocca, V., Whitehill, T.L. and Ng, S.S. (2002) Contour tone production by Cantonese speakers with cerebral palsy. *Journal of Medical Speech-Language Pathology* 10, 243–248.

Ciocca, V., Whitehill, T.L. and Ma, J.K-Y. (2004) The impact of cerebral palsy on the intelligibility on pitch-based linguistic contrasts. *Journal of Physiology and Anthropology* 23, 283–287.

Clumeck, H., Barton, D., Macken, M.A. and Huntington, D.A. (1981) The aspiration contrast in Cantonese word-initial stops: Data from children and adults. *Journal of Chinese Linguistics* 9, 210–224.

Dabul, B.L. (2000) *Apraxia Battery for Adults – Second Edition (ABA-2)*. Austin, TX: Pro-Ed.

Darley, F.L., Aronson, A.E. and Brown, J.R. (1969a) Differential diagnostic patterns of dysarthria. *Journal of Speech and Hearing Research* 12, 246–269.

Darley, F.L., Aronson, A.E. and Brown, J.R. (1969b) Clusters of deviant speech dimensions in the dysarthrias. *Journal of Speech and Hearing Research* 12, 462–497.

Darley, F.L., Aronson, A.E. and Brown, J.R. (1975) *Motor Speech Disorders*. Philadelphia, PA: Saunders.

Duffy, J.R. (2005) *Motor Speech Disorders: Substrates, Differential Diagnosis, and Management* (2nd edn). St. Louis, MO: Mosby.

Fung, R.S-Y. (2009) Characteristics of Chinese in relation to language disorders. In S-P. Law, B.S. Weekes and A.M-Y. Wong (eds) *Language Disorders in Speakers of Chinese* (pp. 1–17). Bristol: Multilingual Matters.

Fukusake, Y., Monoi, H., Tatsume, I.F., Kumai, I., Hijikata, N. and Hirose, H. (1983) Analysis of characteristics of dysarthric speech based on auditory impression. *Japanese Journal of Logopedics and Phoniatrics* 24, 149–164.

Hashimoto, M. (1970) Notes on Mandarin phonology. In R. Jakobson and S. Kawamoto (eds) *Studies in General and Oriental Linguistics* (pp. 207–220). Tokyo: TEC.

Hua, Z. (2002) *Phonological Development in Specific Contexts: Studies of Chinese-speaking Children*. Clevedon: Multilingual Matters.

Jacques, R.D., Rastatter, M. and Sullivan, J. (1985) Some effects of congenital spasticity on fundamental frequency. *Perceptual and Motor Skills* 61, 75–80.

Jeng, J.Y., Weismer, G. and Kent, R.D. (2006) Perception and production of Mandarin tone in adults with cerebral palsy. *Clinical Linguistics and Phonetics* 20, 67–87.

Kent, R.D., Weismer, G., Kent, J.F. and Rosenbek, J.C. (1989) Toward phonetic intelligibility testing in dysarthria. *Journal of Speech and Hearing Disorders* 54, 482–499.

Kertesz, A. (1982) *Western Aphasia Battery*. New York: The Psychological Corporation.

Kwan, K.W-Y. (1998) A phonetic study of the motor speech disorders in Hong Kong Cantonese. MPhil thesis, City University of Hong Kong.

Ladefoged, P. and Maddieson, I. (1996) *The Sounds of the World's Languages*. Oxford: Blackwell.

Lau, C.C. and So, K.W. (1988) Material for Cantonese speech audiometry constructed by appropriate phonetic principles. *British Journal of Audiology* 22, 297–304.

Lee, W-S. and Zee, E. (2003) Standard Chinese (Beijing). *Journal of the International Phonetics Association* 33, 109–112.

Liu, H-M., Tseng, C-H. and Tsao, F-M. (2000) Perceptual and acoustic analysis of speech intelligibility in Mandarin-speaking young adults with cerebral palsy. *Clinical Linguistics and Phonetics* 14, 447–464.

Lowit-Leuschel, A. and Docherty, G. (2001) Prosodic variation across sampling tasks in normal and dysarthric speakers. *Logopedics, Phoniatrics, Vocology* 26, 151–164.

Ma, J.K-Y. (2009) Lexical tone production by Cantonese speakers with Parkinson's disease. *Proceedings of Interspeech 2009 (INTERSPEECH 2009)* (pp. 1691–1694). Red Hook, NY: Curran Associates.

Ma, J.K-Y., Ciocca, V. and Whitehill, T.L. (2006) Effect of intonation on Cantonese lexical tones. *Journal of the Acoustical Society of America* 120, 3978–3987.

Ma, J.K-Y. and Whitehill, T.L. (2008) Quantitative analysis of intonation patterns produced by Cantonese speakers with Parkinson's disease: A preliminary study. In *9th Annual Conference of the International Speech Communication Association 2008 (INTERSPEECH 2008)* (pp. 1749–1752). Red Hook, NY: Curran Associates.

Ma, J.K-Y., Whitehill, T.L. and So, S.Y-S. (2010) Intonation contrast in Cantonese speakers with hypokinetic dysarthria associated with Parkinson's disease. *Journal of Speech, Language, and Hearing Research* 53, 836–849.

Ma, J.K-Y., Ciocca, V. and Whitehill, T.L. (2011) The perception of intonation questions and statements in Cantonese. *Journal of the Acoustical Society of America* 129, 1012–1023.

Mathews, S. and Yip, V. (1994) *Cantonese: A Comprehensive Grammar*. London: Routledge.

Platt, L.J., Andrews, G. and Howie, P.M. (1980) Dysarthria and adult cerebral palsy: II. Phonemic analysis of articulation errors. *Journal of Speech and Hearing Research* 23, 45–55.

Ramig, L.O., Sapir, S., Fox, C. and Countryman, S. (2001) Changes in vocal loudness following intensive voice treatment (LSVT®) in individuals with Parkinson's disease: A comparison with untreated patients and normal age-matched controls. *Movement Disorders* 16, 79–83.

Sapir, S., Spielman, J.L., Ramig, L.O., Story, B.H. and Fox, C. (2007) Effects of intensive voice treatment (the Lee Silverman Voice Treatment [LSVT]) on vowel articulation in dysarthric individuals with idiopathic Parkinson disease: Acoustic and perceptual findings. *Journal of Speech, Language, and Hearing Research* 50, 899–912.

Sun, T-K., Chiu, S-C., Yeh, S-H. and Chang, K-C. (2006) Assessing reliability and validity of the Chinese version of the stroke scale: Scale development. *International Journal of Nursing Studies* 43 (4), 457–463.

Tseng, C.Y. (2000) 漢語神經語言學的新方向：以巴金森症病患的語音現象為例 [New direction in Chinese neurolinguistics: Using speech characteristics of Parkinson's disease as an example]. *Chinese Study* 18, 443–472.

Vance, T.J. (1976) An experimental investigation of tone and intonation in Cantonese. *Phonetica* 33, 368–392.

Whitehill, T.L. (1994) Cantonese Speech Materials (CSM). Paper presented at the Annual Convention of the American Speech-Language-Hearing Association, New Orleans.

Whitehill, T.L. (1995) *Cantonese Speech Intelligibility Test (CSIT) – Research Edition*. Hong Kong: University of Hong Kong.

Whitehill, T.L. (2003) *Cantonese Sentence Intelligibility Test – Research Edition*. Hong Kong: University of Hong Kong.

Whitehill, T.L. (2010) Studies of Chinese speakers with dysarthria: Informing theoretical models. *Folio Phoniatrica et Logopedica* 62, 92–96.

Whitehill, T.L. and Ciocca, V. (2000a) Perceptual-phonetic predictors of single-word intelligibility: A study of Cantonese dysarthria. *Journal of Speech, Language, and Hearing Research* 43, 1451–1465.

Whitehill, T.L. and Ciocca, V. (2000b) Speech errors in Cantonese speaking adults with cerebral palsy. *Clinical Linguistics and Phonetics* 14, 111–130.

Whitehill, T.L., Ciocca, V. and Chow, D.T-Y. (2000) Acoustical analysis of lexical tone contrasts in dysarthria. *Journal of Medical Speech-Language Pathology* 8, 337–344.

Whitehill, T.L., Ciocca, V. and Lam, S.L-M. (2001) Fundamental frequency control in connected speech in Cantonese speakers with dysarthria. In B. Maassen, W. Hulstijn and R. Kent (eds) *Speech Motor Control in Normal and Disordered Speech* (pp. 228–231). Nijmegen: University of Nijmegen Press.

Whitehill, T.L., Ma, J.K-Y. and Lee, A.S-Y. (2003) Perceptual characteristics of Cantonese hypokinetic dysarthria. *Clinical Linguistics and Phonetics* 17, 265–271.

Whitehill, T.L., Ciocca, V. and Yiu, E.M-L. (2004) Perceptual and acoustic predictors of intelligibility and acceptability in dysarthria. *Journal of Medical Speech-Language Pathology* 12, 229–233.

Whitehill, T.L., and Wong, C.C-Y. (2006) Contributing factors to listener effort for dysarthric speech. *Journal of Medical Speech-Language Pathology* 14, 335–341.

Whitehill, T.L. and Wong, L-N. (2007) Effect of intensive voice treatment on tone language speakers with Parkinson's disease. *Clinical Linguistics and Phonetics* 21, 919–925.

Whitehill, T.L., Kwan, L., Lee, F.P-H. and Chow, M.M-N. (2011) Effect of LSVT® on lexical tone in speakers with Parkinson's disease. *Parkinson's Disease* 2011, 897494.

Wong, P.C-M. and Diehl, R.L. (1998) Effect of spectral distance on vowel perception. *Proceedings of the 16th International Congress on Acoustics and the 135th Meeting of the Acoustical Society of America* (pp. 2015–2016). New York: American Institute of Physics.

Wong, P.C-M. and Diehl, R.L. (1999) The effect of reduced tonal space in Parkinsonian speech on the perception of Cantonese tones. *Journal of the Acoustical Society of America* 105, 1246.

Xie, Y., Zhang, Y, Zheng, A., Liu, A., Wang, X., Zhuang, P., Li, Y. and Wang, X. (2011) Changes in speech characters of patients with Parkinson's disease after bilateral subthalamic nucleus stimulation. *Journal of Voice* 25, 751–758.

Yiu, E.M-L. (1992) Linguistic assessment of Chinese-speaking aphasics: Development of a Cantonese aphasia battery. *Journal of Neurolinguistics* 7, 379–424.

Yorkston, K.M. and Beukelman, D.R. (1981) *Assessment of Intelligibility of Dysarthric Speech*. Tigard, OR: C.C. Publications.

Zee, E. (1991) Chinese (Hong Kong Cantonese). *Journal of the International Phonetic Association* 21, 46–48.

# 11 Diagnosis and Therapy in Adult Acquired Dysarthria and Apraxia of Speech in Dutch

Roel Jonkers, Hayo Terband
and Ben Maassen

## Introduction

We start with a short overview of the phonology of Dutch. We will then describe the diagnostic and therapeutic materials that are used in the Netherlands for dysarthria and apraxia of speech (AOS). In the final part of this chapter, we will address some language-specific aspects of Dutch that are interesting for the study of people with these disorders.

Dutch is the native language of a population of 30 million people, living mainly in the Netherlands and Flanders (the northern part of Belgium). In standard Dutch, about 40 different phonemes are used. Consonants comprise plosives (/p,b,t,d,k,g/), fricatives (/f,v,s,z,x,ɣ,h/), nasals (/m,n,ŋ/), liquids (/l,r/) and semivowels (/j,w/). Dutch has a rich vowel system with 13 monophthongs, comprising both lax vowels (/ɑ,ɛ,ɪ,ɔ,ʏ,ə/) and tense vowels (/a,e,i,o,u,y,ø/) and 3 diphthongs (/ɛi,œy,ɔu/). Dutch also has a range of typical phonological processes, many shared with other languages. Assimilation of voicing is often present and can be both progressive and regressive. In contrast to e.g. English, the occurrence of voicing assimilation is not context dependent. Obstruent clusters always agree in voicing, and final devoicing of obstruents is found throughout. Prevoicing also constitutes a typical Dutch phonological process. Voiceless plosives in Dutch are unaspirated and oppositions such as /b/:/p/ are accomplished by means of a voice onset time (VOT) of approximately zero in the voiceless counterpart. In the realisation of prevocalic plosives, vocal cord vibration starts before the release burst of the plosive, which means that VOT attains negative values. English and German do not exhibit prevoicing, but several Slavic languages such as Russian and Polish do.

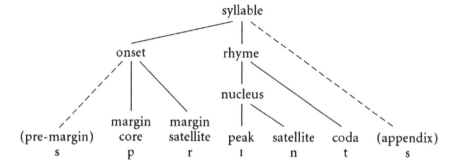

**Figure 11.1** Syllable structure of Dutch (example from Den Ouden, 2002)

In Dutch, the syllable template can be very complex (e.g. CCCVCCC), including the extrasyllabic pre-margin and appendix positions. Onsets and coda satellites can only be filled with sonorant consonants, the pre-margin only with the phoneme /s/ and the appendix with coronal voiceless obstruents (see Den Ouden [2002] for a more elaborate description).

Concerning prosody, Dutch, like German and English but in contrast to French and Spanish, is described as a stress-timed language in which stressed syllables occur at even intervals (Rietveld & Van Heuven 2001). Stressed syllables are longer than unstressed syllables and vowel reduction takes place in unstressed syllables. In Dutch, syllables are grouped into bounded trochaic feet in which the syllable in the weak non-initial position is often reduced to a schwa.

## Diagnostic and Therapeutic Materials in Dutch

Until some years ago, no valid diagnostic materials had been available in the Netherlands for the diagnosis of AOS and dysarthria. In 1996, Dharmaperwira-Prins published a book on the diagnosis and therapy of dysarthria and AOS. This book is widely used in the education of speech and language therapists (SLTs). It gives a theoretical background to the different types of dysarthria and AOS based on the Mayo Clinic classification (Darley *et al.*, 1975), a differential diagnostic test (the test for dysarthria and verbal apraxia [DYVA]) and suggestions for therapy. The DYVA consists of a general case history; a general analysis of spontaneous speech including intelligibility, speech rate and prosody; reading and writing (to observe problems with hand motorics); diadochokinesis; and items to test respiration, resonance and phonation.

In 2009, the fourth modified edition of this book was published. The DYVA, currently known as TEDYVA (TE for textbook, which is integrated in this edition), is still widely used in clinical practice, although mainly for the diagnosis of dysarthria. In 2008, Feiken *et al.* published the results of a questionnaire that had been sent to SLTs to find out what materials are used in the diagnosis and therapy of AOS. The outcome was that all SLTs used test scores from general diagnostic aphasia test batteries in combination with their clinical judgment to diagnose AOS. Only 25% of the SLTs additionally used the DYVA, showing that the DYVA is not generally used for the diagnosis of AOS. Furthermore, although the DYVA is not a statistically valid test, it might be suitable for the overall diagnosis of dysarthria, but it remains non-specific in terms of studying the symptoms of the different types of dysarthria (Kalf & De Swart, 2007).

In addition to the DYVA, a Dutch translation of the original *Frenchay Dysarthria Assessment* (Enderby, 1983) is regularly used for the diagnosis of dysarthria. No validation or norms for this adaptation are available though.

Recently, more specific diagnostic tests have been developed for the diagnosis of both dysarthria and AOS. Knuijt and De Swart (2007) published the *Radboud Dysartrieonderzoek* and Feiken and Jonkers (2012) the *Diagnostic Instrument for Apraxia of Speech (DIAS)*. Both are described in more detail below.

## The diagnosis of dysarthria

The *Radboud Dysartrieonderzoek* aims to standardise the quantitative and qualitative analysis of all aspects of speech. Both objective and subjective measures are used. Five levels of analysis are observed: respiration, voicing, articulation, resonance and prosody. The preferred method for the analysis of speech quality is a standardised reading text and a diadochokinetic test. Movements of the articulators; production of consonants, vowels and clusters; nasality; speech rate; syllabification; and diadochokinesis are scored on a four-point scale, varying from impossible (0), clearly deviant (1), slightly deviant (2) to normal (3). Voice quality is determined from running speech and the maximum duration of phonation. The same four-point scale is used to score voice quality, loudness, dynamics, intonation (prosody), amplitude, vocal range and vocal volume. Finally, different aspects of breathing are analyzed. Given the scoring system, most speech deficit symptoms can be scored based on the numerical scales. The *Radboud Dysartrieonderzoek* has been used not just in clinical practice, but also in scientific research. No indications, however, are provided for a differential diagnosis between the different types of dysarthria, AOS and aphasia.

## The diagnosis of apraxia of speech

As mentioned, no specific materials are used in clinical practice for the diagnosis of AOS. Feiken *et al.* (2008), however, revealed that SLTs clearly expressed the need for valid materials, not only to differentially diagnose AOS from other speech disorders, but also to be able to evaluate therapy. In 2012, the DIAS (Feiken and Jonkers) was published.

This consists of four subtests. In the *subtest for orofacial apraxia*, the participant is asked to consciously make use of the articulators in nonverbal tasks. These tasks permit the diagnosis of orofacial apraxia, given that it often co-occurs with AOS, and may be important for certain therapy approaches. In the subtest *articulation of phonemes*, participants repeat consonants and vowels three times in a row. The test consists of 30 items – 15 consonants and 15 vowels. The consonants differ according to place or manner of articulation. The addition of a schwa is permitted where it would be natural in saying the sound in isolation (e.g. /p/, /t/). The vowels are chosen with respect to their position in the vowel triangle. The place of articulation of the consonants was varied to circumvent perseveration, e.g. labial /m/ is followed by alveolar /d/. The role of this task is to find out whether an individual is able to consistently produce three identical phonemes in a row, and to establish whether more errors are made on consonants compared to vowels.

The third task comprises diadochokinetic and syllable repetition tasks. It is assumed that participants with AOS will have more difficulty alternating between different phonemes (alternating diadochokinesis), rather than with the repetition of the same phonemes (sequential diadochokinesis) (Ogar *et al.*, 2006; Thoonen *et al.*, 1996). The diadochokinetic and syllable repetition test consists of six sequencing and six alternating items. This subtest progresses according to the level of complexity, starting with simple CV structures, e.g. [pa-pa-pa] vs [pa-ta-ka] and ending with CCVCC structures, e.g. [staŋk-staŋk-staŋk] vs [staŋk-blaŋk-draŋk]. In some of the items, the initial or final consonant changes alternately, whereas in others the consonant clusters change.

The subtest *articulation of words* aims to disclose specific claimed symptoms of AOS, including syllable segmentation, clusters, initiation problems and the influence of articulatory complexity. The test contains 66 items increasing in length and articulatory complexity by the number of syllables, the number of phonemes and articulatory complexity (CV structures, CC clusters within a syllable, CCC clusters within a syllable, abutting consonants (C-C) at the syllable boundary).

Scoring for orofacial apraxia and repetition of words is based on a three- and a four-point scale, respectively, varying from no response (0) to correct (3 or 4; with specific guidelines for scoring on the different scales). A correct-incorrect score is used for the repetition of phonemes and a count by time score for the diadochokinetic test (number of correct repetitions of syllables within eight seconds). The diagnosis of AOS, however, is not based on these scores, but on the presence of symptoms of AOS (see below).

The DIAS was validated on the basis of the scores of a group of control participants, speakers with AOS, with dysarthria and with aphasia. Thirty participants with AOS were tested in the validation phase of the DIAS. Participants were selected as possibly having AOS by the treating speech therapist based on the criteria of the Academy of Neurologic Communication Disorders and Sciences (ANCDS) list (Wambaugh, 2006). This judgment was then confirmed by an independent clinical linguist. Twenty individuals without AOS but with aphasia or dysarthria were also tested. Aphasia was diagnosed with the Aachen Aphasia Test (Graetz *et al.*, 1992). Dysarthria was diagnosed with the Radboud Dysartrie Onderzoek (RDO; Knuijt & De Swart, 2007).

The diagnosis of AOS in the DIAS was not based on the test scores, but on the presence of eight specific symptoms of AOS. In the literature, there is at least some agreement that these symptoms are characteristic of AOS. This does not mean that there is consensus that these eight symptoms are the only manifestations of AOS, or that they must all be present to diagnose AOS. Nevertheless, it was decided to take these symptoms as a starting point. The eight indicative symptoms were: inconsistency of errors; more errors with consonants than with vowels; more difficulty with alternating diadochokinesis than with sequential diadochokinesis; visible or audible groping; initiation problems; syllable segmentation; segmentation of consonant clusters; and effects of articulatory complexity. Individuals without speech and language disturbances rarely showed these symptoms. In participants with AOS, the symptoms were present, but with considerable variation. Nevertheless, when any three of the eight symptoms were present, a diagnosis of AOS could be secured. In 26 out of 30 speakers tested with AOS, three or more symptoms were present. Three of the remaining four individuals could not be categorised as they were severely affected and unable to complete all subtests. The fourth participant had less than three symptoms. Although originally included as having AOS, the individual was decided not to have AOS based on the test.

None of the 10 participants with dysarthria but two of the 10 speakers with aphasia showed three or more symptoms. Although these two aphasic speakers were not originally classified as participants with AOS by the SLT, this could mean that they were suffering from AOS as well according to the diagnostic criteria employed.

With respect to the subtest scores, the participants with AOS scored significantly lower than the groups with aphasia and dysarthria on all subtests. A logistic regression led to a correct division into a group of participants with and without AOS in 90% of the cases. In a further study with 10 participants with AOS, the DIAS was able to measure improvement, based on the critical differences provided for the different subtest scores. These outcomes indicate that in the near future the DIAS may be used for the diagnosis of AOS as well as an outcome measure for the evaluation of therapy.

## Therapy

No specific therapy program is available for treating dysarthria or AOS in adults in the Dutch language. The DYVA (Dharmaperwira-Prins, 1996) provides suggestions for training the different components of speech (posture, breathing, voice, articulation, intonation and specific movements of the tongue, lip or cheeks), but these are not evidence based.

More general programs for speech deficits promote the use of music or melody in therapy. In 1987, melodic intonation therapy (MIT; Albert *et al.*, 1973) was adapted for the Dutch language (Lugt van der-Wiechen & Verschoor, 1987). The Rehabilitation Centre 'Rijndam' in Rotterdam recently performed an evaluation study of MIT in both the acute and the chronic phase using neuroimaging techniques to study the underlying neural reorganisation processes of recovery from AOS, and showed the positive therapeutic effects of MIT (Van der Meulen *et al.*, 2012).

A therapy program that was recently developed in the Netherlands, in which music plays an important role, is speech-music therapy for aphasia (SMTA) (De Bruijn *et al.*, 2005). SMTA is a combination of speech and music therapy used to remediate fluency problems associated with phonological deficits in aphasia. SMTA is also used to treat people with dysarthria or AOS. SMTA consists of two interwoven treatment approaches: a speech therapy approach focusing on sounds, words and sentences; and music therapy focusing on singing, emphasising rhythmic speech and finally the intended normal speech. In more severely disordered speakers, training emphasises the production of commonly used words and phrases in unison and at later stages through question-answer sequences, including repetition. Every exercise has its own specifically written melody and is practised in the sequence singing-rhythmic speech-speech. Rhythmic speech is supported for example by clapping. Finally, patients have to speak without musical assistance. SMTA is administered at least twice a week in half-hour sessions. Therapy ends if the target improvement is attained or if no more improvement is seen. The difference between SMTA and MIT is that MIT uses fixed and stylised melodies, whereas SMTA is based on music that specifically fits the individual, both with respect to their musical preference and their speech problems. The melodic and rhythmic patterns in MIT are simple: melodies of two tones (high and low), long or short. The rhythmic pattern and melody in SMTA are much more elaborate and contain different musical elements such as meter and dynamics.

So far, about 100 speakers have been treated using this program. Practice-based evidence is therefore sufficiently available. The authors of the program are currently conducting a formal evaluation of the efficacy of the program employing controlled methods.

The Pitch Limiting Voice Treatment (PLVT) (De Swart *et al.*, 2003) is widely used in the Netherlands in patients with hypokinetic dysarthria due to Parkinson's disease. This treatment, like the Lee Silverman Voice Treatment (LSVT) (Ramig *et al.*, 1994), encourages individuals to speak loud, but importantly adds 'while keeping your voice low' (i.e. low pitch) to the instruction (in short: 'loud and low'). Maintaining vocal pitch at an appropriate level limits the increase in laryngeal muscle tension, preventing a strained or pressed voice and fatigue. Although the PLVT is aimed at voice, it is widely used by SLTs to increase or maintain speech intelligibility in general in patients with Parkinson's disease. Apart from an increase in the volume and clarity of the voice, the treatment also leads to improved (deeper) breathing and articulation. Although at this moment, no large-scale efficacy study has been carried out, a comparative, non-treatment study with 32 patients showed that both the LSVT and the PLVT instructions resulted in a similar increase in loudness on an investigatory task, but in the case of the PLVT this was not accompanied by an increase in vocal pitch and laryngeal muscle tension (De Swart *et al.*, 2003).

Although not in the scope of this chapter, since it was developed for children rather than adults, we briefly describe the 'Dyspraxia Programme' (Dutch: 'Dyspraxie Programma') (Erlings *et al.*, 1993), which offers a systematic combination of diagnostic assessment followed by treatment of childhood apraxia of speech (CAS). The program, based on the Nuffield Dyspraxia Programme (Connery, 1985), has two starting points. First of all, the treatment program is constructed according to the stages of normal speech (motor) development, starting from pre-speech oral motor skills, single speech sounds, combining speech sounds in syllables and words of increasing length and complexity, to sentences and connected speech. This not only offers a natural program for children, but it also gives a structure to the program that is relatively transparent for SLTs. Second, treatment is preceded by extensive diagnostic assessment, which in the philosophy of the authors adds to its effectiveness and efficiency. The two starting points combined result in a program that follows the specific phonological and syllabic structure of Dutch, in which a particular order of speech sounds is trained, with systematic build-up of syllabic complexity.

## Language-Specific Aspects for Dutch

There are two distinct characteristics of Dutch that make it an interesting language for the study of AOS and dysarthria. First, typical aspects of Dutch phonology might play a role in foreign accent syndrome (FAS), a syndrome that is often seen as a specific outcome of AOS (cf. Miller *et al.*, 2006; Moen, 2000). Gilbers *et al.* (2013) describe the data of two Dutch FAS speakers. According to them, many characteristics of FAS relate to force of articulation. They discuss some parameters of hyperarticulation, or fortition such as longer, negative VOT for prevoiced plosives or altered vowel quality, the latter for example seen in less vowel reduction. If these symptoms are present, speakers no longer sound Dutch, but may sound for example German. They also describe a change in prosody, specifically a tendency toward 'syllable timing', whereas Dutch is a 'stress-timed' language, leading to the perception of for example French. According to the authors it is expected that listeners will perceive the accent of a language that is characterised by a larger amount of fortition compared to their native speech. This assumption predicts that people may hear e.g. a German, Spanish or Arabic accent in a Dutch FAS speaker, but not a Dutch accent in e.g. a Spanish or German FAS speaker. This prediction is currently being further investigated in relation to other speakers with AOS.

Secondly, Dutch is characterised by a large number of consonant clusters, which can be complex. As a result, AOS in Dutch is characterised by high rates of perceived phonological omission and substitution errors (Den Ouden, 2002). This permits a more sophisticated quantitative analysis of error patterns than simply calculating the overall percentage of correctly produced consonants. It provides the opportunity to determine the percentages of particular phonemes or phoneme classes in relation to the phonotactic context. This type of analysis has not yet been conducted in adult AOS, but the paradigm has been used successfully in research into CAS. Thoonen *et al.* (1994) conducted a paradigmatic and syntagmatic feature value analysis of the consonant substitution and omission errors in the speech of 11 children with CAS compared to age-matched controls (paradigmatic: feature retention; syntagmatic: feature assimilation. For example in /taka/ for /taga/, place of articulation is retained while manner of articulation is assimilated). Although children with CAS showed a higher rate of almost all error types, when compared to control children, with both paradigmatic and syntagmatic errors, the relative number of errors (i.e. after correction for the overall higher error rate) appeared identical for both groups. Error profiles showed only very few differences between groups, suggesting that the speech of children with CAS can be characterised by a high rate of 'normal' slips of the tongue.

As in many languages, consonant clusters in Dutch can occur both within and across syllable boundaries (so called 'abutting' consonants). This provides an interesting window for the study of motor speech disorders. Speech motor planning is thought to involve the retrieval of the spatial and temporal goals of the articulatory movements from sensorimotor storage. These are currently postulated to involve syllable-sized chunks stored in a so-called syllabary (e.g. Aichert & Ziegler, 2004; Cholin *et al.*, 2005; Levelt & Wheeldon, 1994; Ziegler *et al.*, 2010). If no matching syllable-sized chunks are available, the system is forced to use the 'indirect route' and assembles the syllables from smaller, phoneme-sized units – at least according to the view expounded in the model of Levelt *et al.* (1999). This dual-route hypothesis though has been challenged by other work. Aichert and Ziegler (2004) in particular, have proposed a different view. Based on the effects of syllabic complexity and syllable frequency on error rate in patients with AOS, they argued that the impairment does not entail a complete loss of the syllabary, but entails a defective process of retrieving the syllabic motor programs. The experimental results would indicate that syllabic representations can be accessed, at least to some degree.

Further work in Dutch, which also has within and across syllable clusters could help address this issue further – for instance, by manipulating syllable structure in an otherwise unchanged phonetic context (such as the English phrases 'fell table' vs 'felt able'). The Dutch language provides ample opportunities for this. Assuming that in normal speech the use of syllable-sized chunks has the effect of preserving the coherence of the spatial and temporal scaling aspects of speech movements, a deficiency in speech motor planning could cause deviant coarticulation and durational patterns. Such experiments have been carried out in children with CAS. Nijland *et al.* (2003) compared coarticulation and durational structure in Dutch phrases like 'zus giet' (/zʉs-xit/, meaning: sister pours) vs 'ze schiet' (/zə-sxit/, meaning: she shoots). Interestingly, the majority of the children with CAS produced much more consonant omissions in cases where the two medial consonants formed a cluster, as in /zə-sxit/, than in cases where they were abutting consonants, as in /zʉs-xit/. Apparently, the syllabic structure influences the quality of consonant production.

In contrast, no effects of syllable structure were found on coarticulation, neither in the normally speaking children nor in the children with CAS, although the children with CAS did show an overall larger variability of vowel and consonant quality, irrespective of syllable structure. With respect to the durational patterns, the normally speaking children showed systematic durational adjustments to syllabic structure in the segments of the stressed syllable in the sense that both [s] and the second vowel were shorter in /zə-sxit/ compared to /zʉs-xit/. Such systematic durational patterns were not found in the speech of children with CAS. The normally speaking children also showed inter-syllabic effects in durational structure in the form of prosodic differences between the phrases, which were not found for the children with CAS. This lack of a consistent intra- and inter-syllabic temporal structure in the speech of children with CAS suggests that motor planning in children with CAS is poorly organised at the syllabic level.

These experiments have not yet been carried out in adult AOS, and could provide important insight in the motor planning impairments involved. An important comparison here would be contrasting speech motor output in a developing system, where syllable-level programming may not yet have been established vs a system where there has been impairment to a previously intact, fully developed system.

# Concluding Remarks

There is a strong base for clinical research regarding dysarthria and AOS in Dutch speakers. Apart from the development and evaluation of diagnostic instruments and treatment programs, a large body of research is focused on the development of computerised or web-based assessment methods, including full test batteries and treatment programs (e.g. Beijer *et al.*, 2010a, 2010b; Maassen *et al.*, in press; Van Haaften *et al.*, 2011; Van Nuffelen *et al.*, 2009). We expect that in the Netherlands and Flanders, such automated aids will play an important role in the diagnosis and treatment of dysarthria and AOS in the near future.

Overall, dysarthria and AOS in Dutch are very similar to English, but not to many other languages such as Spanish or Cantonese, with much simpler syllabic structures and/or much simpler vowel systems. Dutch contains complex consonant clusters in syllable initial as well as in syllable final position. In AOS, these complex syllable structures elicit many speech errors, which can be of different types in initial and final position. A speech error in AOS that is typical for Dutch is prevoicing in voiced plosives, which could play a role in speech that is perceived as being spoken with a foreign accent. In addition, AOS in Dutch seems to be predominantly characterised by high rates of perceived phonological omission and substitution errors; however, future cross-linguistic research is necessary to support this claim.

Similar to English, Dutch also features a rich vowel system compared to languages like Spanish. Although errors in vowel production have not been found to be typical for dysarthria or AOS in Dutch, this does mean that vowel centralisation could affect intelligibility more than in languages with simpler vowel systems.

## References

Aichert, I. and Ziegler, W. (2004) Syllable frequency and syllable structure in apraxia of speech. *Brain and Language* 88, 148–159.

Albert, M.L., Sparks, R.W. and Helm, N.A. (1973) Melodic intonation therapy for aphasia. *Archives of Neurology* 29, 130–131.

Beijer, L.J., Rietveld, T.C.M., Hoskam, V., Geurts, A.C.H. and De Swart, B.J.M. (2010a) Evaluating the feasibility and the potential efficacy of e-learning-based speech therapy (EST) as a web application for speech training in dysarthric patients with Parkinson's disease: A case study. *Telemedicine and e-Health* 16, 732–738.

Beijer, L.J., Rietveld, T.C.M., Van Beers, M.M.A., Slangen, R.M.L., Van den Heuvel, H., De Swart, B.J.M. and Geurts, A.C.H (2010b) E-learning-based speech therapy: A web application for speech training. *Telemedicine and e-Health* 16, 177–180.

Bruijn de, M., Zielman, T. and Hurkmans, J. (2005) *Speech-Music Therapy for Aphasia, SMTA*. Beetsterzwaag: Revalidatie Friesland.

Cholin, J., Schiller, N.O. and Levelt, W.J.M. (2005) The preparation of syllables in speech production. *Journal of Memory and Language* 50, 47–61.

Connery, V. (1985) *Nuffield Dyspraxia Programme*. London: Nuffield Hearing and Speech Centre.

Darley, F.L., Aronson, A.E. and Brown, J.R. (1975) *Motor Speech Disorders*. Philadelphia, PA: Saunders.

De Swart, B.J.M., Willemse, S.C., Maassen, B.A.M. and Horstink, M.W.I.M. (2003) Improvement of voicing in patients with Parkinson's disease by speech therapy. *Neurology* 60, 498–500.

Den Ouden, D.B. (2002) *Phonology in Aphasia: Syllables and Segments in Level-Specific Deficits*. Groningen Dissertations in Linguistics 39. Rijksuniversiteit Groningen.

Dharmaperwira-Prins, R. (2009) *Dysartrie en Verbale Apraxie – DYVA onderzoek*. Lisse: Pearson Assessment.

Enderby, P. (1983) *Frenchay Dysarthria Assessment*. Austin, TX: Pro-Ed.

Erlings-van Deurse, M., Freriks, A., Goudt-Bakker, K., Van der Meulen, S.J. and de Vries, L. (1993) *Dyspraxie Programma*. Lisse: Swets & Zeitlinger.

Feiken, J., Hofstede, D. and Jonkers, R. (2008) De diagnostiek van verbale apraxie. *Logopedie en Foniatrie* 7/8, 228–234.

Feiken, J.F. and Jonkers, R. (2012) *Diagnostisch Instrument voor Apraxie van de Spraak (DIAS)*. Houten: Bohn, Stafleu & Van Loghum.

Gilbers, D., Jonkers, R., van der Scheer, F. and Feiken, J. (2013) On the force of articulation in the foreign accent syndrome. In C. Gooskens and R. Van Bezooijen (eds) *Phonetics in Europe* (pp. 11–33). Hamburg: Peter Lang.

Graetz, P., De Bleser, R. and Willmes, K. (1992) *Akense Afasietest*. Lisse: Swets & Zeitlinger.

Kalf, J.G. and de Swart, B.J.M. (2007) *Handleiding 'Radboud Oraal Onderzoek'*. Nijmegen: UMC St Radboud. See https://www.radboudumc.nl/Informatievoorverwijzers/Verwijzersinformatie/Documents/Logopedie_Handleiding%20Radboud%20Oraal%20onderzoek.pdf (accessed March 2014).

Knuijt, S. and de Swart, B.J.M. (2007) *Handleiding 'Radboud Dysartrieonderzoek'*. Nijmegen: UMC St Radboud.

Levelt, W.J.M. and Wheeldon, L. (1994) Do speakers have access to a mental syllabary? *Cognition* 50, 239–269.

Lugt van der-van Wiechen, K.L. and Verschoor, J. (1987) *Melodic Intonation Therapy. Nederlandse Bewerking*. Rotterdam: Stichting Afasie Rotterdam.

Maassen, B., van Haaften, L., Diepeveen, S., de Swart, B., van der Meulen, S. and Nijland, L. (in press) *Computer Articulation Instrument (CAI)*. Amsterdam: Boom test uitgevers.

Miller, N., Lowit, A. and O'Sullivan, H. (2006) What makes acquired foreign accent syndrome foreign? *Journal of Neurolinguistics* 19, 385–409.

Moen, I. (2000) Foreign accent syndrome: A review of contemporary explanations. *Aphasiology* 14, 5–15.

Nijland, L., Maassen, B., Van der Meulen, S., Gabreels, F., Kraaimaat, F.W. and Schreuder, R. (2003) Planning of syllables in children with developmental apraxia of speech. *Clinical Linguistics and Phonetics* 17, 1–24.

Ogar, J., Willock, S., Baldo, J., Wilkins, D., Ludy, C. and Dronkers, N. (2006) Clinical and anatomical correlates of apraxia of speech. *Brain and Language* 97, 343–350.

Ramig, L.O., Bonitati, C., Lemke, J. and Horii, Y. (1994) Voice treatment for patients with Parkinson disease: Development of an approach and preliminary efficacy data. *Journal of Medical Speech-Language Pathology* 2, 191–209.

Rietveld, A.C.M. and Van Heuven, V.J. (2001) *Algemene fonetiek*. Bussum: Coutinho.

Thoonen, G., Maassen, B., Gabreels, F. and Schreuder, R. (1994) Feature analysis of singleton consonant errors in developmental verbal dyspraxia (DVD). *Journal of Speech and Hearing Research* 37, 1424–1440.

Thoonen, G., Maassen, B., Wit, J., Gabreëls, F. and Schreuder, R. (1996) The integrated use of maximum performance tasks in differential diagnostic evaluations among children with motor speech disorders. *Clinical Linguistics and Phonetics* 10, 311–336.

Van der Meulen, I., Van de Sandt-Koenderman, M.E. and Ribbers, G.M. (2012) Melodic intonation therapy: Present controversies and future opportunities. *Archives of Physical Medicine and Rehabilitation* 93, 46–52.

Van Haaften, L., Diepeveen, S., de Swart, B. and Maassen, B. (2011) Standardization of a Computer Articulation Instrument (CAI). *Stem-, Spraak- en Taalpathologie* 17 (Suppl), 88.

Van Nuffelen, G., Middag, C., De Bodt, M. and Martens, J.P. (2009) Speech technology-based assessment of phoneme intelligibility in dysarthria. *International Journal of Language and Communication Disorders* 44, 716–730.

Wambaugh, J.L. (2006) Treatment guidelines for apraxia of speech: Lessons for future research. *Journal of Medical Speech Language Pathology* 14, 317–321.

Ziegler, W., Staiger, A. and Aichert, I. (2010) Apraxia of speech: What the deconstruction of phonetic plans tells us about the construction of articulate language. In B. Maassen and P. Van Lieshout (eds) *Speech Motor Control: New Developments in Basic and Applied Research* (pp. 3–22). Oxford: Oxford University Press.

# 12 Some Segmental and Prosodic Aspects of Motor Speech Disorders in French

## Danielle Duez

In their classical study, Darley *et al.* (1969) defined dysarthrias as 'speech disorders resulting from disturbances in muscular control over the speech mechanism due to damage to the central or peripheral nervous system'. They hypothesized that a correlation exists between the different kinds of abnormality of motor functioning, different speech disorders and perceptual impressions. Five types of dysarthria were delineated on the basis of certain perceptual dimensions of voice and speech (e.g. prosody, articulation): flaccid (in bulbar palsy), spastic (in pseudobulbar palsy), ataxic (in cerebellar disorders), hypokinetic (in parkinsonism) and hyperkinetic (in dystonia and chorea); there was also mixed dysarthria (spastic-flaccid) resulting from amyotrophic lateral sclerosis (ALS). In addition, a hierarchy in the clusters of dimensions was established and the most prominent cluster was identified in each dysarthria type.

The study has been a source of inspiration for acoustic, physiological and perceptual studies on motor speech disorders. For example, it led to the search to identify phonetic distortions specific to different neurological pathologies, thereby improving our knowledge of motor speech disorders and our understanding of normal speech production (Kent *et al.*, 2000).

However, the influence of Darley *et al.* (1969) has been somewhat constraining. Their all-embracing assertion that 'speech pathology reflects neuropathology' has hampered subsequent evaluation of speech production deficits. For example, O'Dwyer and Neilson (1988), in contradiction to Darley *et al.*'s conclusion, found no strict relationship between the symptoms of certain neurological diseases and aberrant speech production characteristics; furthermore, certain normal sounding patients who underwent acoustic analysis were shown to have production anomalies (Weismer, 1984). Another important limiting factor resulted from the identification of different types of dysarthria being exclusively based on evaluations by American experts of speech samples produced by American patients. Although the results give valuable information on the perceptual characteristics of the different dysarthrias, they ignored or underestimated speech disorders specific to other languages.

For this reason, this chapter is devoted to describing aspects of dysarthria in spoken French. The first part is a rapid presentation of the main aspects of the French linguistic system (segmental and prosodic), with comparisons to the English linguistic system in order to better highlight the characteristics of French. The second part consists of a survey of the literature concerned with the segmental and prosodic characteristics of dysarthria in French speech. To better focus on specificities in dysarthria, the results for French are compared with those obtained for English. Analysing divergences between French and English is of particular interest because, although strongly related at the lexical level since William the Conqueror (11th century), they are highly divergent in the phonetic domain. According to Delattre (1966), they occupy the two phonetic extremes in the table of world languages.

# Some General Characteristics of French Speech

## Segmental characteristics of French

### French vowel system

Traditionally, vowels are classified according to their aperture, their place of articulation, the position of the lips, their duration and the level of fundamental frequency (F0). Concerning the aperture (i.e. the vertical distance which separates the dome of the tongue from the palate), it can be seen in Table 12.1 that in French there are 11 oral vowels which are classified as closed, mid-closed, mid-open or open. It can also be seen that the place of articulation (which refers to the place on the top of the dome of the tongue in relation to the palatal vault) distinguishes front (palatal) and back (velar) vowels. The lips can be spread, rounded or protruded in varying degrees, depending partly on the height of the tongue and the place of articulation (for more details, see Marchal, 2009). In French, all back vowels are rounded; in addition, there is a set of front labialized vowels.

French also possesses a set of nasal vowels produced with velum lowering, thus allowing air to pass through both the nasal and oral cavities. Tongue and lip positions are approximately the same as those required for their oral counterparts (see Table 12.1).

Vowels have intrinsic duration directly related to jaw position and tongue body height (House & Fairbanks, 1953; Lehiste, 1970). In French, nasal vowels are 40% longer than low vowels which are 13% longer than mid-high vowels, which in turn are 15% longer than high vowels (Di Cristo, 1985). The differences between high and low vowels are greater in English than in French (for more details, see also Di Cristo, 1985). Vowels also have intrinsic fundamental frequency (IF0) that is a function of aperture.

**Table 12.1** Articulatory description of French vowels

| Aperture | | | Place of articulation | | | Nasality |
|---|---|---|---|---|---|---|
| | | | Front | | Back | |
| Small (closed) | | | i | y | u | − |
| Mid | Mid Closed | | e | ø | o | |
| | Mid Open | | ɛ | œ | ɔ | |
| | | | ɛ̃ | œ̃ | ɔ̃ | + |
| Large (open) | | | a | | ɑ | − |
| | | | | | ɑ̃ | + |

| − | + |
|---|---|
| Labiality | |

Source: Marchal (2011)

The difference between the IF0 of high /i y and u/ and low vowels /a/ is about 10 Hz (Di Cristo & Hirst, 1986).

The French vowel system has a certain number of specificities which appear clearly when they are compared to the English vowel system. For example, all French vowels are monophthongal, they are not reduced during their emission nor do they change quality and they tend to be relatively short, especially in open syllables (Delattre, 1966); in English, diphthongs containing a long segment with two successive targets are common. Another interesting specificity in French is the high number of rounded vowels due to rounded front vowels, something inexistent in English vowels. Nasal vowels are another important specific aspect of French; these have a phonological role and allow meaning distinctions among words.

### French consonant system

Traditionally, consonants are classified according to their voicing, manner of articulation and place of articulation. As can be seen in Table 12.2, French possesses six oral stops, which are voiceless (/p, t, k/) or voiced (/b, d, g/). There are also three voiced nasal stops. Out of the 11

**Table 12.2** Articulatory description of French consonants

| Place of articulation | | Stops | | | Constrictives | | | | Articulatory organ |
|---|---|---|---|---|---|---|---|---|---|
| | | Orals | | Nasals | Without complete oral constriction | | | Laterals | |
| | | | | | | Without lip protusion | With lip protusion | | |
| | | | | | Medium | | | | |
| | | **Voicing** | | | **Voicing** | | | | |
| | | − | + | | − | + | − | + | |
| Laryngal | | | | | | | | | Vocal folds |
| Uvular | Palatal vault | | | | | | | ʁ | Dorsal |
| Velar | | k | g | | | | | | |
| Labiovelar | | | | | | | w | | |
| Labiopalatal | | | | | | | ɥ | | |
| Palatal | | | | ɲ | | j | | | Tongue |
| Alveopalatal | | | | | ʃ | ʒ | | | Pre dorsal |
| Alveolar | | | | | s | z | | l | Apex |
| Dental | | t | d | n | | | | | |
| Labiodental | | | | | f | v | | | Lip |
| Bilabial | | p | b | m | | | | | |

Source: Marchal (2011)

constrictives, 5 are produced with a weak constriction and are voiced such as the 3 glides (/j, ɥ/ and /w/), the liquid /l/ and the so-called Parisian /ʁ/; the remaining six constrictives are /f, v, s, z, ʃ, ʒ/.

The French consonant system diverges from the English system in that it has a smaller number of constrictives, i.e. it is missing the three constrictives /h, θ/ and /ð/ and the two affricates /tʃ/ and /dʒ/, none of which exists in French. Another difference can be found in the nasals: French possesses the palatal /ɲ/ whereas English has the velar /ŋ/.

Like vowels, consonants can be phonologically similar yet have important phonetic differences. For example, in French, voiceless stops are not aspirated and are often thought to exclude voice onset time (VOT; the interval between stop release and vowel voicing), contrary to English stops. In addition, there is a strong tendency in French to anticipatory assimilation, unlike in English (Delattre, 1966).

## Prosodic characteristics of French

Prosody consists of intonation, accentuation, rhythm and temporal variables. Prosody governs stress, tone and quantity oppositions in numerous languages and contributes to the identity of words (for more details, see Hirst, 2006). At the sentence, paragraph and discourse level, prosody rules intonation, accentuation and phenomena associated with duration control (pauses, final lengthening and speech rate and tempo variations), characterises the way individual words are combined into larger speech units and governs the relative prominence of different words and the grouping of syntactic and semantic units and informational units. Besides linguistic information, prosody also transmits paralinguistic and extralinguistic characteristics (as defined by Laver, 1991). These prosodic functions are expressed differently in the various languages of the world through specific variations and interactions of F0, intensity, speech segment duration and pauses. In the following section, the prosodic characteristics of French are examined.

## Intonation in French

French intonation is of the rising type whereas English is viewed as of the falling type. In French, major and minor continuation rises and 'finality fall' prevail in the F0 curves for simple declarative sentences (Delattre, 1961). Even in monosyllabic or disyllabic utterances, the rising-falling pattern is often present (Di Cristo, 1998). Contrary to English, finality in French is not indicated by a local fall on the final syllable but involves the last two words of the sentence. Martin (1982) and Vaissière (1974, 2002) confirmed that finality is achieved by combining a high or high-rising tone at the end of the penultimate word with a contrasting falling tone on the very last word.

Intonation contributes to the identification of the syntactic structure: minor continuation rises mostly coincide with minor phrase boundaries and major continuation rises coincide with major phrase boundaries. Content words exhibit high tone, realised either at their onset, offset or both (most frequently at offset) whereas function words have a low target anchored at the very end of the last of a series of function words. As function words are particularly numerous in French (significantly more than in English), one may conclude that there is a contrast between content words associated with a high tone and function words associated with a low tone (for more details, see Vaissière, 2002).

As in many other languages, intonation in French has many functions, such as the expression of interrogation. Interrogation can be marked with partial or total questions (i.e. not syntactically marked or by means of the expression *Est ce que?* Is it true that?). Concerning the latter, there is a certain controversy over the general shape of the pitch pattern; however, most studies agree that the use of final rise is a characteristic of total questions. Compared to continuatives, this rise has greater range (Rossi, 1981), higher final pitch (Boë & Contini, 1975) and steeper slope (Léon & Bhatt, 1987). Intonation has also a crucial role in focalization and expressivity. French speakers can use focal accents for intensification or for contrast. In the first case, a word or a lexical item is highlighted by an extra pitch prominence; in the second, an item focused for contrast is characterised by a global rising-falling pitch pattern (Di Cristo, 1998).

### Speech rate, pause time, speech time and articulation rate

Speech rate and its two main components (pause time and articulation rate) reflect the processes involved at the different levels of speech production; they are influenced by factors such as the speech situation, speaker habits and specificities. There is a strong link between speech rate and pause time: a slow rate is often characterised by a long pause time (e.g. in descriptions as shown by Grosjean & Deschamps [1973]); not unsurprisingly, when speech rate increases, pauses tend to disappear and/ or become shorter (Grosjean & Collins, 1979).

Numerous studies of different languages have shown that the frequency and duration of pauses are related to linguistic structure; generally, pauses are more frequent and longer at the end of sentences than within sentences. Grosjean and Deschamps (1975) found, in spontaneous French and English interviews, that about 70% of all pauses occurred at major constituent breaks (defined primarily as clause and sentence breaks) and that these were significantly longer than pauses within constituents.

Although pause distribution is strongly linked to the syntactic structure of the message, it also depends on factors such as the length of constituents. For example, in their study on patterns of silence in American English read speech, Grosjean *et al.* (1979) observed that speakers tend to place pauses between word groups of equal length. A more recent study on structures of performance in French (Monnin & Grosjean, 1993) showed a similar pattern with sentences broken up into groups of words of more or less equal length, thereby maintaining a certain symmetry between the different components of the sentence. In spite of this, important differences exist between the distributional scheme of pauses in French and English. For example, in French, there is a specific prosodic status of postposed adjectives, with a pause occurring between the adjective and the preceding noun, and bundling of function words to heads on the left.

Articulation rate determines the pace at which speech segments are actually produced. It is speaker specific, pertaining to the inherent speed of articulatory movements; it depends on the influence of many physiological, linguistic and social factors (for more details, see Jacewicz *et al.*, 2009). Articulation rate is also highly variable within the production of the same speaker (Miller *et al.*, 1984), being the main source of variability of speech segments (Miller, 1981), and it strongly influences speech rhythm. When articulation rate increases, major boundaries may be replaced by minor boundaries (without a pause), minor boundaries may disappear and final-phrase syllables (which are more variable than non-final syllables) shorten significantly (Duez, 1987).

### Stress in French

French is a fixed stress language where the stressed syllable is the final full syllable (i.e. not containing a schwa) of the last lexical item of a rhythmic group. The optional schwa (or mute-e [ə]) is an unstable vowel which is dropped at the end of words, except in southern French. Its pronunciation within words and groups depends on various factors such as speech style, number of syllables within groups and number of consecutive consonants within words. More details can be found in Delattre (1966), Léon (1971) and Tranel (1987).

The last lexical item is usually a content word (see Example 1), occasionally a clitic (see Example 2). The stress group may be equivalent to a clause, a phrase or a word, explaining why French stress, which has an important grouping function, is often named 'group stress' or 'phrase stress' (Delattre, 1939; Garde, 1968; Grammont, 1933; Marouzeau, 1956).

(1)  VIENS (come) Viens VITE (come quickly)
(2)  Cuisez-LE à feu DOUX (cook it slowly)

In addition to final stress, there is an optional non-emphatic initial stress (Di Cristo, 1998; Fónagy, 1980; Pernot, 1929-1930; Scherck, 1912; Vaissière, 1974) which has been traditionally specific to public speech styles (Vaissière, 1974) but is now spreading to less formal speech styles (Fónagy, 1980). Initial stress is highly probabilistic because its realisation depends on style, word length, word class and syllable structure (Fónagy, 1980; Fónagy & Fónagy, 1976), as well as the number of syllables in a group.

Initial and final stressed syllables are characterised by pitch prominence and differential lengthening patterns. Emphasis is given to greater lengthening towards the beginning of the syllable (onset consonant) for initial stress and greater lengthening towards the end of the syllable (nucleus and coda consonant) for final stress (Hirst *et al.*, 1998). The reinforcement of the initial syllable contributes to identifying the beginning of content words whereas the prominence given to the final syllable reinforces phrase boundary.

In English there are three stress levels: primary, secondary and unstressed (Hayes, 1995). Stressed syllables tend to have higher pitch excursion, higher intensity and longer duration (Ladefoged, 1975). However, there are different acoustic characteristics for stress lengthening and phrase-final lengthening (Edwards & Beckman, 1988). Segments lengthened for stress reasons are lengthened uniformly throughout the syllable whereas segments in sentence-or-phrase-final position undergo greater lengthening in the peak and coda than at the onset (Campbell, 1992).

In French, the conjunction of final F0 rise and final lengthening reinforces boundaries, explaining why French is considered a 'boundary language' (Vaissière, 1991) or a 'non-stress language' (Vaissière & Michaud, 2006). English, on the contrary, is considered a true 'stress language' (Vaissière, 1991).

### Rhythm in French

Rhythm is based on grouping, regularity and repetition of structures (Fraisse, 1974). In French, the rhythmic organisation is based on the repetition of groups consisting of a stressed syllable preceded by a sequence of non-stressed syllables. French is usually termed a 'right-headed language' whereas English is labelled a 'left-headed language' (see Hirst & Di Cristo, 1998). This distinction is strongly related to the typology proposed by Pike (1945) who distinguished syllable-timed languages (such as French) and stress-timed languages (such as English). In French, syllables give the impression of being of equivalent duration although there is no strict syllabicity but an alternating and (slightly) increasing duration pattern (Duez & Nishinuma, 1985). In English, the stressed syllables are perceived as occurring at regular intervals, whatever the number of intervening unstressed syllables.

In fact, the rhythm of a language appears to be the result of specific phonological phenomena such as the variety of syllable types, the presence or absence of phonological vowel length distinctions, the presence or absence of vowel reduction and the salience of word stress (Dasher & Bolinger, 1982; Dauer, 1983). In French, syllables tend to be mostly of the CV type, vowels tend to keep their quality (Delattre, 1966), there is no lexical distinction of quantity and the prominence pattern relies mostly on the significant lengthening given to final-phrase syllables. In English, syllables are mostly CVC (Delattre, 1966), unstressed syllables are strongly reduced and the prominence pattern mainly relies on pitch accents.

# Characteristics of the Dysarthria in French

This section presents the studies (mostly perceptual and acoustic) made on dysarthria in French. It is to note, however, that these studies are mainly concerned with hypokinetic dysarthria that has inspired the greatest amount of research.

## Segmental aspects of dysarthria in French

Articulatory incompetence and inaccuracy have been reported in many articulatory and kinematic studies of dysarthric speech in various languages. At the acoustic level, this has been shown to be reflected by vowel distortion and consonant imprecision.

### Vowel distortion

In early oscillographic analyses of the speech produced by bulbar or pseudocerebellar and parkinsonian patients, Gremy (1958) observed frequency variations from one phoneme to another, and even within phonemes, which would suggest vowel alterations. However, there was no information on the type of alteration. More recently, in the application of the paired-word Intelligibility Test for the assessment of intelligibility in French (Gentil, 1992), the author examined the impact of Friedreich's ataxia on the speech produced by nine patients. Perceptual data obtained for vowels revealed an alteration of the high/low contrast such as in 'riz/rat' (rice/rat) and front/back vowels such as in 'lit/loup' (bed/wolf).

The distribution of errors within phonetic contrasts represented 23% for the high/low contrast and only 1% for the front/back contrast. This was interpreted as an indication that certain articulatory adjustments are more vulnerable than others to impairment. In the group of ataxic patients, the tongue height contrast was found more difficult to produce than the tongue advancement contrast. Unfortunately, in her paired-word Intelligibility Test, Gentil (1992) did not consider oral/nasal and labialized/non-labialized contrasts that are French specific. The fact that Gentil's Intelligibility Test was based on a phonetic Intelligibility Test developed for English by Kent et al. (1989), may explain this omission. One would naturally imagine, however, that the rigidity or the paralysis of the velum may have a deleterious impact on the production of oral vowels. For example, an electromyographic investigation of the pathological velum in

ALS demonstrated that nasal air leakage is correlated with the subjective perception of rhinolalia and is an indicator of the evolution of the disease (Robert *et al.*, 1995). How this impacts oral/nasal contrasts is of crucial interest. Concerning labialized vowels, high rigidity of the lower lip (Gentil *et al.*, 1998; Hunker *et al.*, 1982) and the resulting reduction in movements may impact their production. This remains to be tested.

Studies on motor speech disorders in American English showed that dysarthric speakers with reduced displacements and velocities often produce individual movements or changes in their overall vocal tract shape (Weismer, 1997). At the acoustic level, this is reflected by compressed vowel space (Weismer *et al.*, 2001) and lower than normal slopes of second formant transitions (Kent *et al.*, 1989; Weismer, 1991; Weismer *et al.*, 1992). Unfortunately, there are no investigations of this type for French dysarthric speech. However, alterations of the different speech production mechanisms have been stressed in studies of the intrinsic characteristics of speech segments. For example, Baudelle *et al.* (2003) compared the impact of Parkinson's and cerebellar ataxia on intrinsic F0 and duration, and observed for parkinsonian speakers a complete disappearance of the IF0 contrast between [i] and [u] and a significant reduction in the contrast between [a] and [u]. This was interpreted as the result of reduced lingual movement amplitude.

On the contrary, in speech produced by cerebellar patients, IF0 contrasts tended to be maintained. Different effects of disease were also observed for durational contrasts. In cerebellar speech, intrinsic durational contrasts were significantly altered, probably because of the major coordination deficit that characterises cerebellar disorders. In parkinsonian speech, intrinsic durational contrasts were maintained between open vowels such as [a] and closed vowels such as [i and u] in spite of a global reduction in vowel duration, this suggesting some forms of contrast transposition. However, in contrast to the aforementioned findings, vowels were found to be lengthened during reading in parkinsonian patients (Duez, 2009); nasals were found to be longer than orals in both parkinsonian speech and control speech whereas high and low vowels were of similar duration. It was assumed that patients either took or needed more time to execute the high vowel tongue gesture or they may have produced high vowels with a lower height gesture.

## Consonant insufficiency

As for vowels, reductions of articulatory displacement and velocity were found to alter the integrity of consonantal gestures. For example, in the already mentioned oscillographic analysis, Grémy (1958) reported a strong alteration of stop vs nasal and voiced vs voiceless contrasts in speech produced by pseudobulbar patients. This author also observed articulatory anomalies for parkinsonian patients with voicing of intervocalic voiceless consonants and devoicing of syllable-initial voiced consonants. Devoicing of voiced initial stops also occurred in cerebellar dysarthric speech; in addition, there was simplification of clusters and assimilation of phonemes (Alajouanine *et al.*, 1958).

Two groups of cerebellar patients were reported in oscillographic and electroglottographic investigations of ataxic dysarthria (Grémy *et al.*, 1967). The 'severe' group was characterised by laryngeal irregularities and specific impairment of articulation such as devoicing of voiced stops and exaggerated explosions of voiceless stop consonants, whereas the 'moderate' group presented mostly articulatory deficiency, more precisely a lack of differentiation between phonemes that lost their distinctive features (see Gentil [1992] for more details). Using the same techniques, an evaluation of the speech of 25 patients with pseudobulbar syndrome and 30 patients with ALS confirmed the vulnerability of certain features and phonetic contrasts, such as voiceless consonant vs voiced consonant, voiced fricative vs voiced stop consonant, voiceless stop vs voiced stop consonant, [l] and [ʀ] vs null and stop vs nasal (Chevrie Muller *et al.*, 1970). In the previously mentioned word Intelligibility Test (Gentil, 1992), underlying phonetic impairments were determined from the intelligibility scores of nine speakers with Friedreich's ataxia. Certain contrasts and features were found more vulnerable than others: they were, in decreasing order: (1) initial voicing, (2) stop vs nasal, (3) final voicing, final consonant vs null, (4) stop vs fricative, (5) alveolar vs palatal, (6) stop place, (7) [ʁ] vs [l] and (8) initial consonant vs null.

Lingual consonant production abnormalities have been described in acoustic studies on stops produced by parkinsonian patients. For example, in spectrographic studies of consonants, Uziel *et al.* (1975) noted the voicing of voiceless stops, the 'hypervoicing of some voiced consonants' and the devoicing of some voiced stops. Some characteristics of stops were also found in spectrographic studies of read texts (Duez, 2007). One of the main characteristics was the spirantization of gaps due to an incomplete closure of the articulators: 12% of stops had visible noise in parkinsonian speech; the corresponding percentage in control speech was 1.8%. Another characteristic was the greater voicing of voiceless stops in parkinsonian speech (5.7% of the total number of voiceless stops) than in control speech (2.3%), this being a consequence of larynx rigidity. A certain number of voiced stops were weakened into approximants: 40% of the /b/'s and 58% of the /g/'s displayed overlapping of occlusion and mid-frequency formants; in control speech the corresponding percentages were 6% and 24%, respectively. Consonant weakening was also characterised by absent bursts, reduced energy, shortened duration, frequent nasalization of voiced stops preceded by a nasal vowel, and omissions of consonants (especially in clusters and at the coda where segments are produced with less articulatory force and precision [Straka, 1964]). Interestingly, these data explain the

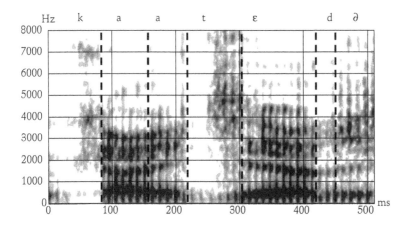

**Figure 12.1** Wide-band spectrogram of the intended sequence /kaʁaktɛʁ də/ produced by a parkinsonian speaker. There is no occlusion and no burst for the omitted /k/ in /ʁak/, continuous voicing for the /t/, overlapping of occlusion and mid-frequency formants for the /d/ and no /ʁ/

alteration or loss of phonetic contrasts reported in intelligibility tests (Gentil, 1992).

Examples of consonant weakening for the sequences 'caractère de' (character of) are shown in Figure 12.1. The spectrogram for a patient with Parkinson's disease in Figure 12.1 shows evidence of [k] omission with the absence of occlusion and burst, continuous voicing for the [t] with visible low frequencies, and change into approximant for the [d] that is shortened and has mid-frequency formants.

Articulatory deficits have a similar impact on the production of speech segments in other languages, such as in English. For example, Weismer (1997) observed that motor speech disorders often disrupt segmental distinctions. An inability among patients with ALS to stop vocal fold vibration at the interface of a voiceless obstruent and vowel, also the spirantization of stop gaps and voicing of voiceless stops and voiceless fricatives in the speech of Parkinson's patients, may cause errors in the detection of the obstruent voicing feature and contribute to intelligibility deficits (Weismer, 1984). Concerning parkinsonian speech, it also seems that articulatory undershoot and the failure of articulators to reach their target position in time contribute to the perception of accelerated speech (Kent & Rosenbek, 1982).

## Prosodic aspects of dysarthric French speech

An examination of the clusters determined by Darley *et al.* (1969) clearly demonstrate prosodic disturbances in each type of dysarthria.

These disturbances were grouped into 'prosodic excess' and 'prosodic insufficiency'. Prosodic excess mainly relied on the distortion of rhythmic patterns, including the dimensions of excess and equal stress, prolonged phonemes, prolonged intervals and slow rate; prosodic insufficiency was characterised by flattened F0 and reduced loudness, reduced stress contrasts and fast rate.

## Intonation

Manipulation of the stiffness and length of the vocal folds, raising or lowering of the larynx and change in sub-glottal pressure allow speakers to vary the periodicity of vocal fold vibration and control the temporal course of modulation, F0 range and F0 height, and the size and direction of F0 movements (Vaissière, 2005). Therefore, it is fair to think that deficits in F0 control cause an alteration of intonation. Studies indicated that intonation impairment is one of the most striking prosodic characteristics of dysarthria. For example, in a perceptual study of the speech of 22 French-speaking patients suffering from Friedreich's ataxia, Joanette and Dudley (1980) observed that the most severely affected dimension was pitch level, the second being pitch breaks. The authors also noted that the subjective pitch level of voice was influenced by many variables such as harsh voice and rapid oscillations of amplitude, not just by F0. More recently, Gentil (1990) observed a high F0 variability and sudden F0 changes in repeated productions of the syllable /pa/ and the sustained vowel /i/ for cerebellar patients. For these patients, coefficients of variability were always greater than for normal subjects. Exaggerated modulations of F0 and aberrant line of F0 were also found by Baudelle et al. (2003).

On the contrary, a clear tendency for less F0 variability was observed in parkinsonian speech. In a correlational study of vocal and clinical symptoms in 81 French parkinsonian patients, monopitch was found to be one of the speech impairments bearing a close relationship to clinical symptoms (Seguier et al., 1974). This was confirmed in a series of acoustic studies of parkinsonian speech prosody that showed a significant reduction in F0 variability caused mainly by loss of the high part of the range (see Viallet et al., 2000, 2003). Hypomelody in parkinsonian speech is probably the consequence of muscular rigidity (Weismer, 1984), especially in the cricothyroid muscles responsible for controlling pitch change (Aronson, 1990).

An illustration of these tendencies can be seen in Figures 12.2a and 12.2b. In the sentence 'Monsieur Seguin n'avait jamais eu de bonheur avec ses chèvres' (Mr Seguin was never lucky with his goats) read by a control subject the intonation phrasing contributes to the identification of the syntactic structure and segmentation (see Ex1). There are three major and one minor continuation rises associated with the boundaries of major and minor phrases, respectively. In the sentence produced by a

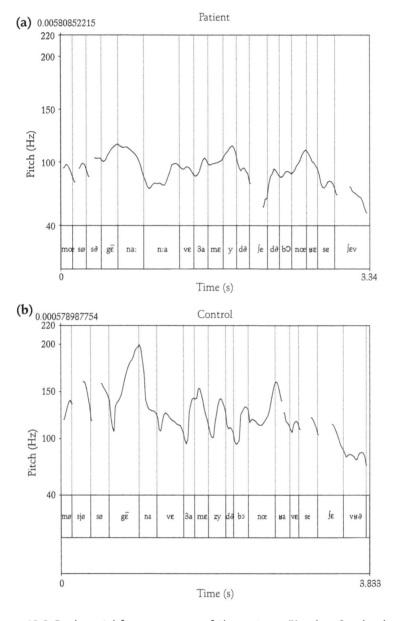

**Figure 12.2** Fundamental-frequency curve of the sentence 'Monsieur Seguin n'avait jamais eu de bonheur avec ses chèvres' produced by a patient (a) and a control (b). There is a reduction of F0 for the patient. For example, there is a slow rise in the final syllable of the phrase 'monsieur SeGUIN' going from 105 Hz to 113 Hz whereas for the control speaker there is a steep rise going from 138 Hz to 195 Hz. One can also observe dysfluencies in the sentence produced by the patient such as the repetition of the syllable 'na' and the syllable 'de'

parkinsonian patient, there is loss of F0 rises and peaks and flattening of the F0 curve.

Ex1.

[Monsieur SeGUIN] [n'avait jamais EU de boNHEUR] [avec ses CHEvres]
[møsjøsəgɛ̃]          [navɛʒamɛzydəbɔnœʁ]          [avɛkseʃevʁə]

Acoustic investigations of statements and total questions produced by 20 native speakers of Quebec French (10 dysarthric speakers of various aetiologies and 10 controls) also indicated performance deficits for the dysarthric group. Dysarthric subjects had lower F0 differences between the last syllable of the statement and the last syllable of the question than non-dysarthric speakers (Le Dorze et al., 1994). Differences were also observed between the different types of dysarthria. The lowest differences were found for the two patients with flaccid dysarthria (3.5 Hz) and the two patients with mixed dysarthria (14.25 Hz) whereas the highest differences were for the two patients with hypokinetic dysarthria (56 Hz). The differences reported for the three ataxic speakers and the hyperkinetic patient were 26.3 Hz and 14.25 Hz, respectively. The values obtained for the different patients were correlated with the severity of dysarthria. The results indicated that dysarthric speakers are less capable of generating the particular prosodic contrast that distinguishes declarative from interrogative sentences. To explain this deficit, the authors referred to Lieberman's (1967) breath-group theory of intonation, according to which laryngeal tension needs to increase near the end of a question in order to compensate for the reduction in pulmonary air occurring naturally at the end of a sentence. They assumed that the reduced intonation difference in dysarthric speakers was caused by a loss of control in speech breathing or a reduced ability of the laryngeal structures to respond to the requirements of interrogatives. On the contrary, the expression of emotions and attitudes has not been investigated in dysarthric French speech; however, as acoustic and perceptual attributes of vocal expressions of 'basic' emotions in speech are largely unaffected by language or linguistic similarity (Pell et al., 2009), one may assume that the expression of some emotions in French (in particular those which require increased articulatory efforts) will be compromised as in English. This needs to be tested in both acoustic and perceptual studies.

Anomalies in the curve of F0 were also observed in other languages. For example, acoustic investigations of different speech samples produced by normal American speakers and 17 American parkinsonian patients demonstrated reduced (F0) mean, range and variability in parkinsonian speech, in syllable production and in read speech and monologues (Canter, 1963, 1965; Goberman et al., 2005; Kegl et al., 1999; Pell et al., 2006); in contrast, the acoustic measure of F0 was shown to be elevated in the parkinsonian samples (Illes *et al.*, 1988; Metter & Hanson, 1986). Abnormalities in the production of terminal question rises by parkinsonian patients (Kegl *et al.*, 1999) and expressions of different emotions such as anger, disgust and happiness (Cheang & Pell, 2007; Pell & Leonard, 2003) were also observed. As for French, the intonation patterns in dysarthria associated with cerebellar lesions were characterised by a generally flat F0. However, as syllables tend to be dissociated in ataxic speech, the phrase-level intonation usually observed in normal speech disappeared and was replaced by a tendency to produce each syllable in a series with a monotypic intonation (for more details, see Kent & Rosenbek, 1982).

## Temporal organisation

The temporal organisation of speech reflects the different processes involved at all levels of speech production. Dysregulation in the temporal organisation of speech may thus reveal information on impairments of the speech production system. This has been the basis of perceptual and acoustic investigations on dysarthria in various languages.

However, although it is well known that better knowledge of the dysregulation of the temporal organisation of speech allows improved understanding of motor speech disorders, there are relatively few studies on this subject in French. In the 'batterie d'évaluation Clinique de la dysarthrie' (BECD), which was based on the *Frenchay Dysarthria Assessment* (Enderby, 1983), the following dimensions were used to evaluate the temporal organisation of dysarthric speech: slow and fast speech rate, fluctuations of speech rate, fluency breaks and inappropriate silences (Auzou & Rolland-Monnoury, 2006). However, the perceptual data obtained were mostly used for the evaluation and follow-up of dysarthric patients, not for the characterisation of different types of dysarthria.

In the acoustic study mentioned earlier (Le Dorze *et al.*, 1994), dysarthric speech (3.1 syll/sec) was found to be significantly slower than non-dysarthric speech (4.7 syll/sec). As for intonation, there were differences between dysarthric speakers. A hyperkinetic patient and two patients with flaccid dysarthria had the slowest speech rates (1.9 syll/sec and 2.1 syll/sec, respectively), two patients with mixed dysarthria produced 3.1 syll/sec, three ataxic patients 2.9 syll/sec, and two hypokinetic patients 4.6 syll/sec. These results were confirmed in acoustic studies of hypokinetic and ataxic dysarthria. For example, the speaking rate in parkinsonian speech was found to be slightly slower than in control speech, due to longer pause time, articulation rate being similar in parkinsonian speech and control speech (Duez, 2005). In contrast, speech rate was found to be irregular and slow in ataxic dysarthria, compared to control speech (Baudelle *et al.*, 2003; Bell-Berti & Chevrié-Muller, 1991; Gremy *et al.*, 1967). In ataxic speech, slowness of speech rate leads to elongation and distortion of speech segments (especially of fricatives), creating a negative impact on speech intelligibility. However, with the temporal acceleration of speech, there is a clear improvement of perceived intelligibility, the effect being greater when the speed is more than 50% of control speakers (Woisard *et al.*, 2010).

Pauses and articulation rate, the two main components of speech rate, have inspired several studies. Interestingly, in their analysis of ataxic dysarthria, Gremy *et al.* (1967) observed two forms of bradylalia: the first was related to the elongation of phonemes or syllables, the second was characterised by the repetition of phonemes or syllables and the presence of frequent silent pauses unrelated to the context. Unfortunately, the authors did not provide information on the distribution of pauses. More recently, the analysis of paragraphs read by parkinsonian patients indicated two sorts of pauses (Duez, 2005). There were syntactic pauses located at syntactic breaks and non-syntactic pauses occurring within phrases and words (the latter being less frequent). As in control speech, the frequency and duration of syntactic pauses were strongly correlated with the syntactic structure of the paragraph, indicating that the distributional scheme of pauses was intact and that the syntactic function of prosody was preserved by the patients.

In contrast, non-syntactic pauses were often associated with a dysfluency such as a repetition or a false start. It was assumed that their occurrence resulted from difficulties in initiating or producing the right movements. More generally, it seems that short and frequent pauses in parkinsonian speech result from a respiratory deficit. Interestingly, these can be used as a strategy to combat a rigid chest wall (a type of hypertonia) and decreased breath support (Solomon & Hixon, 1993). Contrary to ataxic dysarthria, there was no syllable elongation in parkinsonian dysarthria and articulation rate was similar to control speech.

How within-phrase pauses impact the perception of the prosodic structure of the message is a question of interest. This may partly depend on the prosodic characteristics of languages. In French, within-phrase pauses may have a deleterious effect on the perception of the rhythmic organisation of sentences since right-headed languages do not allow pauses in the middle of rhythmic groups (Wenk & Wioland, 1982). Further analysis should investigate the impact of within-phrase pauses on the perception of rhythm in French parkinsonian speech.

Comparisons with results obtained for speech rate and articulation rate in English partly confirm those obtained for French. For example, parkinsonian patients were shown to experience speech acceleration (Canter, 1963; Hammen & Yorkston, 1996) and to speak more slowly (Goberman *et al.*, 2005; Ludlow *et al.*, 1987) but to have mean speaking rates consistent with normal controls (Caligiuri, 1989). Concerning articulation rate, Hammen and Yorkston (1996), Mac Rae *et al.* (2002) and Solomon and Hixon (1993) found that subjects with Parkinson's disease had a faster articulation rate, produced fewer syllables and spoke for less time per breath, whereas Nishio and Niimi (2002) and Goberman *et al.* (2005) reported similar duration in parkinsonian and control speech but large individual differences. There is more agreement in the results obtained for pause time. In general, pause time was greater, being related to longer and more frequent pauses (see e.g. Goberman *et al.*, 2005; Hammen & Yorkston, 1996; Metter & Hanson, 1986; Solomon & Hixon, 1993) and inappropriate pauses occurred within phrases (Hammen & Yorkston, 1996; Solomon & Hixon, 1993).

### Stress and rhythm

Rhythmic patterns of speech are influenced by factors such as speech rate, number of syllables and the position of syllables and segments within an utterance. Concerning the number of syllables, it has been shown that syllables and segments occurring early in an utterance are progressively shortened as the length of the utterance is increased by adding syllables (Lindblom & Rapp, 1973). This 'compensatory shortening' is mostly a word-level shortening effect, but it can also operate within a higher-level domain like a phrase. Another timing phenomenon is 'final lengthening', which refers to the increased duration of syllables that occurs in phrase and utterance-final position. How motor disorders affect these two basic timing phenomena was examined in the speech of two dysarthric French subjects suffering from Friedreich's ataxia by Bell-Berti and Chevrie-Muller (1991). They observed final lengthening and compensatory shortening effects for controls and dysarthric subjects, even though the dysarthric speakers produced acoustic segments with significantly greater durations than the control speakers. These results were interpreted as an indication of the preservation of the linguistic/motor planning level.

Final lengthening has also been investigated in speech produced by patients suffering from Parkinson's disease (Duez *et al.*, 2009). A normal production of final lengthening was observed for the patients, pre-pausal final syllables were found to be longer than non-pre-pausal final syllables, in conformity with the literature for normal speech (Klatt, 1975). The analysis of the duration of vowels and consonants also revealed that final-syllable vowels were lengthened proportionally more than final-syllable consonants, suggesting a progressive lengthening in final syllables. The fact that patients with Parkinson's disease respected the lengthening pattern of French suggests that they had no difficulty with the production of final lengthening, probably because final lengthening is like a localised change in speaking tempo, which does not require stronger movements or increased effort and amplitude of articulators (Edwards *et al.*, 1990).

The similarity of the duration pattern of control speech and parkinsonian speech is shown in Figures 12.3a and 12.3b. In the sentence '*Et là-HAUT le LOUP les manGEAIT*' (And up there the wolf ate them), the phrase-final syllables of the sentence are lengthened similarly by the patient and the control speaker; the pause also has the same distribution.

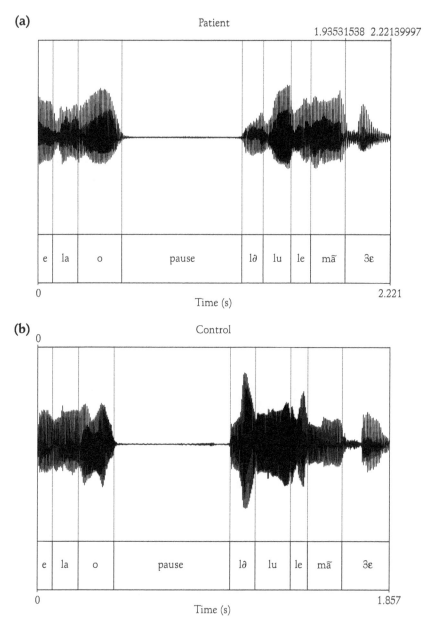

**Figure 12.3** Oscillograms of the sentence 'et la-haut le loup les mangeait' produced by a parkinsonian patient (a) and a control (b). There is similar lengthening of the final-phrase syllables [o], [lu] and [ʒɛ] and a silent pause occurring at the same place in the sequence produced by the patient and the control

As already mentioned, there is no lexical stress in French and the perception of the prominence pattern relies mainly on phrase-final and utterance-final lengthening. Therefore, the preservation of final lengthening in parkinsonian and ataxic speech is of crucial importance for the marking of prosodic boundaries. In normal speech, lengthened syllables are often superimposed with F0 variations while parkinsonian speech is characterised by a flattened F0 and ataxic speech by an aberrant F0 line. This may partly weaken the strength of phrase boundaries in parkinsonian speech, an assumption that remains to be controlled. Concerning initial prominence, which is characterised by melodic rise and consonant lengthening, it may also be seriously compromised, a hypothesis that needs to be tested.

The situation is different in English. Contrary to French ataxic patients, American ataxic patients were inconsistent in their durational adjustments of the stem syllable as the number of syllables in a word was varied; furthermore, they generally made smaller reductions than normal subjects when suffixes were added. In addition, they did not demonstrate normal final lengthening (Kent *et al.*, 1979). These disturbances of the normal timing pattern, with prolongation of a variety of segments and a tendency toward equalized syllable durations, were accompanied by abnormal contours of fundamental frequency, particularly monotone and syllable-falling patterns. All these alterations, resulting from a failure in motor control, may have a deleterious effect on the production and perception of lexical stress, and consequently on lexical access; this may also affect the production and the perception of rhythm.

In hypokinetic dysarthria, 'reduced stress' has also been shown to degrade the production of lexical contrasts. For example, in a prosodic analysis of noun phrases and noun compounds, Darkins *et al.* (1988) reported that parkinsonian patients were unable to produce a F0 drop in the noun compound or a pause between the elements of the noun phrase. However, as there was no significant loss of prosodic comprehension, the authors assumed that the knowledge of linguistic rules necessary to differentiate noun compounds from noun phrases was retained in parkinsonian patients. Interestingly, poverty of prosodic information has been recently confirmed in an acoustic and perceptual investigation of phonemic and contrastive stress in parkinsonian speech – the linguistic-prosodic features of parkinsonian speech were perceived as abnormal by healthy listeners, underscoring an important functional deficit (Cheang & Pell, 2004).

# Concluding Remarks and Perspectives for Future Research

This brief review of the literature on segmental and prosodic aspects of speech motor disorders in French, and their comparison with results published for English, illustrates how motor disorders affect the two languages similarly. For example, the spirantization of stops in parkinsonian speech gives us valuable indications for articulatory behaviour in patients suffering from Parkinson's disease: reductions of articulatory displacement and velocity result in incomplete stop consonant obstructions to the vocal tract airstream. At the acoustic level, this is reflected by the presence of frication noise. Although the spirantization of stops is frequent in speech disorders, it is sometimes considered as a 'signature' of parkinsonian dysarthria (for more details, see Weismer, 1997). Similarly, the strong correlation between pause pattern and syntactic structure in French and English parkinsonian speech is a clear indication that the syntactic function of prosody is preserved in parkinsonian dysarthria. The convergence of this finding with the fact that there is no loss of prosodic comprehension for American patients, who can differentiate noun compound from noun phrase, agrees with the conception that basal ganglia do not control motor programmes but rather contribute to the specification of individual movements and their fluent execution. We can therefore suppose that Parkinson's disease does not impair motor programming but instead affects the performance of movement (see Kent et al., 2000 for more details).

Most studies of the different dysarthrias have focused on characteristics common to different languages. One of their main objectives was to provide information on speech disorders resulting from neurologic diseases. Even so, there is a crucial lack of knowledge on the way motor disorders affect the phonology of different languages. As already mentioned, the incapacity of dysarthric patients to mark the pitch prominence in stressed syllables (or to lengthen them) has important consequences for intelligibility in lexical-stressed languages such as English. Similarly, velar insufficiency in ALS may have dramatic consequences for intelligibility in French where oral/nasal vowel contrast has a phonological role. More acoustic and perceptual studies on dysarthric speech are required to examine the impact of motor disorders on characteristics specific to different languages. In French, phonetic intelligibility tests (such as Gentil, 1992) should be updated; for example, they should include words containing oral and nasal vowels, also front-rounded and non-rounded vowels. Furthermore, the already mentioned BECD (Auzou & Rolland-Monnoury, 2006) should include recent data such as those on prominence patterns and final lengthening in French dysarthric speech. This speech assessment method, which replaces 'l'évaluation Clinique de la dysarthrie' (Auzou & Rolland-Monnoury, 1998), includes a complete evaluation of the severity of dysarthria, a phonetic and acoustic analysis of the speech produced by patients, a motor evaluation and a self-evaluation. Even though the main objective of the BECD was to propose clinical evaluations and evaluations of existing therapeutic protocols, one may suppose that further analysis of listener responses would provide a 'phonetic error profile' showing the impact of neurological diseases on the linguistic structure of the language. This would contribute significantly to the understanding of overall speech intelligibility deficit and, more specifically, to speech intelligibility deficit in French.

Speech production is strongly dependent on the speech situation. It is well known that read and conversational speech require different brain resources: in conversational speech, speakers simultaneously plan their sentences, search for words and speak; in speech read aloud, readers have advance access to the structure of the whole sentence, they are guided by punctuation and can organise their production. It is therefore normal that read and conversational speech have different acoustic-phonetic patterns. For example, in read speech, sounds are more clearly articulated than in conversational speech (Lindblom, 1990; Picheny *et al.*, 1986), there is less reduction and contextual assimilation (Duez, 1992; Krull, 1989; Picheny *et al.*, 1986), syllables tend to be longer (Duez, 1987), rhythm is more regular (Fraisse, 1974) and dysfluencies are mostly absent (Duez, 1982).

Until now, most descriptions of French dysarthric speech have been based mainly on short sequences or paragraphs produced in highly controlled situations, probably because of the high variability of pathological speech and the necessity to obtain a large set of acoustic, physiological and clinical data (for more details, see Ghio *et al.*, 2012). However, it is everyday conversations that make up the great bulk of linguistic exchanges; therefore, it is of prime importance to develop further studies of conversational dysarthric speech in various languages, as these will give us a better and a more global knowledge of production and intelligibility deficits.

## Acknowledgements

I am very grateful to Anja Lowit and and Nicholas Miller for their invitation to write this chapter and their helpful comments on an earlier version, and to Anthony Scrimgeour for style improvement. The samples used in the current study are part of the AHN corpus (Ghio *et al.*, 2012).

## References

Alajouanine, T., Scherber, J., Sabouraud, O. and Gremy, F. (1958) Etude oscillographique de la parole cérébelleuse. *Revue Neurologique* 98, 708–714.

Aronson, A. (1980) *Clinical Voice Disorders: An Interdisciplinary Approach.* New York: Thieme.

Auzou, P. and Rolland-Monnoury, V. (1998) *Evaluation Clinique de la dysarthrie.* Isbergues: Ortho Edition.

Auzou, P. and Rolland-Monnoury, V. (2006) *BECD Batterie d'évaluation clinique de la dysarthrie.* Isbergues: Ortho Edition.

Baudelle, E., Vaissière, J., Renard, J.L., Roubeau, B. and Chevrie-Müller, C. (2003) Caractéristiques vocaliques intrinsèques et co-intrinsèques dans les dysarthries cérébelleuse et parkinsonienne. *Folia Phoniatrica Logopaedica* 55, 137–146.

Bell-Berti, F. and Chevrie-Muller, C. (1991) Motor levels of speech timing: Evidence from studies of ataxia. In H.F.M. Peters, W. Hulstijn and W.C. Starkweather (eds) *Speech Motor Control and Stuttering* (pp. 293–301). Amsterdam: Elsevier Science.

Boë, L.J. and Contini, M. (1975) Etude de la phrase interrogative. *Travaux de l'Institut de Phonétique de Grenoble* 4, 85–102.

Caligiuri, M.P. (1989) The influence of speaking rate on articulatory hypokinesia in parkinsonian dysarthria. *Brain and Language* 36, 493–502.

Campbell, W.N. (1992) Syllable-based segmental duration. In G. Bailly and C. Benoît (eds) *Talking Machines: Theories, Models and Design* (pp. 211–224). Amsterdam: Elsevier.

Canter, G.J. (1963) Speech characteristics of patients with Parkinson's disease: I. Intensity, pitch and duration. *Journal Speech Hearing Disorders* 28, 221–229.

Canter G.J. (1965) Speech characteristics of patients with Parkinson's disease: III. Articulation, diadochokinesis, over-all speech adequacy. *Journal Speech Hearing Disorders* 30, 217–224.

Cheang, H.S. and Pell, M.D. (2004) Impact of Parkinson's disease on the production of contrastive and phonemic stress from the listener's perspective. *Brain and Language* 9, 21–22.

Cheang, H.S. and Pell, M.D. (2007) An acoustic investigation of Parkinsonian speech in linguistic and emotional contexts. *Journal of Neurolinguistics* 20, 221–241.

Chevrie-Muller, C., Dordain, M. and Grémy, F. (1970) Etude phoniatrique clinique et instrumentale des dysarthries. II Résultat chez les malades présentant des syndromes bulbaires et pseudobulbaires. *Revue Neurologique* 122, 123–138.

Darkins, A.W., Fromkin, V. and Benson, D.F. (1988) A characterization of the prosodic loss in Parkinson's disease. *Brain and Language* 34, 315–327.

Darley, F.L., Aronson, A.E. and Brown, J.R. (1969) Differential diagnostic patterns of dysarthria. *Journal of Speech and Hearing Research* 12, 249–269.

Dasher, R. and Bolinger, D. (1982) On pre-accentual lengthening. *Journal of the International Phonetic Association* 12, 58–69.

Dauer, R.M. (1983) Stress-timing and syllable-timing re-analysed. *Journal of Phonetics* 11, 51–62.

Delattre, P. (1939) L'accent final en francais: accent d'intensité, accent de hauteur, accent de durée. *The French Review* 12, 141–145.

Delattre, P. (1961) La leçon d'intonation de Simone de Beauvoir: Etude d'intonation déclarative comparée. *The French Review* 35, 59–67.

Delattre, P. (1966) Studies in French and comparative phonetics. *Selected Papers in French and English by Pierre Delattre*. Mouton: The Hague.

Di Cristo, A. (1985) *De la microprosodie à l'intonosyntaxe*. Aix en Provence: Publications Université de Provence.

Di Cristo, A. (1998) Intonation in French. In D. Hirst and A. Di Cristo (eds) *Intonation Systems: A Survey of Twenty Languages* (pp. 195–218). Cambridge: Cambridge University Press.

Di Cristo, A. and Hirst, D. (1986) Modelling French micromelody: Analysis and synthesis. *Phonetica* 43, 11–30.

Duez, D. (1982) Silent and non silent pauses in three speech styles. *Language and Speech* 25, 11–28.

Duez, D. (1987) Contribution à l'étude de la structuration temporelle de la parole en français. Thèse de Doctorat d'Etat, University of Aix en Provence.

Duez, D. (1992) Second formant locus-nucleus patterns: An investigation of spontaneous French speech. *Speech Communication* 11, 417–427.

Duez, D. (2005) Organisation temporelle de la parole et dysarthrie parkinsonienne. Les troubles de la parole et de la déglutition dans la maladie de Parkinson. In C. Ozsancak and P. Auzou (eds) *Les troubles de la Parole et de la Déglutition et Dysarthrie Parkinsonienne* (pp. 195–213). Marseille: Solal.

Duez, D. (2007) Acoustic analysis of occlusive weakening in Parkinsonian French speech. *Proceedings of the 16th International Congress of Phonetic Sciences* (pp. 1–4) Cederom. Saarbrücken: University of Saarbrücken.

Duez, D. (2009) Segmental duration in parkinsonian French speech. *Folia Phoniatrica Logopaedica* 61, 239–246.

Duez, D. and Nishinuma, Y. (1985) Evidence on the rhythm of spoken French. *Phonetic Experimental Research, Institute of Linguistics, University of Stockholm (PERILUS)*, 25–35.

Duez, D., Legou, T. and Viallet, F. (2009) Final lengthening in Parkinsonian French speech: Effects of position in phrase on the duration of CV syllables and speech segments, *Clinical Linguistics and Phonetics* 23, 781–793.

Edwards, J., Beckman, M.E. and Fletcher, J. (1990) The articulatory kinematics of final lengthening. *Journal of the Acoustical Society of America* 89, 369–382.

Edwards, J. and Beckman, M.E. (1988) Articulatory timing and the prosodic interpretation of syllable duration. *Phonetica* 45, 156–174.

Enderby, P.M. (1983) *Frenchay Dysarthria Assessment*. Austin, TX: ProEd.

Fónagy, I. (1980) L'accent français: accent probabilitaire. In I. Fónagy and P. Léon (eds) *L'accent en Français Contemporain* (pp. 123–233). Didier: Montreal, Paris, Bruxelles.

Fónagy, I. (1980) L'accent français: accent probabilitaire. In I. Fónagy, P. Léon and F. Carton (eds) *L'accent en Français Contemporain* (Studia Phonetica 15) (pp. 123–233). Paris: Didier.

Fraisse P. (1974) *Psychologie du Rythme*. Paris: Presses Universitaires de France.

Garde, P. (1968) *L'accent*. Paris: Presses Universitaires de France.

Gentil, M. (1990) Dysarthria in Friedreich disease. *Brain and Language* 38, 438–448.

Gentil, M. (1992) Phonetic intelligibility testing in dysarthria for the use of French language clinicians. *Clinical Linguistics and Phonetics* 6, 179–189.

Gentil, M., Tournier, C.L., Perrin, S. and Pollak, P. (1998) Effects of Levodopa on finger and orofacial movements in Parkinson's disease. *Progress in Neuro-Psychopharmacology and Biological Psychiatry* 22, 1261–1274.

Ghio, A., Pouchoulin, G., Teston, B., Pinto, S., Fredouille, C., De Looze, C., Robert, D., Viallet, F. and Giovanni, A. (2012) How to manage sound physiological and clinical data of 2500 dysphonic and dysarthric speakers. *Speech Communication* 54, 664–679.

Goberman, A.M., Coelho, C.A. and Robb, M.P. (2005) Prosodic characteristics of Parkinsonian speech: The effect of levodopa-based medication. *Journal of Medical Speech Language Pathology* 13, 51–68.

Grammont, M. (1933) *Traité de Phonétique*. Paris: Delagrave.

Grémy, F. (1958) Contribution à l'étude oscillographique de certaines dysarthries. Thèse de Médecine, Paris. See https://www.karger.com/Article/Pdf/263774

Grémy, F., Chevrié Muller, C. and Garde, E. (1967) Etude phoniatrique clinique et instrumentale des dysarthries. Technique I. Résultats chez les malades présentant un syndrome cérébelleux. *Revue Neurologique* 116, 401–424.

Grosjean, F. and Deschamps, A. (1973) Analyse des variables temporelles du français spontané. *Phonetica* 28, 191–226.

Grosjean, F. and Deschamps, A. (1975) Analyse contrastive des variables temporelles de l'anglais et du français: vitesse de parole, variables secondaires et phénomènes d'hésitation. *Phonetica* 31, 144–184.

Grosjean, F. and Collins, M. (1979) Breathing, pausing and reading. *Phonetica* 36, 98–114.

Grosjean, F., Grosjean, L. and Lane, H. (1979) The patterns of silence: Performance structures in sentence production. *Cognitive Psychology* 11, 58–81.

Hammen, V. and Yorkston, K. (1996) Speech and pause characteristics following speech rate reduction in hypokinetic dysarthria. *Journal of Communication Disorders* 29, 429–445.

Hayes, B. (1995) *Metrical Stress Theory: Principles and Case Studies.* Chicago, IL: University of Chicago Press.

Hirst, D. (2006) Phonetics: The prosody of speech and language. In K. Brown (ed.) *Encyclopaedia of Language and Linguistics* (pp. 167–178). Oxford: Oxford University Press.

Hirst, D., Astésano, C. and Di Cristo, A. (1998) Differential lengthening of syllabic constituents in French: The effect of accent type and speaking style. In *Proceedings of International Conference on Spoken Language Processing* (ICSLP), Sydney, Australia (pp. 3309–3312). Cederom. Sydney: Australian Speech and Technology Association.

Hirst, D. and Di Cristo, A. (1998) A survey of intonation systems. In D. Hirst and A. Di Cristo (eds) *Intonation Systems* (pp. 1–44). Cambridge: The Cambridge University Press.

House, A. and Fairbanks, F. (1953) The influence of consonant environment upon the secondary acoustical characteristics of vowels. *Journal of the Acoustical Society of America* 25, 105–113.

Hunker, C.J., Abbs, J.H. and Barlow, S.M. (1982) The relationship between parkinsonian rigidity and hypokinesia in the orofacial system. A quantitative analysis. *Neurology* 32, 749.

Illes, J., Metter, E.J., Hanson, W.R. and Iritani, S. (1988) Language production in Parkinson's disease: Acoustic and linguistic considerations. *Brain and Language* 33, 146–160.

Jacewicz, E., Fox, R., O'Neill, C. and Salmons, J. (2009) Articulation rate across dialect, age, and gender. *Language Variation and Change* 21, 233–256.

Joanette, Y. and Dudley, J.G. (1980) Dysarthric symptomology of Friedreich's ataxia. *Brain and Language* 10, 39–50.

Kegl, J., Cohen, H. and Poizner, H. (1999) Articulatory consequences of Parkinson's disease: Perspectives from two modalities. *Brain and Cognition* 40, 355–386.

Kent, R., Netsell, R. and Abbs, J.H. (1979) Acoustic characteristics of dysarthria associated with cerebellar disease. *Journal of Speech and Hearing Research* 22, 627–648.

Kent, R. and Rosenbek, J.C. (1982) Prosodic disturbance and neurological lesion. *Brain and Language* 15, 259–291.

Kent, R.D., Weismer, G., Kent, J.F. and Rosenbek. J.C. (1989) Toward phonetic intelligibility testing in dysarthria. *Journal of Speech and Hearing Disorders* 54, 482–499.

Kent, R.D., Kent, J.F. and Weismer, G. (2000) What dysarthrias can tell us about the neural control of speech. *Journal of Phonetics* 28, 273–302.

Klatt, D.H. (1975) Vowel lengthening is syntactic determined in a connected discourse. *Journal of Phonetics* 3, 129–140.

Krull, D. (1989) Second formant locus patterns and consonant-vowel coarticulation in spontaneous speech. *Phonetic Experimental Research, Institute of Linguistics, University of Stockholm (PERILUS)* X, 87–108.

Ladefoged, P. (1975) *A Course in Phonetics.* New York: Harcourt Brace Jovanovich.

Laver, J. (1991) *The Gift of Speech: Readings in the Analysis of Speech and Voice.* Edinburgh: Edinburgh University Press.

Le Dorze, G., Ouellet, L. and Ryalls, J. (1994) Intonation and speech rate. *Journal of Communication Disorders* 27, 1–18.

Lehiste, I. (1970) *Suprasegmentals.* Cambridge, MA: Massachusetts University Press.

Léon, P. (1971) *Essais de Phonostylistique*, Studia Phonetica 4. Montréal, Paris: Nathan.

Léon, P. R. and Bhatt, P. (1987) Structures prosodiques du questionnement radiophonique. *Études de Linguistique Appliquée* 66, 88–105.

Lieberman, P. (1967) *Intonation, Perception and Language* (Research Monograph No. 38). Cambridge, MA: The MIT Press.

Lindblom, B. (1990) Explaining phonetic variation: A sketch of the H&H theory. In W. Hardcastle and A. Marchal (eds) *Speech Production and Speech Modelling* (NATO ASI Series) (pp. 403–439). Dordrecht: Kluwer Academic.

Lindblom, B. and Rapp, K. (1973) Some temporal regularities of spoken Swedish. *Papers in Linguistic from the University of Stockholm (PILUS)* 21, 1–59.

Ludlow, C.L., Connor, N.P. and Bassich, C.J. (1987) Speech timing in Parkinson's and Huntington's disease. *Brain and Language* 32, 195–214.

Mac Rae, P.A., Tjaden, K. and Schoonings, B. (2002) Acoustic and perceptual consequences of articulatory rate change in Parkinson's disease. *Journal Speech Hearing Research* 45, 35–50.

Marchal, A. (2009) *From Speech Physiology to Linguistics Phonetics*. London, New York: Wiley.

Marchal, A. (2011) *Précis de Physiologie de la Production de la Parole*. Marseille: Solal.

Marouzeau, J. (1956) Accent de mot et accent de phrase. *Le Français Moderne* 24, 241–248.

Martin, P. (1982) Phonetic realisations of prosodic in French. *Speech Communication* 1, 283–294.

Metter, E.J. and Hanson, W.R. (1986) Clinical and acoustical variability in hypokinetic dysarthria. *Journal of Communications Disorders* 19, 347–366.

Miller, J.L. (1981) Effects of speaking rate on segmental distinctions. In P.D. Eimas and J.L. Miller (eds) *Perspectives on the Study of Speech* (pp. 39–70). Hillsdale, NJ: Erlbaum Associates.

Miller, J., Grosjean, F. and Lomanto, C. (1984) Articulation rate and its variability in spontaneous speech: A reanalysis and some implications. *Phonetica* 41, 215–225.

Monnin, P. and Grosjean, F. (1993) Les structures de performance en français: caractérisation et prédiction. *L'Année Psychologique* 9, 9–30.

Nishio, M. and Niimi, S. (2001) Speaking rate and its components in dysarthric speakers. *Clinical Linguistics and Phonetics* 15, 309–317.

O'Dwyer, N.J. and Neilson, P.D. (1988) Voluntary muscle control in normal and athetoid dysarthric speakers. *Brain* 111, 877–899.

Pell, M.D. and Leonard, C.L. (2003) Processing emotional tone from speech in Parkinson's disease: A role for the basal ganglia. *Cognitive, Affective & Behavioral Neuroscience* 3, 275–288.

Pell, M.D., Cheang, H.S. and Leonard, C.L. (2006) The impact of Parkinson's disease on vocal-prosodic communication from the perspective of listeners. *Brain and Language* 97, 123–134.

Pell, M.D., Paulmann, S., Dara, C., Alasseria, A. and Kotz, S. (2009) Factors in the recognition of vocally expressed emotions: A comparison of four languages. *Journal of Phonetics* 37, 417–435.

Pernot, H. (1929-1930) L'intonation. *Revue de Phonétique* 6, 273–289.

Picheny, M.A., Durlach, N.I. and Braida, L.D. (1986) Speaking clearly for the hard of hearing II: Acoustic characteristics of clear and conversational speech. *Journal of Speaking and Hearing Research* 29, 434–446.

Pike, K. (1945) *The Intonation of American English*. Ann Arbor, MI: University of Michigan.

Robert, D., Sangla, I., Azulay, J.P., Giovanni, A., Cannoni, M. and Pouget, J. (1995) Diagnostic et suivi de l'insuffisance vélaire dans les formes bulbaires des maladies du motoneurone. In *Actes du Congrès sur le voile pathologique* (pp. 63–68). Lyon: Société française de Phoniâtrie.

Rossi, M. (1981) Continuation et question. In M. Rossi, A. Di Cristo, D. Hirst, P. Martin and Y. Nishinuma (eds) *L'intonation: de l'acoustique à la sémantique* (pp. 149–187). Paris: Klinscsieck.

Scherk, O. (1912) *Über den französischen Akzent*. Dissertation. Berli, Schersow, Kirchain, N.L.

Seguier, N., Spira, A., Dordain, M., Lazar, P. and Chevrier-Muller, C. (1974) Etude des relations entre les troubles de la parole et les autres manifestations cliniques dans la maladie de Parkinson. *Folia Phoniatrica* 26, 108–126.

Solomon, N.P. and Hixon, T.J. (1993) Speech breathing in Parkinson's disease. *Journal of Speech and Hearing Research* 36, 294–310.

Straka, G. (1964) L'évolution phonétique du latin au français sous l'effet de l'énergie et de la faiblesse articulatoire. *T.L.L., Centre de Philologie Romane, Strasbourg II*, 17–28.

Tranel, B. (1987) *The Sounds of French: An Introduction.* Cambridge, MA: Cambridge University Press.

Uziel, A., Bohe, M., Cadilhac, J. and Passouant, P. (1975) Les troubles de la voix et de la parole dans les syndromes parkinsoniens. *Folia Phoniatrica Logopaedica* 27, 166–176.

Vaissière, J. (1974) On French prosody. *MIT Quarterly Progress Report* 114, 212–223.

Vaissière, J. (1991) Rhythm, accentuation and final lengthening in French. In J. Sundberg, L. Nord and R. Carlson (eds) *Music, Language and Brain* (pp. 108–120). Houndsmills: Macmillan.

Vaissière, J. (2002) Cross-linguistic prosodic transcription: French vs. English. In N.B. Volskaya, N.D. Svetozarova and P.A. Skrelin (eds) *Problems and Methods of Experimental Phonetics. In Honour of the 70th Anniversary of Pr. L.V. Bondarko* (pp. 147–164). St Petersburg: St Petersburg State University Press.

Vaissière, J. (2005) Perception of intonation. In D.B. Pisoni and R.E. Remez (eds) *The Handbook of Speech Perception* (pp. 236–263). Oxford: Blackwell.

Vaissière, J. and Michaud, A. (2006) Prosodic constituents in French: A data-driven approach. In I. Fónagy, Y. Kawaguchi and T. Moriguchi (eds) *Prosody and Syntax* (pp. 47–64). Amsterdam: John Benjamins.

Viallet, F., Meynadier, Y., Lagrue, B., Mignard, P. and Gantcheva, R. (2000) The reductions of tonal range and of average pitch during speech production in "off" parkinsonians are restored by L. dopa. *Movement Disorders* 15, 131.

Viallet, F., Teston, B., Jankowski, L., Purson, A., Meynadier, Y. and Lagrue, B. (2003) Analyse acoustique de la production vocale: Contribution à l'évaluation de la dysprosodie parkinsonnienne. *Revue Neurologique* 159, 1S16–1S18.

Weismer, G. (1984) Articulatory characteristics of Parkinsonian dysarthria: Segmental and phrase-level timing spirantization and glottal-supraglottal coordination. In M.R. McNeil, J.C. Rosenbek and A.E. Aronson (eds) *The Dysarthrias* (pp. 101–130). San Diego, CA: College-Hill.

Weismer, G. (1991) Assessment of articulatory timing. *NIDCD Monograph* 1, 84–95.

Weismer, G. (1997) Motor speech disorders. In W.J. Hardcastle and J. Laver (eds) *The Handbook of Phonetic Sciences* (pp. 191–219). Oxford: Blackwell.

Weismer, G., Martin, R., Kent, R.D. and Kent, J.F. (1992) Formant trajectory characteristics of males with ALS. *Journal of the Acoustical Society of America* 91, 1085–1098.

Weismer, G., Jeng, J., Laures, J.S., Kent, R.D. and Kent, J.F. (2001) Acoustic and intelligibility characteristics of sentence production in neurogenic speech disorders. *Folia Phoniatrica Logopaedica* 53, 1–18.

Wenk, B.J. and Wioland, F. (1982) Is French really syllable-timed? *Journal of Phonetics* 10, 193–216.

Woisard-Bassols, V., Espesser, R., Ghio, A., Nguyen, N. and Duez, D. (2010) Effet de l'accélération artificielle du signal de parole sur la perception des dysarthries cérébelleuses: à propos de deux cas. *Folia Phoniatrica Logopaedica* 62, 185–194.

# 13 German Language Contributions to the Understanding of Acquired Motor Speech Disorders

## Bettina Brendel and Ingrid Aichert

This chapter begins with a brief overview of selected topics dealing with the phonology/phonetics of modern standard German (MSG). Following this, three different aspects of motor speech disorders in German speakers are summarised: a short review of acoustic-perceptual studies of speech production in patients with various types of dysarthria followed by a description of the latest developments in dysarthria assessment and recent research results related to the nature, assessment and treatment of apraxia of speech (AOS).

## Some Features of German Phonology

### German consonant system

The overall sound inventory of MSG comprises 25 consonants assigned to 6 sound categories. Stops comprise /p/, /b/, /t/, /d/, /k/, /g/ and /ʔ/. In MSG there is no voicing lead; voiced plosives are realised unaspirated with a voice onset time (VOT) of 0–30 milliseconds, whereas the voiceless cognates are aspirated with a VOT of >30 milliseconds. The fricatives are /f/, /v/, /s/, /z/, /ʃ/, /ʒ/, /ç/, /x/ /h/, /χ/ and /ʁ/, the nasals /n/, /m/ and /ŋ/, the approximant /j/, the lateral approximant /l/, as well as the trills /r/ and /ʀ/. Additionally, four different affricates occur in MSG: /pf/, /ts/, /tʃ/ and /dʒ/. Not all of the listed consonants are true phonemes. For example, the glottal stop is generally not accepted as a phoneme and the phoneme status of the affricates and the sounds /ʒ/, /h/ and /ŋ/ in MSG is under discussion (see Wiese, 2006). The phones /r/, /ʀ/ and /ʁ/ are allophones of the r-sound (Duden, 2005) and /ç/, /x/ or /χ/ are allophones of the dorsal fricative (dorsal consonants are produced by contact of the dorsum, i.e. mid body of the tongue and hard palate, velum or uvula). Therefore, the number of consonantal phonemes in MSG varies between 18 and 24 (see Wiese, 2006) – depending on the author and without considering the glottal stop.

## German vowel system

The German vowel system is composed of 3 diphthongs (/aɪ/, /aʊ/ and /ɔʏ/) and 17 monophthongs, including rounded front vowels which do not exist in English. Vowel quality in terms of vowel length or 'tenseness' is a distinctive feature in MSG, e.g. *Hüte* (/hyːtə/, 'hats') vs *Hütte* (/hʏtə/, 'huts'), Miete (/miːtə/, 'rent') vs *Mitte* (/mɪtə/, 'middle') or *Rate* (/raːtə/, 'installment') vs *Ratte* (/ratə/, 'rat'). The short (lax) vowels occur only in closed syllables, i.e. when the coda position within a syllable is occupied. The vowels are /iː/, /ɪ/, /yː/, /ʏ/, /eː/, /ɛ/, /ɛː/, /ø/, /œ/, /aː/, /a/, /oː/, /ɔ/, /uː/, /ʊ/, /ɐ/ and /ə/. The schwa, only present in unstressed syllables, is typically not considered to be a phoneme. The vowel /ɐ/ is an allophonic, vocalised variant of /r/ in postvocalic (word final) position, such as *Uhr* (/uːɐ/, 'clock') or *Kinder* (/kɪndɐ/, 'children').

## Syllable structure and phonological rules

### Syllable structure constraints

Syllable structure constraints in MSG state that the minimum unit necessary for creating a monosyllabic word is a vowel (monophthong or diphthong), e.g. *Ei* (/aɪ/, 'egg'). The onset of a monosyllabic word can be composed of up to three consonants, e.g. *Mai* (/maɪ/, 'may'), *Brei* (/braɪ/, 'porridge') or *Stroh* (/ʃtroː/, 'straw'). The coda can comprise up to four consonants (recall, each of the four affricates /pf/, /ts/, /tʃ/ and /dʒ/ is considered as one phoneme in MSG): *Tat* (/tatʰ/, 'deed'), *Takt* (/taktʰ/, 'beat'), *kommst* (/kɔmst/, 'you come'), *schrumpfst* (/ʃrumpfst/, 'you shrink') or *plantschst* (/plantʃst/, 'you splash'). Taking into account additional possible clusters in word initial position, MSG can include words with a high 'consonantal density', like *strolchst* (/ʃtrɔlçst/, 'you roam about').

Complex syllables are built up according to the sonority hierarchy or sonority sequencing principle. Starting with the highest sonority, the hierarchy is vowels (open vowels have a higher sonority than closed vowels), /r/, /l/, nasals, fricatives and plosives (Hall, 2000; Wiese, 2006). The centre of a syllable – the vowel – shows the highest sonority which degrades to the left and right boundary. Thus, certain consonant clusters are not possible within a syllable, either in initial or final position, respectively. For example, the cluster /lk/ is not possible in initial (/*lk-/) but in final position (*Volk*, 'folk'). The other way round, /kl/ will only be initial (*Klang*, 'sound') but not final (/*-kl/).

*Final devoicing rule*

In contrast to English, MSG is characterised by a final devoicing rule for obstruents meaning that final obstruents are always realised as voiceless sounds irrespective of their orthographic realisation. This implies that minimal pairs like 'dog' vs 'dock' do not exist in German. For example, the written words *Bund* ('union') and *bunt* ('colourful') or *Rad* ('wheel') or *Rat* ('advice') are homophones in MSG.

*Dorsal fricative assimilation*

Another rule within the consonantal system is the dorsal fricative assimilation: the allophones of the voiceless dorsal fricatives /ç/ and /x/ or /χ/ assimilate to the tongue position of the preceding vowel: the palatal allophone follows after front vowels, the velar fricative occurs after non-low back tense vowels and low vowels precede the uvular fricative (see Wiese, 2006).

## German word stress pattern

MSG is, like English, a stress-timed language meaning that strong/stressed and weak/unstressed syllables are alternating. In phonology, the concept of metrical foot is assumed to account for this alternating stress pattern. Syllable stress is realised by a combination of increased duration, altered (normally raised) fundamental frequency and higher intensity on vowels in stressed compared to unstressed syllables. Although word stress in MSG can vary across syllable positions, there is a preference for trochaic stress (trochee: first syllable strong, second weak) or more generally a preference for penultimate stress patterns (Domahs *et al.*, 2008). This stands, for example, in contrast with French where the word stress is relatively fixed to the last syllable within multisyllabic words.

# Characterisation of Dysarthric Speech in German-speaking Patients

Since the mid-1980s, a couple of acoustic or combined acoustic-perceptive studies investigated the speech production of German-speaking patients with dysarthria. The studies focused predominately on disorders of the cerebellum (Ackermann *et al.*, 1997, 1999; Ackermann & Hertrich, 1993, 1994, 1997; Ackermann & Ziegler, 1991a, 1994; Brendel *et al.*, 2013; Hertrich & Ackermann, 1993, 1999; Ziegler & Wessel, 1995) and the basal ganglia (Ackermann *et al.*, 1997; Ackermann & Ziegler, 1991b; Hertrich & Ackermann, 1994; Skodda, 2011; Skodda *et al.*, 2012; Skodda & Schlegel, 2008). Patient sample size varied between 3 and 20 individuals and included mostly a neurologically unimpaired control group. The earlier studies were carried out by two clinical research groups working closely together, thus the techniques and materials were largely the same: speakers were obliged to produce phonotactically legal pseudowords /geC1V.C2e/ where C1 and C2 were /p/, /t/ or /k/ and V was /i/, /y/, /u/ or /a/. These pseudowords were embedded in the carrier sentence *Ich habe ____ gehört* ('I heard ____'), resulting for example in *Ich habe getate gehört*.

Generally speaking, the performed acoustic analyses of the speech signal concentrated mainly on various durational measurements such as speech rate, vowel and/or syllable duration, VOT as well as closure times. By and large, the results are in line with studies investigating English-speaking dysarthric patients. For example, compared to healthy control speakers, a markedly reduced speech rate, prolonged segment duration and slowed movement execution could be documented for patients with cerebellar lesions (Ackermann *et al.*, 1997, 1999; Ackermann & Hertrich, 1993, 1994, 1997; Ackermann & Ziegler, 1991a, 1994; Brendel *et al.*, 2013; Hertrich & Ackermann, 1993), spastic dysarthria (Ackermann *et al.*, 1997; Ziegler & von Cramon, 1986) or Huntington disease (Ackerman *et al.*, 1997; Hertrich & Ackermann, 1994) but not for patients with Parkinson's disease (Ackermann & Ziegler, 1991b; Skodda & Schlegel, 2008).

One study (Ackermann *et al.*, 1999) investigated the distinctive tense-lax contrast in two German minimal pairs (*Gram* vs *Gramm*, 'grief' vs 'gram' and *Rate* vs *Ratte*, 'instalment' vs 'rat') in a group of control speakers, eight patients with ataxic dysarthria and nine individuals with Parkinson's disease. Whereas the control speakers and the Parkinson group did not differ from each other, the results were not consistent for the cerebellar group: the vowel duration for *Rate–Ratte* was within the normal range but the realisation of the other pair was compromised. The authors hypothesised that an aberrant vowel length contrast might depend on the articulatory complexity which is assumed to be higher for *Gram–Gramm* compared to *Rate–Ratte*.

Concerning the stress pattern, the German studies showed that cerebellar patients produced less durational contrasts between stressed and unstressed syllables (Ackermann & Hertrich, 1993, 1994). However, despite the prolongation of unstressed syllables, a general syllable isochrony could not be observed in contrast to the well-known findings of American studies (Darley *et al.*, 1975; Duffy, 2005; Kent *et al.*, 2000).

The reported German studies investigated relatively universal speech parameters, whereas analyses of more unique features of MSG are lacking. One small exception is the already mentioned work from Ackermann and coworkers (1999). Unfortunately, this single study is not sufficient to make a reliable general statement about the tense-lax realisation in patients with (cerebellar) dysarthria. Consequently, there are no data concerning whether, or in what way, patients with dysarthria violate rules/constraints on the segmental and suprasegmental levels of speech which are specific for German. For example, there is no information about which sound categories/consonant clusters or which metrical structures are more or less error prone.

# Dysarthria Assessment in German-speaking Patients

For the German-speaking area there has been a lack of diagnostic instruments allowing on the one hand a detailed and systematic characterisation of dysarthric speech, which are, on the other hand, still practicable during the clinical routine. Recently, two different assessment tools have been developed by the Clinical Neuropsychology Research Group (EKN) in Munich.

## Munich Intelligibility Profile

The telediagnostic online Intelligibility Test, the Munich Intelligibility Profile (MVP, 'Münchner Verständlichkeitsprofil', http://www.mvp. phonlab.de/) (Ziegler & Zierdt, 2008) is based on a word identification task yielding an index of the efficiency of vocal communication. The administration of the MVP takes about 15–20 minutes. On a computer screen, 72 words will be presented randomly, one half in isolation, the other half embedded in carrier sentences differing in syllable number and positioning of the target word. Overall, there is a pool of 2784 content words from which the target words and their possible alternatives (see below) are selected. The pool contains as many monosyllabic words as disyllabic trochees. The MVP includes a number of randomisation procedures (for details, see Ziegler & Zierdt, 2008) for the selection of the 72 items to avoid listeners' familiarisation with the test items.

Patients either read or repeat the items in imitation of the clinician. Speech recordings are stored on a data server. Later on, selected listeners evaluate the patient's productions. A pool of listeners, qualified speech and language therapists, perform the ratings for which an expense allowance is paid. As a rule, each recording session is evaluated by three different raters. The allocation of the recordings to listeners is organised and administered centrally by the Clinical Neuropsychology Research Group. This procedure ensures that listeners are unfamiliar with a patient, which is an important precondition for a valid intelligibility measurement. By applying a multiple choice task, the listeners have to identify each produced item out of a visually presented set of 12 phonetically similar words. Carrier phrases are presented only auditorily, not orthographically. Hence, listeners have solely to mark the word they hear.

The ratings from the listeners are averaged, giving the overall percentage of correctly identified words (values above the cut-off score of 95% are considered to be in the normal range; see Ziegler & Zierdt, 2008).

In addition, the intelligibility profile includes an error analysis differentiating between sound categories (single consonants, clusters and vowels), articulators (labial, apical, dorsal), resonating chamber (oral/nasal) and articulatory mode (plosive/fricative). Finally, a judgement regarding speech rate and mean F0 is also provided.

### Bogenhausener Dysarthria Scales

With the Bogenhausener Dysarthria Scales (BoDyS) (Nicola *et al.*, 2004) a detailed and systematic profile of the patient's speech characteristics can be created. The profile is based on the perceptual ratings performed by experts. It should be pointed out that BoDyS capture only speech relevant dimensions; in other words, the examination of non-speech vocal tract movements, e.g. isolated movements of the lips or tongue movements, is not included.

The BoDyS comprise the auditory perceptual rating of 12 speech samples (3 interview questions, 3 sentence repetition tasks, 3 reading passages and 3 picture descriptions). The test examination takes about half an hour and should be recorded with an audio tape or even better a video tape. Each of the 12 speech probes is rated on a total number of 28 variables, e.g. increased inspiration frequency, lengthening of expiration period, excessive or insufficient loudness, uncontrolled alteration in pitch and loudness, harsh voice, hypo-articulation, decreased or increased speech rate and reduced pitch variation. These variables are assigned to nine scales: (1) respiration, (2) absolute pitch/loudness, (3) voice regularity, (4) voice quality, (5) articulation, (6) resonance, (7) speech tempo, (8) fluency and (9) prosodic modulation. Perceptual ratings are based on a two-step approach. First, each speech probe is rated for whether a variable is present or not. Second, each variable is judged regarding its severity on a five-point scale (0 = very severe, 4 = no impairment).

Individual severity scores on each scale are averaged across the 12 speech samples and a BoDyS total score is obtained as an overall measure of dysarthria severity by averaging the scores across all nine scales. The BoDyS profile gives a detailed description of possible dysarthric symptoms and provides information about the consistency and severity of a given variable. Both aspects are essential for the planning and administration of a goal-directed therapy.

# German Language Contributions to Understanding the Nature, Assessment and Treatment of Apraxia of Speech

For AOS, a number of studies have been conducted with German patients. Most of this research has been undertaken by the Clinical Neuropsychology

Research Group (EKN) in Munich. Investigations have addressed what is the underlying pathological mechanism in AOS (e.g. Aichert & Ziegler, 2004), what factors influence error rate in apraxic speakers (e.g. Staiger & Ziegler, 2008) and the efficacy of treatment methods (e.g. Brendel & Ziegler, 2008). Furthermore, materials for diagnosis and treatment of patients with AOS have been developed by this group (e.g. Liepold et al., 2003). In the following, we will give a short overview of these.

## Factors influencing the error pattern in AOS

### Syllable frequency and complexity

The starting point for several investigations was the speech production model of Levelt et al. (1999), where apraxic impairment can be attributed to the phonetic encoding stage (e.g. Code, 1998). At this point, the authors assumed that speakers access a long-term store of motor patterns for the frequently occurring syllables of their language, the 'mental syllabary'. These syllable gestures are assumed to be holistically represented. Furthermore, it is postulated that infrequent or new syllables have no holistically stored phonetic code and must therefore be assembled online from smaller, subsyllabic units like single segments.

Two studies investigated the influence of syllable frequency on the error production of German patients with AOS (Aichert & Ziegler, 2004; Staiger & Ziegler, 2008). The results revealed that patients were more accurate on frequent syllables than on infrequent ones. The syllable inventory in German comprises (similar to English) about 11,000 syllables. However, also comparable to English, it is possible to produce almost 80% of all speech with only the 250 most frequent syllables (Aichert et al., 2005). Both studies showed that in particular these 200–250 most frequent syllables, which are very highly overlearned motor speech patterns, appeared to be the least vulnerable ones to break down in apraxic speakers (for syllable frequency effects in English-speaking patients with AOS, see Laganaro, 2008).

Other studies with German patients have reported an influence of syllable complexity on apraxic speech (e.g. Aichert & Ziegler, 2004; Engl-Kasper & Ziegler, 1993; Ziegler, 2005; for similar results in the English-speaking literature, see e.g. Romani & Galluzzi, 2005). Complex syllables with consonant clusters (e.g. Brett, board) were produced with a higher error rate compared to simple syllables (e.g. Bett, bed). Regarding the pathological mechanism of AOS, it was concluded that due to the influences of syllabic factors (i.e. syllable frequency and syllable structure) there is still access to the mental syllabary in patients with AOS, but that the syllabic programmes appear to be partly destroyed.

Besides the influence of syllable frequency and syllable structure, there are further factors which appear to have an impact on the error pattern in German patients with AOS. In line with the English-speaking literature (e.g. Odell *et al.*, 1990), it is assumed, for example, that patients have a prominent problem initiating utterances. Aichert and Ziegler (2004) report higher error rates on the onset consonants of monosyllabic words compared to the coda consonants (see also Aichert & Ziegler, 2013). With regard to word length, consistent results could not be determined (e.g. Aichert *et al.*, 2012; Engl-Kasper & Ziegler, 1993) and point to individual differences between patients with AOS (for a discussion of this factor, see Ziegler, 2005).

### Influence of word stress

A particular language-specific parameter is word stress, which has been addressed recently (Aichert *et al.*, 2011). As already mentioned, German has a regular metrical pattern, the trochaic form. In their investigation, the authors compared bisyllabic trochaic words (e.g. *'Puma*, puma) with bisyllabic iambic (weak-strong) words (e.g. *Me'nü*, menu). The results revealed that trochaic words were produced with less segmental and prosodic errors compared to iambic words. It is assumed that the regular metrical pattern in German has a facilitating effect on word production abilities in patients with AOS. To our knowledge, there are no studies in other languages which systematically investigated the influence of word stress in apraxic speakers. We speculate that in languages like French, where iambic stress is the default stress pattern, the opposite error pattern will occur (i.e. more errors on trochaic compared to iambic words).

## Assessment of AOS

For the systematic assessment of German patients with AOS, the 'Hierarchische Wortlisten (hierarchical wordlists) are available (Liepold *et al.*, 2003). The repetition test includes 96 items which are systematically controlled for 'syllable complexity' (items with and without consonant clusters), 'syllable number' (one to four syllables) and 'lexicality' (words and non-words). Each item is analysed for phonemic errors, phonetic errors and impaired fluency (e.g. searching behaviour, intersyllabic pauses). After having analysed all items, an error profile shows if the production abilities of a patient are influenced by the factors of syllable complexity, syllable number and/or lexicality. The test does not provide a clear diagnosis of AOS. However, to our knowledge there are also no tests in other languages that unequivocally diagnose a speech apraxic impairment. This is probably due to the problem of differentiating AOS from phonological aphasic impairments and from specific dysarthrias (e.g. Croot, 2002). Nevertheless, a systematic assessment can reveal which factors influence the error pattern of an individual patient. This diagnostic information provides the basis for the interpretation of a patient's impairment and furthermore guides treatment.

## Treatment of AOS

Studies of the error patterns and the underlying pathology in AOS have also led to learning and treatment studies in German patients. Two studies focused on the role of the syllable as a target unit. In patients with severe AOS, the effectiveness of learning single segments was compared to the effectiveness of learning whole syllables (Aichert & Ziegler, 2008a). Syllabic learning was clearly superior to segmental learning. These results may be due to the fact that single consonants are rather artificial entities of articulation whereas the syllable is a more natural unit of speech motor programming and can therefore be reacquired more easily than single phonemes. A further study that investigated patients with moderate and mild AOS revealed that the learning of phonologically simple syllables, which were derived from complex target syllables, showed generalisation effects to the untrained target syllables (Aichert & Ziegler, 2008b). Therefore, speech apraxic patients show not only improvements on the syllables they have learned, but also on phonologically related syllables. These effects cannot be explained by the assumption of holistically stored syllable programmes (see above, Levelt et al., 1999). In contrast, the results suggest that syllabic motor programmes comprise an internal phonological structure. This architecture may be represented as a kind of phonetic network, where phonetically similar syllables may share motor programme units at different subsyllabic levels (Ziegler, 2005). Within such a model, training of a set of syllables also leads to a strengthening of structurally related syllable programmes.

A treatment study by Brendel and Ziegler (2008) applied a rhythmical cueing technique using acoustic stimulation, the metrical pacing therapy (MPT), and compared this method with a non-rhythmical control treatment. The study revealed that both methods lead to an improvement of segmental accuracy. However, the MPT intervention, but not the control treatment, also enhanced the suprasegmental abilities of the patients, namely, their speaking rate and fluency.

The variety of cueing techniques that has been described in the English literature on AOS treatment (e.g. visual or tactile cues; for an overview see Wertz et al., 1984) is also recommended in the German literature (e.g. Staiger & Aichert, 2010). Additionally, some language-specific adaptations of the methods are available. For example, the Prompts for Restructuring Oral Muscular Phonetic Targets (PROMPT) system, a specified set of tactile-kinaesthetic cues for English sounds, was adapted for German consonants and vowels (Birner-Janusch, 2001). The 'Speech Trainer' (Funk et al., 2006) software permits visualisation of speech movements for single German sounds and connected speech (syllables, words). However, the effectiveness of the Speech Trainer has still to be proved. Generally, independent of a specific language, future research is needed to guide evidence-based treatment decisions in patients with AOS (see also Wambaugh *et al.*, 2006).

# Conclusion

This overview of German language contributions to understanding dysarthria and AOS reveals a rich number of research activities dealing with the theoretical and therapeutic aspects of the disorders. Whereas studies analysing dysarthric speech in respect of the unique features of MSG are lacking, language-specific aspects (e.g. influence of word stress) have been addressed in AOS. However, also for AOS, cross-language studies are required to evaluate language-specific findings. In general, we need cross-language comparisons to other Germanic languages that exhibit similar features to German (e.g. English or Dutch) as well as comparisons to diverging systems (e.g. Romance or Semitic languages).

## References

Ackermann, H. and Ziegler, W. (1991a) Cerebellar voice tremor: An acoustic analysis. *Journal of Neurology, Neurosurgery, and Psychiatry* 54, 74–76.

Ackermann, H. and Ziegler, W. (1991b) Articulatory deficits in Parkinsonian dysarthria: An acoustic analysis. *Journal of Neurology, Neurosurgery, and Psychiatry* 54, 1093–1098.

Ackermann, H. and Hertrich, I. (1993) Dysarthria in Friedreich's ataxia: Timing of speech segments. *Clinical Linguistics & Phonetics* 7, 75–91.

Ackermann, H. and Hertrich, I. (1994) Speech rate and rhythm in cerebellar dysarthria: An acoustic analysis of syllabic timing. *Folia Phoniatrica et Logopaedica* 46, 70–78.

Ackermann, H. and Ziegler, W. (1994) Acoustic analysis of vocal instability in cerebellar dysfunctions. *Annals of Otology, Rhinology and Laryngology* 103, 98–104.

Ackermann, H. and Hertrich, I. (1997) Voice onset time in ataxic dysarthria. *Brain and Language* 56, 321–333.

Ackerman H., Hertrich, I., Daum, I., Scharf, G. and Spieker, S. (1997) Kinematic analysis of articulatory movements in central motor disorders. *Movement Disorders* 12, 1019–1027.

Ackermann, H., Gräber, S., Hertrich, I. and Daum, I. (1999) Phonemic vowel length contrasts in cerebellar disorders. *Brain and Language* 67, 95–109.

Aichert, I. and Ziegler, W. (2004) Syllable frequency and syllable structure in apraxia of speech. *Brain and Language* 88, 148–159.

Aichert, I., Marquardt, C. and Ziegler, W. (2005) Frequenzen sublexikalischer Einheiten des Deutschen: CELEX-basierte Datenbanken. *Neurolinguistik* 19, 5–31.

Aichert, I. and Ziegler, W. (2008a) Segmentales und silbisches Lernen bei Sprechapraxie: eine Studie zur Erhebung von Lern- und Transfereffekten. *Forum Logopädie* 3, 10–17.

Aichert, I. and Ziegler, W. (2008b) Learning a syllable from its parts: Cross-syllabic generalisation effects in patients with apraxia of speech. *Aphasiology* 22, 1216–1229.

Aichert, I., Büchner, M. and Ziegler, W. (2011) Why is ['ju:do] easier than [ju've:l]? Perceptual and acoustic analyses of word stress in patients with apraxia of speech. *Stem-, Spraak- en Taalpathologie* 17, 15.

Aichert, I., Wunderlich, A. and Ziegler, W. (2012) Einflussfaktoren bei Sprechapraxie: Gruppeneffekte und individuelle Variation. *Sprachheilarbeit* 57, 136–146.

Aichert, I. and Ziegler, W. (2013) Word position effects in apraxia of speech: Group data and individual variation. *Journal of Medical Speech-Language Pathology* 20, 7–11.

Birner-Janusch, B. (2001) Die Anwendung des PROMPT Systems im Deutschen – eine Pilotstudie. *Sprache, Stimme, Gehör* 25, 174–179.

Brendel, B. and Ziegler, W. (2008) Effectiveness of metrical pacing in the treatment of apraxia of speech. *Aphasiology* 22, 77–102.

Brendel, B., Ackermann, H., Berg, D., Lindig, T., Schölderle, T., Schöls, L., Synofzik, M. and Ziegler, W. (2013) Friedreich ataxia: Dysarthria profile and clinical data. *Cerebellum* 12, 475–484.

Code, C. (1998) Major review: Models, theories and heuristics in apraxia of speech. *Clinical Linguistics and Phonetics* 12, 47–65.

Croot, K. (2002) Diagnosis of AOS: Definition and criteria. *Seminars in Speech and Language* 23, 267–280.

Darley, F.L., Aronson, A.E. and Brown, J.R. (1975) *Motor Speech Disorder*. Philadelphia, PA: WB Saunders.

Der Duden (2005) *Das Standardwerk zur deutschen Sprache; Bd. 6, Aussprachewörterbuch*. Mannheim-Leipzig-Wien-Zürich: Dudenverlag.

Domahs U., Wiese, R., Bornkessel-Schlesewsky, I. and Schlesewsky, M. (2008) The processing of German word stress: Evidence for the prosodic hierarchy. *Phonology* 25, 1–36.

Duffy, J.R. (2005) *Motor Speech Disorders: Substrates, Differential Diagnosis and Management* (2nd edn). St. Louis, MO: Mosby Elsevier.

Engl-Kasper, E.M. and Ziegler, W. (1993) Wodurch können sprechapraktische Symptome beeinflusst werden? *Aphasie und verwandte Gebiete* 6, 4–15.

Funk, J., Montanus, S. and Kröger, J. (2006) Therapie von neurogenen und kindlichen Sprechstörungen mit dem PC-Programm "Speech Trainger". *Forum Logopädie* 20, 6–13.

Hall, T.A. (2000) *Phonologie. Eine Einführung*. Berlin: De Gruyter.

Hertrich, I. and Ackermann, H. (1993) Dysarthria in Friedreich's ataxia: Syllable intensity and fundamental frequency. *Clinical Linguistics & Phonetics* 7, 177–190.

Hertrich, I. and Ackermann, H. (1994) Acoustic analysis of speech timing in Huntington's disease. *Brain and Language* 47, 182–196.

Hertrich, I. and Ackermann, H. (1999) Temporal and spectral aspects of coarticulation in ataxic dysarthria: An acoustic analysis. *Journal Speech, Language, Hearing Research* 42, 367–381.

Kent, R.D., Kent, J.F., Duffy, J.R., Thomas J.E., Weismer, G. and Stuntebeck, S. (2000) Ataxic dysarthria. *Journal of Speech, Language, and Hearing Research* 43, 1275–1289.

Laganaro, M. (2008) Is there a syllable frequency effect in aphasia or in apraxia of speech or both? *Aphasiology* 22, 1191–1200.

Levelt, W.J.M., Roelofs, A. and Meyer, A.S. (1999) A theory of lexical access in speech production. *Behavioral and Brain Sciences* 22, 1–75.

Liepold, M., Ziegler, W. and Brendel, B. (2003) *Hierarchische Wortlisten. Ein Nachsprechtest für die Sprechapraxiediagnostik*. Dortmund: Borgmann.

Nicola, F., Ziegler, W. and Vogel, M. (2004) Die Bogenhausener Dysarthrieskalen (BODYS): Ein Instrument für die klinische Dysarthriediagnostik. *Forum Logopädie* 18, 14–22.

Odell, K., McNeil, M., Rosenbek, J.C. and Hunter, L. (1990) Perceptual characteristics of consonant production by apraxic speakers. *Journal Speech Hearing Disorders* 55, 345–359.

Romani, C. and Galluzzi, C. (2005) Effects of syllabic complexity in predicting accuracy of repetition and direction of errors in patients with articulatory and phonological difficulties. *Cognitive Neuropsychology* 22, 817–850.

Skodda, S. (2011) Aspects of speech rate and regularity in Parkinson's disease. *Journal of the Neurological Sciences* 310, 231–236.

Skodda, S. and Schlegel, U. (2008) Speech rate and rhythm in Parkinson's disease. *Movement Disorders* 23, 985–992.

Skodda, S., Grönheit, W. and Schlegel, U. (2012) Impairment of vowel articulation as a possible marker of disease progression in Parkinson's disease. *PLoSONE* 7: e32132. doi: 10.1371.

Staiger, A. and Ziegler, W. (2008) Syllable frequency and syllable structure in the spontaneous speech production of patients with apraxia of speech. *Aphasiology* 22, 1201–1215.

Staiger, A. and Aichert, I. (2010) Therapie der Sprechapraxie. *Aphasie und verwandte Gebiete* 25, 27–46.

Wambaugh, J.L., Duffy, J.R., McNeil, M.R., Robin, D.A. and Rogers, M.A. (2006) Treatment guidelines for acquired apraxia of speech: A synthesis and evaluation of the evidence. *Journal of Medical Speech-Language Pathology* 14, xv–xxxiii.

Wertz, R.T., La Pointe, L.L. and Rosenbek, J.C. (1984) *Apraxia of Speech in Adults: The Disorder and Its Management.* Orlando, FL: Grune & Stratton.

Wiese, R. (2006) *The Phonology of German.* New York: Oxford University Press. (Reprinted: original from 1996.)

Ziegler, W. (2005) A nonlinear model of word length effects in apraxia of speech. *Cognitive Neuropsychology* 22, 603–623.

Ziegler, W. and von Cramon, Y. (1986) Spastic dysarthria after acquired brain injury: An acoustic study. *British Journal of Disorders of Communication* 21, 173–187.

Ziegler, W. and Wessel, K. (1995) Speech timing in ataxic disorders: Sentence production and rapid repetitive articulation. *Neurology* 47, 208–214.

Ziegler, W. and Zierdt, A. (2008) Telediagnostic assessment of intelligibility in dysarthria: A pilot investigation of MVP-online. *Journal of Communication Disorders* 41, 553–577.

# 14 Motor Speech Disorders in Languages of the Indian Subcontinent: Some Perspectives from Hindi and Kannada

## R. Manjula and Naresh Sharma

## Languages of the Indian Subcontinent: Hindi and Kannada

Among the languages of South Asia, Hindi and Kannada are two significant languages. Hindi is spoken predominantly in the Hindi belt, an area across north-central India, which includes the states of Uttar Pradesh, Madhya Pradesh, Rajasthan, Himachal Pradesh, Bihar, Haryana and the Delhi region. It is an Indo-European language, being a descendant of Sanskrit. Kannada is a major literary language of the Dravidian language family, and is predominantly spoken in the southern Indian state of Karnataka and parts of Andhra Pradesh. According to the 2001 Census of India, there were over 400 million speakers of Hindi and approximately 40 million speakers of Kannada.

A number of regional varieties of both Hindi and Kannada exist, yet the forms considered here are primarily based on the current literary language and the day-to-day language used by educated urban speakers.

### The sound systems of Hindi and Kannada

Traditionally, the arrangement of the Hindi and Kannada alphabets categorises the letters of the alphabets phonetically according to the classification developed by the Sanskrit grammarian *Pāṇini* in the 5th century BC. Pāṇini's classification is based on the manner and place of articulation of the vocalic and consonantal sounds that the individual letters of the alphabet represent, and it is this system which other major Indian languages also adhere to.

## Vowels

Hindi has a 10-vowel system. It consists of three short vowels /ə/, /ɪ/, /ʊ/; 7 long vowels /a:/, /i:/, /u:/, /e:/, /æ:/, /o:/, /ɔ:/; and the vowel length is phonemic. In certain varieties of Hindi, the vowel /æ:/ may have a diphthongal pronunciation with a range from [əɪ] to [aɪ], whereas /ɔ:/ may display pronunciation ranging from [əʊ] to [aʊ].

The Kannada vowel system comprises five short and five long vowel phonemes. The traditional classification of the Kannada alphabet is similar to that of Hindi, with manner and place of articulation informing the order of the vowels.

According to the traditional arrangement of the alphabets, the vowels are ordered as shown in Table 14.1. In addition, 2 diphthongs ಐ /ai/ and ಔ /əu/ occur in Kannada.

The tongue position during articulation of vowels may result in high, mid or low, and front or back vowels. In addition, the position of the lips results in rounded or unrounded vowels. Nasalisation of vowels occurs in Hindi and is distinctive. In general, vowel articulation is unchanged when nasalised, yet /e:/ and /o:/ tend to be articulated at a slightly lower point when nasalised.

Ohala (1999) illustrates the position of the 10 vowels in Hindi as shown in Figure 14.1. The position of the vowels in Kannada is shown in Table 14.2.

In Kannada, all vowels can occur word initially, yet when high front and back vowels are in initial position following a pause they are preceded by a /j/ glide and a /ʋ/ (or [w]) glide, respectively.

**Table 14.1** Hindi and Kannada vowels

| Hindi | Kannada | IPA |
|-------|---------|-----|
| अ | ಅ | /ə/ |
| आ | ಆ | /a:/ |
| इ | ಇ | /ɪ/ |
| ई | ಈ | /i:/ |
| उ | ಉ | /ʊ/ |
| ऊ | ಊ | /u:/ |
| ए | ಎ | /e:/ |
| ऐ | ಏ | /æ:/ |
| ओ | ಒ | /o:/ |
| औ | ಓ | /ɔ:/ |

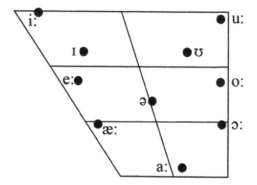

**Figure 14.1** Hindi vowel articulation

## Consonants

Each letter or symbol for the Hindi and Kannada consonants represents a distinct phoneme. In addition, both alphabets are syllabic to the extent that each letter or symbol represents the consonant plus an inherent schwa, therefore making it a CV configuration. In word final position, however, the schwa is not pronounced. For example, the Hindi symbol क represents /k/ plus the schwa. However, the word कब, made up of the letters क /kə/ and ब /bə/, is pronounced /kəb/ rather than /kəbə/ since the schwa is not pronounced in word final position.

The traditional arrangement of the Hindi and Kannada syllabic alphabets categorises the first 25 consonantal sounds according to the phonetic principles of place of articulation, aspiration, voicing and nasalisation.

Table 14.3 illustrates the symbols for the first 25 consonants along with their relevant international phonetic alphabet (IPA) symbols, in alphabetical order.

In addition to the consonants shown in Table 14.3, Hindi possesses two retroflex taps: /ɽ/ which is unaspirated and /ɽʱ/ which is aspirated.

**Table 14.2** Kannada vowel articulation

|  | Front | Central | Back |
|---|---|---|---|
|  | Oral | Oral | Oral |
| High | /ɪ/ |  | /ʊ/ |
|  | /iː/ |  | /uː/ |
| Mid | /e/ |  | /o/ |
|  | /eː/ |  | /oː/ |
| Low |  | /ə/ |  |
|  |  | /aː/ |  |
| Diphthongs |  | /ai/, /əu/ |  |

**Table 14.3** Hindi and Kannada consonants

| | Voiceless non-aspirate | | | Voiceless aspirate | | | Voiced non-aspirate | | | Voiced aspirate | | | Nasal | | |
|---|---|---|---|---|---|---|---|---|---|---|---|---|---|---|---|
| | Hindi | Kannada | IPA | Hindi | Kannada | IPA | Hindi | Kannada | IPA | Hindi | Kannada | IPA | Hindi | Kannada | IPA |
| Velar | क | ಕ | /k/ | ख | ಖ | /kʰ/ | ग | ಗ | /g/ | घ | ಘ | /gʰ/ | ङ | ಙ | /ŋ/ |
| Palatal | च | ಚ | /tʃ/ | छ | ಛ | /tʃʰ/ | ज | ಜ | /dʒ/ | झ | ಝ | /dʒʰ/ | ञ | ಞ | /ɲ/ |
| Retroflex | ट | ಟ | /ʈ/ | ठ | ಠ | /ʈʰ/ | ड | ಡ | /ɖ/ | ढ | ಢ | /ɖʱ/ | ण | ಣ | /ɳ/ |
| Dental | त | ತ | /t̪/ | थ | ಥ | /t̪ʰ/ | द | ದ | /d̪/ | ध | ಧ | /d̪ʱ/ | न | ನ | /n/ |
| Labial | प | ಪ | /p/ | फ | ಫ | /pʰ/ | ब | ಬ | /b/ | भ | ಭ | /bʱ/ | म | ಮ | /m/ |

The voiced consonants can occur as geminate consonants. The velar, palatal and retroflex nasals do not occur initially and generally occur before a homorganic stop. Retroflex consonants generally do not occur in initial position except in some loanwords. English loanwords which contain alveolar /t/ and /d/ are perceived as retroflex by many Hindi and Kannada speakers, and occur almost always with retroflex articulation. Aspirated consonants in Kannada tend to occur primarily in Indo-European loanwords, yet most speakers tend to replace the aspirated sound with its unaspirated counterpart.

In the traditional arrangement of the alphabet, the first 25 consonants are followed by 4 approximants /j, r, l, ʋ/ which tend to be listed together:

- /j/ is a palatal approximant.
- /ʋ/ is an unrounded labio-dental; however, following a consonant in the same syllable, a rounded bilabial /w/ sound may be produced rather than an unrounded labio-dental sound. Both unrounded labio-dental and rounded bilabial sounds are orthographically represented by the same character.
- /l/ is a voiced alveolar or post-dental lateral approximant.
- /r/ is a voiced alveolar or post-dental with a mild roll or tap.

The four approximants are followed by three voiceless sibilant fricatives and a voiced glottal fricative:

- /s/ is an alveolar or post-dental fricative;
- /ʃ/ is a prepalatal fricative;
- /ʂ/ is a retroflex fricative;
- /ɦ/ is the voiced glottal fricative.

In Kannada, sibilant contrasts tend to be eliminated to some extent by many speakers.

Two further consonantal sounds /f/ and /z/ occur in both Hindi and Kannada, mainly in Perso-Arabic loanwords, but are often replaced by contrasting yet phonetically similar free variations. Many Hindi speakers replace the voiceless labio-dental fricative /f/ by [pʰ], whereas in Kannada /f/ is often replaced by [pʰ] or [p]. The voiced alveolar or post-dental fricative /z/ is often replaced by [dʒ] in both Hindi and Kannada, or sometimes by [s] in Kannada.

Within the Hindi phonemic inventory there are the consonantal sounds /q, x, ɣ/ which also occur primarily in Perso-Arabic loanwords.

- /q/ is a non-aspirated voiceless uvular stop;
- /x/ is a voiceless velar fricative;
- /ɣ/ is a voiced velar or post-velar fricative.

Many Hindi speakers tend to replace the above three sounds with the contrasting yet phonetically similar free variations [/k], [kʰ] and [g]. Finally, Kannada possesses a voiced retroflex lateral /ɭ/. This does not occur in initial position.

## Syllable structure and stress

The majority of Hindi and Kannada words have a syllable structure that consists minimally of a single short or long vowel, preceded or followed by up to three consonants, i.e. a (C)(C)(C)V(C)(C)(C) structure. In Hindi, syllable junctures within a word can occur between successive vowels, between a vowel and a proceeding consonant, or between consonants (Kachru, 2006).

Consonant clusters are frequent in both Hindi and Kannada in the medial position, their formation tending to occur across syllable boundaries. Word initial and word final consonant clusters are less frequent, and tend to occur in Sanskrit, English and Perso-Arabic loanwords. In such cases, certain speakers may simplify clusters by inserting a short vowel. This may commonly occur among less-educated speakers or those who are less knowledgeable in English, and may also depend on the source from which speakers draw most of their vocabulary, be it Sanskrit or Perso-Arabic sources.

Kachru (2006) classifies syllables according to one of three weights: light syllables end in a short vowel; medium syllables end in a long vowel or a short vowel followed by a consonant; and heavy syllables are all other types of syllable. In most cases, Hindi stress patterns are predictable (Agnihotri, 2007). In general, where any one syllable in a word is heavier than any other, it tends to bear the main stress. Where two or more syllables in a word are equally heavy, the penultimate syllable usually bears the main stress. Although some syllables may receive more stress than another syllable, stress is not in phonemic contrast, therefore it does not make a difference to the meaning.

There are limited studies on stress in Kannada, but syllables tend to receive equal stress, and it is generally assumed that, as in Hindi, stress does not have a significant role except when it is used for emphasis.

Studies of intonation in Hindi and Kannada are also very limited, but some general observations can be made. Declarative and imperative sentences in both languages tend to have a falling intonation pattern. Interrogatives in Kannada tend to have a rising intonation, whereas in Hindi closed questions have a rising intonation, and information questions, such as 'what', 'when', 'why', etc., follow a rise-fall pattern with the pitch peaking on the question word.

## Morphophonemics

Various morphophonemic alternations exist in Hindi. Occasionally, medial vowels have a tendency to coalesce when they occur together in adjacent morphemes, therefore giving the sense of a diphthong. In other cases, glide insertion may occur. Kachru (2006) illustrates examples of when a front or central vowel is followed by a mid or low central vowel, a transitional /j/ is pronounced. In addition, when a back vowel within a word is followed by a mid or low back or central vowel, a transitional /ʊ/ or its variant [w] is produced. Which variant is produced depends on the speaker's preference or habit.

In Kannada, when two vowels come together in adjacent morphemes, they do not merge but a glide tends to be inserted. Additionally, as mentioned above, in word initial position following a pause the glides /j/ and /ʊ/ occur before front and back vowels, respectively.

The deletion of the schwa implicit in consonants occurs in certain contexts in Hindi and is discussed by Ohala (1973: 117). As mentioned above, deletion of the schwa occurs always in word final position, yet no exact rule to predict when schwa deletion takes place in word medial position has been defined. In general, when a consonant preceded by a vowel (i.e. VC) is followed by a consonant followed by a vowel (i.e. CV), the schwa inherent in the first consonant is deleted.

In Kannada, deletion of most short vowels following the first syllable of a word generally takes place. However, if the deletion would lead to the formation of an unacceptable consonant cluster, the vowels are reduced to an extremely short sound.

Another feature of Kannada is that all words (except loanwords ending in /n/ or /r/) should end in a vowel before a pause. Therefore, an 'epenthetic' or 'enunciative' vowel, usually a /ʊ/, is added to a final consonant before a pause, or if the final consonant occurring before the pause is a /j/, the vowel /ɪ/ is added instead.

# An Overview of Studies on Motor Speech Disorders in Kannada and Hindi: An Investigative and Rehabilitative Perspective

Development of assessment tools and resource material for the rehabilitation of persons with apraxia of speech (AOS) and dysarthria is challenging in India because of its multilingual nature. In Kannada, standard protocols have been developed for the assessment of AOS, specifically in children, but standard resource materials for rehabilitation are scant and have yet to be standardised for apraxia or dysarthria in adults or children.

Several studies in Kannada on childhood apraxia of speech (CAS) have addressed issues such as subgroups (existence of CAS in isolation or as a comorbid disorder) (Banumathy, 2008), the effects of length of linguistic units on vowel duration (Banumathy & Manjula, 2007), the sensitivity of measures such as diadochokinetic (DDK) rate (Rupela & Manjula, 2010) and relational speech timing tasks in the understanding of temporal dysintegrity in speech atypical phonological processes (Banumathy, 2008; Rupela, 2008; Rupela *et al.*, 2010). These atypical phonological processes did not conform overall with those reported in Western languages such as English.

The same does not hold true for Hindi, for which published studies on apraxia or dysarthria are unavailable. However, there is a resource manual (Rupela & Manjula, 2003) in Hindi for the treatment of children with AOS, which has been based on locally developed techniques. Given the scarcity of studies and materials for acquired motor speech disorders, the brief overview that follows of necessity focuses on developmental disorders.

## Apraxia of speech

In the field of speech-language pathology, the diagnosis of AOS, especially in children, is difficult due to the highly variant nature of the disorder with respect to its verbal features, the developmental issues and the comorbid disorders that often occur with AOS and the possible existence of subgroups in this disorder, particularly overlapping with phonological disorders. Recent consensus is that only three speech features have diagnostic validity in CAS: (1) inconsistent error production on both consonants and vowels across repeated productions of syllables or words, (2) lengthened and impaired coarticulatory transitions between sounds and syllables and (3) inappropriate prosody (American Speech-Language-Hearing Association [ASHA], 2007). Whether this generalises to Indian languages has not been investigated precisely, but studies are available.

## Studies on childhood apraxia of speech in Kannada

Although it is highly debated, clinicians continue to believe that CAS exists in a subgroup of children with speech disorders (Guyette & Diedrich, 1981; Stackhouse, 1992). Banumathy (2008) investigated subgroups in children with other developmental language disorders, along with CAS, by means of exploring the co-occurrence of oral motor, oral praxis and verbal praxis deficits. The study included two study groups of Kannada-speaking children in the age range of 4–14 years. Study Group 1 (CAS) constituted 12 children (4M; 8F) with a mean age of 5.9 years. Study Group 2 included 19 children with suspected AOS (sAOS), with comorbid speech and language disorders, namely, phonological impairment (6), expressive language disorder (6) and autism (7). Inclusion of Study Group 2 was based on clinical observations made through 10–15 individual interactive therapy sessions, performance on a 'screening checklist' and a detailed assessment of speech and language skills by another speech-language pathologist.

In the absence of any standard assessment battery in Kannada, an assessment protocol was developed locally and standardised by Banumathy (2008). This was used to assess oral motor, oral praxis and verbal praxis skills in the two groups. Results revealed that the majority of individuals with sAOS exhibited praxis deficits in speech, along with deficits such as hypotonia in oral structures. Co-occurrence of oral and verbal praxis deficits could be delineated and differentiated from oral motor deficits based on the errors observed during sequential oral and verbal praxis skill tests. There was, however, variability within the groups with respect to the degree of severity across the tasks assessed.

In a similar study, Rupela (2008) analysed the oral motor, oral praxis and verbal praxis skills in Kannada-speaking persons with Down syndrome in the 11.6–14.6 years age range. Study Group 1 ($n$=30) with Down syndrome was compared with Control Group 1 which included mental and chronological age-matched persons with cognitive delay (non-syndromic) ($n$=15) and Control Group 2 including typically developing children matched for the mental age of the study group (4.1 and 6.10 years) ($n$=15). A detailed assessment protocol was developed in Kannada to assess the oral motor, oral praxis and verbal praxis deficits. Results revealed that in all the three domains tested, the study group showed more deficits than the control groups. The oral and verbal praxis deficits could be differentiated from oral motor skills by the use of tasks that evaluated praxis deficits relatively independent of oral motor deficits. While oral praxis deficits were observed in varying degrees in the control groups, distinct verbal praxis deficits were noted in persons with Down syndrome. For example, persons with Down syndrome showed a higher percentage of occurrences of simpler phonotactic patterns than the later acquired complex ones (due to errors such as consonant deletions, syllable deletions and cluster reductions) and attempted certain complex phonotactic shapes, highlighting the importance of assessing the phonotactic deficits in this population.

Using a protocol based on those employed by Rupela (2008) and Banumathy (2008), Radhika and Manjula (2008) studied the development of praxis in Kannada-speaking, typically developing children (2.6–4.0 years). The protocol consists of the following tasks: function of the oral mechanism for speech, isolated speech movements, sequential speech movements, word level praxis assessment (words and non-words), relational speech timing (Lehiste, 1972) in word context (i.e. vowel shortening in relation to word length – sit-city-citizen), DDK assessment, sentence-level assessment and conversational assessment. In addition, the protocol allows the examiner to classify the phonological processes into space, timing and whole-word errors proposed by Velleman (2003). As per this classification, spacing error patterns include for example fronting and vowel deviations; timing error patterns include for example voicing and affrication errors; and whole-word error patterns include for example reduplication and consonant harmony. The children were screened for language development, oromotor function and orostructural anomalies. The protocol was standardised based on the performance of the children with the criterion that if 60% of the typically developing children in that age group could perform the task correctly, then that task was considered to be acquired by children of that age group. The performance of children on some of the sections showed a developmental trend. This protocol provides normative data and hence can help in early identification and intervention of children at risk of praxis failures. The scores obtained by a given child with suspected features of verbal apraxia can be compared with the means of the groups on which norms are established in this study. A child at risk will be scored below the mean bar and a child who crosses the mean bar is not considered at risk of verbal praxis failures.

Among the frequently observed cluster of behavioural correlates in CAS, persistence of vowel errors is a feature that often helps in the diagnosis of persons with CAS. However, reports of acoustic measures in the speech of children with CAS are minimal in contrast to adult speakers with apraxia. Acoustic studies of apraxic adults have measured vowel duration and word duration in relation to varying linguistic stimuli and complexity and have arrived at various conclusions relating to the higher-level processing.

Banumathy and Manjula (2007) attempted to study the effect of the length of linguistic units (ranging from two to four syllable words in Kannada) on vowel durations in children with CAS. There was also an attempt made to determine changes in vowel duration in relation to modes of imitation and elicitation with varying linguistic stimuli which included Kannada words and non-words. Two subjects (one female aged 5 years and one male aged 9 years) who were diagnosed as having CAS participated in the study. Two age- and gender-matched, typically developing subjects participated as the control group. The stimuli consisted of 10 sets of words (each set having three words increasing in syllable number) with each word consisting of the 10 frequently occurring vowels (five short and five long vowels) in Kannada. The speech samples were subjected to acoustic analysis for the vowel duration/length of each of the 10 vowels in all the tokens. The results showed that vowel durations were significantly longer for the apraxic group in comparison to the control group. As the words increased in syllable length, vowel durations reduced for both apraxic and control groups.

Rupela and Manjula (2010) used DDK task assessments in 30 Kannada-speaking persons with Down syndrome in the age range of 11.6–14.6 years. The responses were compared with those of mental age-matched persons with cognitive delay (without Down syndrome) and typically developing children. Other than rate, accuracy, consistency and numbers of attempts were also calculated for the DDK tasks. The study also explored the possible presence of CAS in these individuals using DDK measures. In general, persons with Down syndrome exhibited slower rates, greater errors in accuracy of production, lower consistency and took a greater number of attempts to perform the DDK tasks. The errors that suggested apraxia-like deficits that were based on previous reports in persons with CAS were slower rates for sequential motion rate (SMR) tasks, greater errors in sequential tasks, poorer consistency in SMR tasks and a greater number of attempts taken to complete the task. These results were in support of the findings of McCann and Wrench (2007) in persons with Down syndrome and of Thoonen et al. (1996) in persons with CAS.

In another study by Rupela et al. (2010), phonological process analysis was carried out using a 40-word imitation task with 30 Kannada-speaking persons with Down syndrome (aged 11.6–14.6) and compared with 15 non-verbal mental age-matched, typically developing children. Percentages of occurrence were significantly higher for the Down syndrome group with certain exceptions. Some phonological processes were observed only in the Down syndrome group. Some phonological processes observed in persons with Down syndrome, were similar to those observed in English and Dutch (cluster reduction, stopping, gliding, consonant harmony) and others that differed were attributed to the differences in the phonology of Kannada (e.g. retroflex fronting, degemination).

## Studies of dysarthric speech in Kannada

Prosodic subsystem errors, which characterise dysarthric speech, are considered unique to the different varieties of dysarthrias. These characteristics have been well established perceptually in the speech of people with dysarthria. The 'scanning index' (SI) (Ackermann & Hertrich [1994]) is an acoustic measure that has been used to study the speech of ataxic dysarthric speakers and has yielded evidence for the perceptual characteristic of 'staccato speech'. Mathew and Manjula (2008) attempted to estimate SI and variability measures in different dysarthria subtypes in Kannada speakers with overlapping features of prosodic disturbances, since no study had attempted to determine the effects of 'temporal dysregulation' on types of dysarthria (spastic, flaccid, ataxic, hyperkinetic, hypokinetic and mixed varieties), other than the ataxic, using SI.

Tasks of varying linguistic complexities (such as repetitions of syllables with different combinations of consonants and vowels) and sentences with increasing numbers of syllables and varying consonant and vowel environments were selected, including syllable repetition and sentence repetition, to throw light on the possibilities of differential temporal control, over different tasks in people with dysarthria (Lindblom, 1990).

The results revealed that the phenomenon of syllable isochrony is not an exclusive feature of the ataxic variety of dysarthria since all the subjects speaking Kannada with different types of dysarthria (including ataxic dysarthria) performed in a similar manner and their performance was comparable with that of control speakers without dysarthria.

The assumption that the SI is a sensitive measure for assessing the feature of dysprosody seen in dysarthria is also questioned, since the normal controls also showed tendencies to syllable equalisations. This study also questions the computation of the SI as a measure of temporal dysregulation. This is because of the observation that although variations were seen in the means of the syllable durations in few of the trials for the syllable repetition task (especially in the dysarthric group), this was not reflected in the SI score. The SI score of most of the subjects was '1', for both the experimental and control groups. The point of interest was that the SI was more stable in DDK tasks and sentences with a limited number of syllables, leading to the question of its sensitivity in reflecting the temporal characteristics of lengthy utterances in speech. These differences were explained on the basis that Kannada is a syllable-timed language which is agglutinative without elaborate chains of affixes and flexible word order. It is also possible of course that the SI as a measure is not sensitive to reflect on the temporal dysregulation in any language, irrespective of whether it is a syllable- or stress-timed language, a criticism that has been voiced by several researchers.

## Speech rehabilitation in motor speech disorders and resource material in Hindi

In general, there is a dearth of treatment materials in Indian languages. Notwithstanding, Rupela and Manjula (2003) developed the *Manual for Treatment of Developmental Apraxia of Speech in Hindi (MTDASH)*, which incorporates task hierarchies based on the developmental trends seen in normal children. The manual aims to guide clinicians, parents and caregivers in the treatment of Hindi-speaking children who have been diagnosed with CAS from age of identification onwards.

The manual is based on the following general principles:

(1)  A linguistic task hierarchy, which incorporates the following:
   • Sounds acquired early in development are targeted before those acquired later.
   • Vowels are targeted before consonants.
   • Sounds with high visibility are targeted before those with less visibility.

- Consonants offering maximum contrasts have been targeted first, so that, once established, they can help in the production of other consonants with minimum contrasts.
- Open syllables are targeted before closed syllables.
- Ease in terms of length and complexity of utterance has been kept in mind i.e. short and simple utterances have been taken up first.

(2) Prosodic features are incorporated as part of the total remediation programme.
(3) Repetition of each exercise is stressed.
(4) Meaningful and interesting activities are suggested.
(5) Use of multiple modalities during therapy is incorporated.

MTDASH consists of two main sections, targeting sounds and words, respectively. The section on sound target errors in vowel and consonant production includes exercises for improving oral motor control. The focus is on non-nasalised vowels, as nasalised vowels are thought to be more difficult in the initial stages according to Velleman (2003), and therefore not included. A cross-language perspective on this from a language with more extensive nasal vowel system/contrasts would help confirm this assertion, or not, which is based largely on monolingual English speakers. The consonant section provides thorough exercises for voiceless sounds. This is followed by guidelines on how to extrapolate these exercises for the utterance of the nasal, voiced and aspirated counterparts of the voiceless sounds, for which the place of articulation is the same. The second part of the manual is aimed at children who have acquired most vowels and consonants, and consists of chapters targeting specific errors found in word production in apraxic speech such as silent posturing, substitution and omission of phonemes in words, additions of sounds in words and improper sequencing of sounds in words. The manual has been supplemented with pictures and specific instructions to aid the user in the effective use of the manual.

## Conclusion

This necessarily brief review, given the restricted scope of research into motor speech disorders in Indian languages, has focused on studies of motor speech disorders in Kannada as it has been more extensively studied in comparison to other Indian languages. India, being a multilingual country, with such a vast number of languages and dialects from four major families of languages (Indo-European, Dravidian, Austro-Asiatic and Tibeto-Burman) as well as two language isolates (the Nihali language spoken in parts of Maharashtra and the Burushaski language spoken in parts of Jammu and Kashmir), only reflects the need for collective future plans to develop and standardise tools to evaluate clients with motor speech disorders, at least in the major languages of India. The path to this will benefit from a cross-language perspective, both in terms of developing assessment and intervention materials and in understanding the ways in which different motor speech disorders will show themselves in the different languages.

## References

Ackermann, H. and Hertrich, I. (1994) Speech rate and rhythm in cerebellar dysarthria: An acoustic analysis of syllabic timing. *Folia Phoniatrica* 46, 70–78.

Agnihotri, R.K. (2007) *Hindi: An Essential Grammar*. London: Routledge.

American Speech-Language-Hearing Association (ASHA) (2007) Childhood apraxia of speech (Position Statement). See http://www.asha.org/policy/PS2007-00277.htm (accessed 4 July 2011).

Banumathy, N. (2008) Investigation for subgroups in developmental apraxia of speech. Unpublished doctoral thesis, University of Mysore.

Banumathy, N. and Manjula, R. (2007) Effect of length, mode and type of linguistic units on vowel duration in developmental apraxia of speech. *Journal of Acoustical Society of India* 34, 121–125.

Guyette, T.W. and Diedrich, W.M. (1981) A critical review of developmental apraxia of speech. In N.J. Lass (ed.) *Speech and Language: Advances in Basic Research and Practice* Volume 5 (pp. 1–49). NewYork: Academic Press.

Kachru, Y. (2006) *Hindi*. London: John Benjamins Publishing.

Lehiste, I. (1972) The timing of utterances and linguistic boundaries. *The Journal of the Acoustical Society of America* 51, 2018–2024.

Lindblom, B. (1990) Temporal speech characteristics of individuals with multiple sclerosis and ataxic dysarthria: 'Scanning speech' revisited. *Folia Phoniatrica et Logopaedica* 52, 228–238.

Mathew, M.M. and Manjula, R. (2008) Estimation of scanning index in the speech of dysarthric speakers. *Student Research at AIISH Mysore* 3, 65–81.

McCann, J. and Wrench, A.A. (2007) A new EPG protocol for assessing DDK accuracy scores in children: A Down syndrome study. Paper presented in the XVIth International Congress of Phonetics Sciences (ICPhS 2007), Saarbrücken, 6–10 August 2007. See http://www.icphs2007.de (accessed 31 March 2014).

Ohala, M. (1983) *Aspects of Hindi Phonology*. Delhi: Motilal Banarsidass.

Ohala, M. (1999) Hindi. In International Phonetic Association (ed.) *Handbook of the International Phonetic Association: A Guide to the Use of the International Phonetic Alphabet* (pp. 100–103). Cambridge: Cambridge University Press.

Radhika, S. and Manjula, R. (2008) Protocol for appraisal of verbal praxis in typically developing children. *Student Research at AIISH Mysore* 6, 236–253.

Rupela, V. (2008) Assessment of oral motor, oral praxis and verbal praxis skills in persons with Down Syndrome. Unpublished doctoral thesis, University of Mysore.

Rupela, V. and Manjula, R. (2003) Manual for treatment of developmental apraxia of speech in Hindi (MTDASH). *Student Research at AIISH Mysore* 1, 60–67. http://203.129.241.86:8080/digitallibrary/HomeAtoZ.do?alphabet=M&recordPage=2&currentPage=1 (accessed 31 March 2014).

Rupela, V. and Manjula, R. (2010) Diadochokinetic assessment in persons with Down syndrome. *Asia Pacific Journal of Speech, Language and Hearing* 13, 109–120.

Rupela, V., Manjula, R. and Velleman, S.L. (2010) Phonological processes in Kannada speaking adolescents with Down syndrome. *Clinical Linguistics and Phonetics* 24, 431–450.

Stackhouse, J. (1992) Developmental verbal dyspraxia I: A review and critique. *European Journal of Disorders of Communication* 27, 19–34.

Thoonen, G., Maassen, B., Wit, J., Gabreels, F. and Schreuder, R. (1996) The integrated use of maximum performance tasks in differential diagnostic evaluations among children with motor speech disorders. *Clinical Linguistics and Phonetics* 10, 311–366.

Velleman, S.L. (2003) *Childhood Apraxia of Speech Resource Guide*. Clifton Park, NY: Delmar/Thomson/Singular.

# 15 Dysarthria and Apraxia of Speech in Japanese Speakers

## Masaki Nishio

This chapter starts with an outline of the main sound system features of Japanese. This is followed by an overview of studies relating to the assessment and treatment of dysarthria and apraxia of speech in Japanese. The final section concludes with specific features of dysarthria in Japanese.

## The Main Sound System Features of Japanese

Segmentally there are 5 vowels /a, i, u, e, o/ and 15 consonants/ semivowels in Japanese: /m n ɴ p b t d k ɡ s z h r j w/. /t͡s ɸ β/ occur as allophones in standard Japanese but can be used phonemically in some loanwords. Voiceless stops are slightly aspirated, less so than in English. /t, d, n/ are laminal dental-alveolar and /s z/ are laminal alveolar. /ɴ/ is a moraic nasal with variable pronunciation depending on what follows. /r/ is an apical postalveolar flap. The compressed velar is essentially a non-moraic version of the vowel /u/, but not equivalent to [w], since it is pronounced with lip compression ([ɰᵝ]) rather than rounding. A range of other sandhi, palatalization, affrication and gemination rules which apply in connected speech are not detailed here.

Structurally, Japanese is a moraic or mora-counting language, a feature shared with languages such as Tamil and Hawaiian, in contrast to syllabic or syllable-counting languages, such as English, French and Hungarian. Morae form the rhythmic basis of Japanese, producing phonological isochrony. They also constitute the basis of the Japanese kana writing system that uses one character to represent each mora.

Morae are not the same as segments or syllables, even though occasionally they may coincide. Morae are structured according to vowel length and the presence of certain consonants that may act as nuclei. Thus, a single short vowel, semivowel + short vowel, consonant + short vowel and consonant + semivowel + short vowel all count as one mora. /R/, /Q/ (the so-called choked sound) and /N/ (hatsuon) may act as morae. The difference from syllables emerges with long vowels and diphthongs and the presence of nuclear consonants. A long vowel is counted as two morae – 'aa' is one syllable but two morae, as is 'aN'. 'Kankei' (relationship) has two syllables /kan + kei/ but four morae, ka-N-ke-e. Double consonants (sokuon) count as a mora. Hence, Nippon (meaning Japan), which includes sokuon, possesses two syllables but four morae – ni-p-po-N. The contrast between morae and syllables is illustrated well in the adaptation of foreign loanwords to Japanese morae. Trumpet, two syllables, is adapted as six morae – to-ra-N-pe-t sokuon-to. Notice too that foreign words with closed syllables are reinterpreted as open syllables to reflect the generally open syllable characteristic of Japanese. Street /stri:t/, with a closed syllable is restated as [sɯtori:to] with an open syllable. The number of morae believed to characterise Japanese contrasts according to different investigators, and thus varies widely.

## Suprasegmental Features

As regards rhythm, as Japanese has rhythm involving morae and not syllable units, and each mora is perceived as being repeated isochronously, i.e. at equal time length, Japanese is considered to have a mora-timed rhythm, in contrast to stress- and syllable-accented languages. Morae display pitch accent variation. Specifically, Japanese operates a system of high and low tones or pitch accents. Differences in high and low pitches serve to differentiate the meaning of a spoken word. Word accents are derived from the combination of simple morae involving high and low pitches, with different combinations of these two types of simple morae yielding a variety of accents (below). As will be seen, such differentiation of word meaning by enhancing the adjustment function of pitch is highly useful for the treatment of Japanese speakers with dysarthria (J-SWD).

For words in isolation, pitch accent operates as follows: when the initial mora is accented, pitch starts high, falls abruptly on the second mora and levels out; when the accent falls on a non-initial mora, apart from the word final one, pitch commences low to reach a maximum on the accented mora before subsequently abruptly falling away again. In non-accented words, pitch rises from a low on the first morae and levels out in the speaker's mid-range, but it never attains the high of an accented mora. Combinations involving two high pitches are not allowed. Tones are phonemic. Hashi in isolation may take a high-low or a low-high accent sequence, but *háshi* means chopsticks while *hashí* means edge or bridge.

Taking a more abstract description based on a two pitch-level model where any mora is either high or low, the following generalisations can be made. If the accent falls on the initial mora, then the first syllable is high pitched and the others are low. If the accent falls on a mora other than the first, then the first mora is low, the following morae up to and including the accented one are high, and the rest are low. Where a word is unaccented, the initial mora is low and the others are high, including unaccented final inflections that would receive low pitch on an accented word. The high of an unaccented mora is not as high as an accented one. In connected speech there is a general pitch declination over an utterance in all cases except where there is a final accent. This constitutes a prosodic and not a lexical accent aspect of pitch change.

Prominence is employed in Japanese. This defines the special emphasis a speaker makes on certain parts of their speech by either intensifying and increasing the pitch or allotting more time. Normally a high pitch is used for emphasis in Japanese, although a low pitch may occasionally be purposely produced. Prominence is used in subtle accent-conveyed social protocol/practice and reflects the expressive intention of the speaker.

# An Overview of Assessment and Treatment of Dysarthria and Apraxia of Speech in Japanese

## Assessment

In 1973, Hirose introduced the perceptual assessment system for dysarthric speech established by Darley et al. (1969a, 1969b) to Japanese, and perceptual studies of J-SWD developed from then, including comparative studies of different types of dysarthria (Fujibayashi et al., 1977; Fukusako et al., 1983; Kobayashi et al., 1976; Kumai et al., 1978). A study particularly worth mentioning is that of Fukusako et al. (1983) that yielded useful data concerning the speech characteristics of J-SWD. Many of their findings for Japanese were analogous to those found in English speakers described by Darley et al. (1969a, 1969b). Endo et al. (1986) in their analysis of the speech features of J-SWD were the first in the world to establish the special features of unilateral upper motor neuron dysarthria.

The Japanese Society of Logopedics and Phoniatrics developed an integrated dysarthria assessment system (Itoh et al., 1980a). It was actually an attempt to open up a novel path for dysarthria assessment based on American findings in the 1950s–1970s. However, a more Japanese-directed assessment (Nishio, 1994) is the Asahi Speech Assessment Test (ASMT) aimed at a quantitative evaluation of speech production mechanisms. The ASMT measures a total of 69 items in the subsystems of speech, involving the respiratory, laryngeal, velopharyngeal and oral articulatory (tongue, lips and jaw) systems, with performance on non-speech tasks ranked on a scale of 0–3. The ASMT permits not only the differentiation of a normal from a neurologically impaired performance, but it can also be employed to derive treatment plans based on the relative severity of changes in different features.

A later refined version, appearing as the assessment of motor speech for dysarthria (AMSD) was developed in 2004. It was constructed according to the International Classification of Functioning, Disability and Health (WHO, 2001) and comprises three divisions: (1) history of speech problems; (2) physical examination of the speech mechanism; and (3) perceptual assessment of speech. It was recognised as the first standardised integrated assessment method for dysarthria in Japan. The physical examination of the speech mechanism, assessed using non-speech tasks, includes the assessment of the range, strength and rate of movement for each subsystem (e.g. respiratory, laryngeal). The perceptual assessment includes intelligibility, naturalness, speech characteristics (respiration, loudness, vocal quality, pitch characteristics, articulation and prosody) and speaking rate. Both the physical examination of the speech mechanism and the perceptual assessment of speech characteristics are rated on a four-point scale. As the only standardised integrated assessment method for dysarthria, the AMSD is extensively employed throughout Japan. It has been shown to be reliable, with high sensitivity and specificity, supporting its use and practicality, including in many research and clinical case reports.

Itoh (1992) also developed an objective method for measuring therapeutic effects particularly in dysarthric speakers – the single-word Intelligibility Test (Itoh-SWIT). In 2003, Ozawa et al. developed another SWIT (Ozawa-SWIT). Similarities exist between the Itoh-SWIT and the assessment of intelligibility of dysarthric speech devised by Yorkston and Beukelman (1981). The Ozawa-SWIT overlaps more with the Intelligibility Test developed by Kent et al. (1989), designed more for the assessment of the type of articulatory errors in reduced intelligibility based on phonetic contrasts.

Although Watamori (1984) and Nishio (2002) have separately developed methods for testing apraxia of speech in Japanese speakers, a standardised test has yet to be established. The other world-first assessment tests for physiological evaluation pioneered in Japan and worthy of mention include the X-ray microbeam system (Kiritani & Itoh, 1975) and flexible fibrescopy (Sawashima, 1968).

# Novel Findings Relating to Dysarthria in Japanese

Hirose et al. (1978, 1981, 1986) closely analyzed the neuromuscular mechanism of dysarthric speakers using an X-ray microbeam system to track lead pellet movements in the articulators of dysarthric speakers. Figure 15.1 illustrates the movement patterns of the jaw and lower lip during repetition of the monosyllable /pa/ with maximum utterance speed: a normal subject (44-year-old male) is compared with a patient with ataxic dysarthria. It is apparent that the range and velocity of the

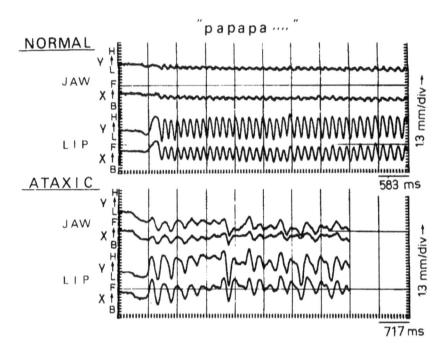

**Figure 15.1** Movement patterns of the jaw and lower lip in a normal subject (upper) and in an ataxic patient (lower) for repetition of the monosyllable /pa/ displayed as time functions of x [back (B) to front (F)] and y [low (L) to high (H)] coordinates

movements of each pellet are markedly inconsistent, and changes in the direction of the movements are often sluggish in the ataxic subject when compared to the normal subject. Figure 15.2 compares the patterns of lip movements for the repetition of the monosyllable /pa/ between a normal and a hypokinetic speaker (59-year-old male) with Parkinson's disease. In this figure, the coordination values for the jaw are subtracted from those of the lip in order to observe the pattern of lip movements independent of that of the jaw. Although the frequency of repetition is similar in both cases (a mean value of 7.7 Hz in the dysarthric speaker vs 7.4 Hz in the speaker without Parkinson's), the range of movements is smaller in the hypokinetic subject, particularly in the y coordinate value. Note also that the range gradually decreases throughout the repetition series until the movement finally ceases.

In other words, these and other findings revealed the typical pathophysiological features that cause abnormal speech characteristics specific to different aetiologies of dysarthria. Furthermore, Hirose (1986) reported on laryngeal function in dysarthric speakers using the flexible fibrescope developed by Sawashima (1986). Imatomi et al. (1997) attempted detailed velopharyngeal fibrescopic studies in dysarthric speakers and

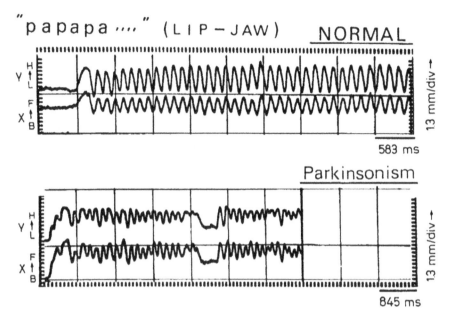

**Figure 15.2** Movement patterns of the lower lip in a normal subject (upper) and in a hypokinetic patient (lower) for repetition of the monosyllable /pa/ displayed as a time function

discovered that different patterns of velopharyngeal closure are displayed when compared with that of the cleft palate. Other physical studies include two dysarthric speakers with amyotrophic lateral sclerosis (ALS) and one ataxic dysarthric speaker with spinocerebellar degeneration by Niimi et al. (1986), where they employed an ultrasonic method specifically for studying tongue movement during speech. Niimi et al. (1986) concluded that the ultrasonic method could be used as a training tool for dysarthric speakers. In recent years, magnetic resonance imaging (MRI) has been used for vocal tract monitoring (Kumada et al., 1992) of normal speakers, though similar studies in dysarthric speakers have yet to be attempted.

Dysarthria-related studies employing acoustic methods include a recent investigation of speaking rate and its components in 72 Japanese patients with various dysarthrias (Nishio & Niimi, 2001a). The data indicate that speaking rate is a sensitive index for detecting/measuring abnormal motor speech performance in all types of dysarthria. Furthermore, in a study in which Nishio and Niimi (2006) correlated the relationship between speaking rate, articulation rate and alternating motion rate (AMR) in 62 Japanese dysarthric speakers, they concluded that AMR disruption is more easily detected in abnormal articulation than either speaking or articulation rate.

# Novel Findings Relating to Apraxia of Speech

With regard to apraxia of speech, fibrescopic observations of velar movements during speech by Itoh *et al.* (1979) demonstrated that repeated utterances of the same word manifest a marked variability in terms of the pattern of velar movements accompanied at times by a phonetic change in the subject with apraxia of speech (55-year-old male). In spite of such variability, the general successive pattern of velar gestures for a given phonetic context approximated the normal pattern. During the production of nasal and non-nasal consonants, the velum tended to take 'neutral' positions. Although anticipatory coarticulation was present, certain degrees of deviation from the normal patterns were observed. These were groundbreaking findings for apraxia of speech at the time in terms of highlighting it as a disorder of motor control and not a phoneme selection breakdown. Furthermore, according to observations on the articulatory movements of a subject with apraxia of speech using the X-ray microbeam system, Itoh *et al.* (1980b) concluded that the temporal organisation among the different articulators of the patient was disturbed in his production of a meaningful Japanese word /deenee/. In addition, the pattern and velocity of the articulatory movements of the patient in repetitions of monosyllables were different from those of typical dysarthric patients.

Based on the findings of this study, Itoh and Sasanuma (1984) proposed an independent schematic model of speech production, rather analogous to that proposed by Darley *et al.* The X-ray microbeam system for studying articulatory movements in apraxia of speech has also been employed by Konno *et al.* (1988a), and time-related and spatial derailments errata have been observed.

With regard to perceptual speech characteristics of apraxia of speech, Sasanuma (1971) calculated that the predominant type of phonemic error was, based on 68 slips, substitution of a syllable or a phoneme (88.2%). She observed that there was no one feature that tended to be more confused with another, whether this was distinctive features, phones, or syllables. This was not in agreement with the contemporary findings of Shankweiler and Harris (1966) or of Johns and Darley (1970) in which consonants were more frequently misarticulated than vowels; and some fricatives, affricates and some consonant clusters were more frequently misarticulated than other consonants or clusters. In two cases with apraxia of speech studied by Sugishita and Konno (1985), apart from perceived substitution being more frequently encountered than other error types in phonemic errors in both subjects, they also noted that consonants errors were more likely to be encountered than vowel errors. In contrast to this finding, distortion errors occurred most frequently independent of time post-onset in a study by Yoshino and Kawamura (1993) examining phonemic errors over time in an individual with apraxia of speech. In another study with five speakers with apraxia of speech, Konno *et al.* (1988b) found that substitution errors were frequently noted early post-onset, and this trend reversed subsequently with predominantly distortion errors, suggesting that the most predominant type of phonemic errors in apraxia of speech is subject to evolution over time. However, studying phonemic errors over time in a case by Tani *et al.* (2002) revealed that data are dependent of the measurement day without a specific error type tendency, i.e. individual variability is a prominent factor. Consequently, the most predominant type of phonemic errors in apraxia of speech in Japanese speakers remains controversial.

# Studies Relating to Treatment and New Findings

## Dysarthria

Historically, with reference to the treatment of dysarthria, systems adopted in the USA from the early half of the 20th century were predominant in Japan. Later, Nishio (1993) proposed a dysarthria management system based on the International Classification of Impaired Disabilities and Handicaps (ICIDH) introduced by the World Health Organization, basing his claims on successful treatment outcomes and providing a broad perspective on the treatment of dysarthria. However, the common concept of treatment for dysarthria in Japan at that time was not evidence based. This vital aspect of pooling of clinical evidence related to J-SWD has only very recently been adopted.

This latter development was spurred on by the establishment of the Japan Clinic of Dysarthria Research in 2002, which has overseen the introduction and adoption of treatment techniques for dysarthria from other countries, principally the USA, and through this, the promotion of relevant research/treatment activities; translations of key foreign language works into Japanese; publication of a standard text by Nishio (2006, 2007) for the treatment of dysarthria; systemic introduction of scientific information from the Academy of Neurologic Communication Disorders and Sciences (ANCDS); and publication of a series dealing with systematic training and drills for dysarthria (Nishio, 2000a, 2000b, 2005a, 2005b).

In a speech treatment (articulation exercises, mora-by-mora finger counting; splitting up of phrases; strengthening exercises) study by Fukusako *et al.* (1989) of 24 cases with spastic dysarthria, improvement in intelligibility was established in 18 (75%) cases. Moreover, in another study using finger counting of each mora in five cases with spastic dysarthria, Fukusako *et al.* (1991) observed that the approach raised intelligibility in all cases. Yamamoto (1996) investigated the effectiveness of using delayed auditory feedback (DAF) in two speakers with Parkinson's hypokinetic dysarthria, with success in both cases.

Nishio and Niimi (2005a) investigated the effectiveness of initial letter cueing in 47 speakers with dysarthria, with intelligibility significantly improved in the first-letter cue condition compared with the no-cue condition. This system is very similar to the alphabet board supplementation system described by Beukelman and Yorkston (1977) (see below). Nishio et al. (2011) have further studied the effectiveness of using speech rate-conversion software by artificially decreasing the sound waveform without changing the pitch in 62 individuals with dysarthria, a method that proved successful for increasing intelligibility.

Based on case reports, pacing board (Abe & Nishio, 2011; Tanaka & Nishio, 2008), voice amplifier (Abe & Nishio, 2011) and Lee Silverman Voice Treatment (LSVT) (Abe & Nishio, 2011) have been found to be effective for treating hypokinetic dysarthria. Tanaka et al. (2008) employed a novel portable pacing board to improve intelligibility in hypokinetic dysarthria in daily life and found that it yielded excellent results in a patient with Parkinson's, even after the pacing board was removed.

Another new approach originally developed in Japan and with accumulating efficacy evidence, concerns constraint-induced movement therapy (CIMT). This has been shown to be effective for the treatment of facial palsy (Nishio, 2006, 2008) and should be effective for facial palsy regardless of language. Recently, mounting evidence has demonstrated the effectiveness of CIMT not only for central nervous system-related facial palsies but also peripherally originating facial palsies.

A study with strong indications for the efficacy of speech-language therapy in dysarthria was conducted by Nishio et al. (2007). It involved 263 Japanese dysarthric speakers with dysarthria from cerebrovascular disease, spinocerebellar degeneration or Parkinson's. After speech therapy, they demonstrated significant improvement in intelligibility while no significant change was observed for the control group (no speech therapy). Among patients with dysarthria caused by cerebrovascular disease, patients who received speech therapy demonstrated significant improvement in articulation regardless of the severity of their disability, and a greater degree of improvement tended to be seen among patients with more severe dysarthria. In addition, significant improvement in intelligibility was observed regardless of the disease stage.

Little has been said of resonance therapy. Michi et al. (1988) demonstrated the effectiveness of palatal lift prostheses (PLP) in 39 dysarthric speakers. The effectiveness of PLP for treating dysarthric speakers has subsequently been replicated by Tachimura et al. (1998), who proposed that a factor in their improvement may be normalization of the input system for sensory information because of PLP.

As for augmentative and alternative communication (AAC) devices, Japan has always been blessed with the best equipment. The eye-gaze communication board was developed by Yuasa in 1979, and the portable electronic typewriter was introduced by Honda et al. in 1977. Since the 1980s, different types of electronic communication aid for severely affected dysarthric speakers have been invented and extensively employed.

In terms of treatment efficacy, it is controversial whether outcomes acquired via speech therapy can be sustained in natural settings. As such, the field of rehabilitation in Japan has recently focused on the correlation between performance ability restored in the clinic and that actually employed in daily life activities. Nishio and Shimura (2005b) examined the relationship between spontaneous speech in a natural setting and speech performance with the speaker applying his/her best efforts (i.e. capacity) in clinic in 97 individuals with dysarthria. Regardless of the type of dysarthria or the level of intelligibility, the results indicated that speech intelligibility deteriorates in an everyday environment compared to that established in a therapy session. Based on these results, Nishio (2005d) emphasises the importance of specific training to carry over speech performance/ability acquired in the speech therapy room into spontaneous speech in a natural setting.

### Treatment: Apraxia of speech

With respect to apraxia of speech, Konno (1988c) demonstrated the effectiveness of using electropalatography (EPG) in two cases. Moreover, Nakazawa (1991) showed the effectiveness of feedback through sense of movement using tactile sensation and intrinsic proprioception. This approach resembles the technique of prompts for restructuring oral muscular phonetic targets (PROMPT). Aizawa *et al.* (1994) have reported that the speech of a patient with aphemia improved remarkably using the mora-by-mora finger-counting method. Others include the traditional motor approach and articulation therapy involving imitation, phonetic derivation and phonetic placement. All in all, although limited cases related to therapeutic efficacy in apraxia of speech have been attempted in Japanese, effectiveness involving a large sample size has not yet been studied in Japan (or anywhere else for that matter).

## Language-Specific Features of J-SWD

Nishio and Niimi (2000a, 2000b) perceptually investigated articulatory function in 58 individuals with dysarthria using an Intelligibility Test involving 100 Japanese monosyllables. The results indicated that among vowel syllables, the highest intelligibility scores are for /a/ while the lowest are for /i/ and /e/, which are classified as front vowels in all severity groups. A confusion matrix shows that /i/ is likely to be replaced by [e], and /e/ tends to be substituted by [i]. With regard to consonants, the following findings have been noted:

(1) With respect to the manner of articulation, intelligibility scores were high for nasal and fricative categories, and low for plosive, affricate and flapped categories in all severity groups and in all types of dysarthria.

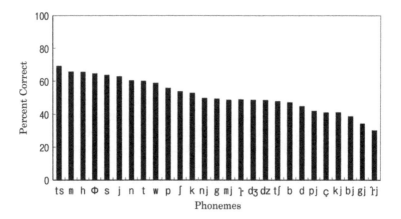

**Figure 15.3** Correct response rates (%) of consonant phonemes in dysarthric speakers with Japanese as their mother tongue (Nishio *et al.*, 2000b)

(2) With respect to the place of articulation, no significant differences in intelligibility scores were found among the six place categories in Japanese in nearly all severity groups and in all types of dysarthria.
(3) Intelligibility scores for unvoiced sounds were higher than those for voiced sounds in almost all severity groups and in all types of dysarthria.
(4) Phonemic analysis showed that a remarkable difference exists among phonemes, with intelligibility scores ranging from 30.08% to 68.39% (Figure 15.3). One finding of note concerns the relative accuracy of /tʃ/ compared to its claimed low accuracy in English dysarthric speakers.

As regards general points which may deserve language-specific comparisons, the following were several important findings by Nishio and Niimi (2001b) in 115 individuals with dysarthria:

(1) Monosyllabic intelligibility scores were far below word intelligibility scores in patients with a moderate level of intelligibility, whereas word intelligibility scores were below monosyllabic intelligibility scores in patients with severe intelligibility scores. The present data can be interpreted as evidence that these two parameters may reflect different aspects of abnormal motor speech performance in J-SWD, though further study invites closer control of stimuli and perceptual ratings.
(2) Intelligibility scores for people who required an AAC system were 20%–30% in monosyllabic word intelligibility, and a scale value of around 3.5 in conversational intelligibility (scale 1 indicates the best while scale 5 indicates the worst; the scoring is at 0.5-point scale intervals, making a total of 9-point scales).

(3)  Speech intelligibility was relatively high and seldom required an AAC system with ataxic and unilateral upper motor neuron dysarthria, whereas speech intelligibility was relatively low and largely necessitated an AAC system in spastic, flaccid and mixed dysarthrias.

## Specific features associated with treatment effects of J-SWD

As a specific feature associated with the treatment effects of J-SWD, the use of the rate control technique is highly effective. The previously mentioned study by Nishio *et al.* (2005a) provides an excellent example. They investigated the effectiveness of initial letter cueing in 47 speakers with dysarthria and intelligibility was significantly higher in the first-letter cue than the no-cue condition, and this applied to each severity level group. The difference was particularly significant in the moderately and severely dysarthric groups. Furthermore, Nishio *et al.* (2007) observed that rhythmic cueing and the pacing board are highly effective for ataxic dysarthria and hypokinetic dysarthria, respectively. It is therefore not uncommon to observe evidence of patients with hypokinetic dysarthria who were unable to perform oral communication, to subsequently carry out oral communication immediately by using the pacing board'.

The fact that rate control techniques are highly useful for establishing therapeutic effects in J-SWD can be interpreted with respect to the points mentioned earlier. The mora or syllable in Japanese displays the following features: (1) a relatively simple structure; (2) a small number of structuring phonemes; and (3) a structure with typically open syllables. All these facilitate the simplification of articulatory complexity and pacing techniques. Therefore, the use of the rate control technique in J-SWD facilitates dramatic intelligibility increases. This actually explains the effectiveness of the mora-by-mora finger-counting method for apraxia of speech as shown by Aizawa *et al.* (1994).

## References

Abe, N. and Nishio, M. (2011) Long-term clinical course of a dysarthric speaker with striatonigral degeneration. *Japanese Journal of Speech, Language, and Hearing Research* 8, 47–54.

Abercrombie, D. (1967) *Elements of General Phonetics.* Edinburgh: Edinburgh University Press.

Aizawa, F., Soma, Y., Nakajima, T., Yoshimura, N. and Otsuki, M. (1994) Remarkable improvement in speech in aphemia using mora-by-mora finger counting method. A case report. *Higher Brain Function Research* 14, 258–264.

Beukelman, D.R. and Yorkston, K.M. (1977) A communication system for severely dysarthric speaker with an intact language system. *Journal of Speech and Hearing Disorders* 42, 265–270.

Darley, F., Aronson, A. and Brown, J. (1969a) Clusters of deviant speech dimension in the dysarthrias. *Journal of Speech and Hearing Research* 12, 462–496.

Darley, F., Aronson, A. and Brown, J. (1969b) Differential diagnostics patterns of dysarthria. *Journal of Speech Hearing Research* 12, 246–269.

Endo, K., Fukusako, Y., Monoi, H., Tatsumi, I., Kumai, K., Kawamura, M. and Hirose, H. (1986) Characteristics of dysarthric speech in unilateral cerebral lesions. *The Japan Journal of Logopedics and Phoniatrics* 27, 129–136.

Fukusako, Y., Monoi, H., Tatsumi, I., Kumai, K., Hijikata, N. and Hirose, H. (1983) Analysis of characteristics of dysarthric speech based on auditory impressions. *The Japan Journal of Logopedics and Phoniatrics* 24, 149–164.

Fukusako, Y., Endo, K., Konno, K., Hasegawa, K., Tatsumi, I., Masaki, S., Kawamura, M., Shiota, J. and Hirose, H. (1989) Changes in speech of spastic dysarthric patients before and after treatment based on perceptual analysis. *Annual Bulletin, Research Institute of Logopedics and Phoniatrics* 23, 119–140.

Fukusako, Y., Monoi, H. and Endo, K. (1991) Treatment for spastic dysarthric speech using the mora by mora method with finger-counting gestures. *The Japan Journal of Logopedics and Phoniatrics* 32, 308–317.

Fujibayashi, M., Fukusako, Y., Monoi, H., Kobayashi, N., Tatsumi, I. and Hirose, H. (1977) Characteristics of dysarthric speech due to cerebellar disorders, pseudobulbar palsy and amyotrophic lateral sclerosis. *The Japan Journal of Logopedics and Phoniatrics* 18, 101–109.

Hirose, H. (1973) Toward differential diagnosis of dysarthrias. In I. Kirikae (ed.) *Approaches to the Disorders of the Central Nervous System* (pp. 214–232). Tokyo: Kanehara Publishers.

Hirose, H. (1986) Pathology of motor speech disorders (dysarthria). *Folia Phoniatrica et Logopaedica* 38, 61–88.

Hirose, H., Kiritani S., Ushijima, T. and Sawashima, M. (1978) Analysis of abnormal articulatory dynamics in two dysarthric patients. *Journal of Speech and Hearing Disorders* 43, 96–105.

Hirose, H., Kiritani, S. and Sawashima, M. (1981) Patterns of dysarthric movement in patients with amyotrophic lateral sclerosis and pseudobulbar palsy. *Folia Phoniatrica et Logopaedica* 34, 106–112.

*The Japan Journal of Logopedics and Phoniatrics* 18, 1–5.

Imatomi, S., Kawahara, A., Shusse, F., Okazaki, K., Kato, M., Ohkubo, F., Sumiya, N. and Ohsawa, F. (1997) Velopharyngeal fiberscopic study of patients with dysarthria. *The Japan Journal of Logopedics and Phoniatrics* 38, 20–28.

Itoh, M. (1992) Single-word intelligibility test for evaluating speech of adults with articulation disorders. *The Japan Journal of Logopedics and Phoniatrics* 33, 227–236.

Itoh, M., Sasanuma, S. and Ushijima, T. (1979) Velar movements during speech in a patients with apraxia of speech. *Brain and Language* 7, 227–239.

Itoh, M., Sasanuma, S., Shibata, S., Takeuchi, I., Tsukuda, I., Nagae, K., Hirose, H., Fukusako, Y. and Funayama, M. (1980a) Dysarthria assessment system. *The Japan Journal of Logopedics and Phoniatrics* 21, 194–211.

Itoh, M., Sasanuma, S., Hirose, H., Yoshioka, H. and Ushijima, T. (1980b) Abnormal articulatory dynamics in a patients with apraxia of speech: X-ray microbeam observation. *Brain and Language* 11, 66–75.

Itoh, M. and Sasanuma, S. (1984) Articulatory movements in apraxia of speech. In A.E. Rosenbek, M.R. McNeil and A.E. Aronson (eds) *Apraxia of Speech: Physiology, Acoustics, Linguistics, Management* (pp. 135–165). San Diego, CA: College-Hill Press.

Jones, D. (1960) *An Outline of English Phonetics*. Cambridge: Cambridge University Press.

Kent, R.D., Weismer, G., Kent, J.F. and Rosenbek, J.C. (1989) Toward phonetic intelligibility testing in dysarthria. *Journal of Speech and Hearing Disorders* 54, 482–499.

Kiritani, S. and Itoh, K. (1975) Tongue-pellet tracking by a computer-controlled x-ray microbeam system. *Journal of the Acoustical Society of America* 57, 1516–1520.

Kobayashi, N., Fukusako, Y., Andoh, M. and Hirose, H. (1976) Characteristic pattern of speech in cerebellar dysarthria. *The Japanese Journal of Communication Disorders* 5, 63–68.

Konno, K., Hirose, H., Kashiwagi, K. and Togashi, O. (1988a) Analysis of apraxia of speech using x-ray microbeam system. *Clinical Neurology* 26, 1460.

Konno, K., Sugishita, M. and Hirose, M. (1988b) Speech characteristics of 5 patient with pure apraxia of speech. *The Japan Journal of Logopedics and Phoniatrics* 29, 107.

Konno, K. and Sugishita, M. (1988c) Treatment of apraxia of speech. *Higher Brain Function Research* 8, 131–137.

Kumada, K., Niitsu, M., Niimi, S. and Hirose, H. (1992) A study on the inner structure of the tongue in the production of the 5 Japanese vowels by tagging snapshot MRI. *Annual Bulletin, Research Institute of Logopedics and Phoniatrics* 26, 1–5.

Kumada, M., Murano, E. and Kobayashi, T. (2001) Botulinum toxin treatment for adductor type spasmodic dysphonia. *The Japan Journal of Logopedics and Phoniatrics* 42, 355–361.

Kumai, K., Ogawa, H., Shiraishi, Y., Monoi, S., Fukusako, Y. and Hirose, H. (1978) Speech characteristics in Parkinsonism. *The Japan Journal of Logopedics and Phoniatrics* 19, 267–273.

Michi, K., Yamashita, Y., Imai, S., Arisawa, Y. and Suzuki, N. (1988) The use of palatal lift prosthesis for patients with velopharyngeal insufficiency resulting from acquired neurologic disease. *The Japan Journal of Logopedics and Phoniatrics* 29, 239–255.

Nakazawa, Y. (1991) Treatment of apraxia of speech. *Higher Brain Function Research* 11, 35.

Niimi, S., Nakayama, H., Masaki, N., Hirose, H. and and Kiritani, S. (1986) A preliminary report on the tongue dynamics of dysarthric patients. *Annual Bulletin, Research Institute of Logopedics and Phoniatrics* 20, 205–210.

Nishio, M. (1993) Speech rehabilitation for dysarthric speaker based on model of chronic disorders. *The Japan Journal of Logopedics and Phoniatrics* 34, 402–416.

Nishio, M. (1994) *Asahi Speech Mechanism Test*. Tokyo: Interuna.

Nishio, M. (2000a) *Speech Rehabilitation Vol. 1*. Tokyo: Interuna.

Nishio, M. (2000b) *Speech Rehabilitation Vol. 2*. Tokyo: Interuna.

Nishio, M. (2002) Motor speech disorders. In M. Ithoh and S. Sasanuma (eds) *Revised Manual for Speech-Language Therapy* (pp. 271–305). Tokyo: Ishiyaku.

Nishio, M. (2004) *Assessment of Motor Speech for Dysarthria (AMSD)*. Tokyo: Interuna.

Nishio, M. (2005a) *Speech Rehabilitation. Vol. 3*. Tokyo: Interuna.

Nishio, M. (2005b) *Speech Rehabilitation. Vol. 4*. Tokyo: Interuna.

Nishio, M. (2006) *Dysarthria: Principles and Practice Vol. 3*. Tokyo: Interuna.

Nishio, M. (2007) *Standard Textbook for Clinical Dysarthria*. Tokyo: Ishiyaku.

Nishio, M. (2008) *Case Studies in Dysarthria*. Tokyo: Interuna.

Nishio, M. and Niimi, S. (2000a) A study of articulatory function in dysarthric speakers: Analysis of intelligibility of vowels. *The Japan Journal of Logopedics and Phoniatrics* 41, 365–370.

Nishio, M. and Niimi, S. (2000b) A study of articulatory function in dysarthric speakers: Analysis of intelligibility of consonants. *The Japan Journal of Logopedics and Phoniatrics* 41, 371–378.

Nishio, M. and Niimi S. (2001a) Speaking rate and its components in dysarthric speakers. *Clinical Linguistics and Phonetics* 15, 309–317.

Nishio, M. and Niimi, S. (2001b) Speech intelligibility in dysarthric speakers. *Japan Journal of Logopedics and Phoniatrics* 42, 9–16.

Nishio, M. and Niimi, S. (2005a) Effects of initial letter cueing on intelligibility of Japanese speakers with dysarthria. *Journal of Multilingual Communication Disorders* 3, 183–193.

Nishio, M. and Shimura, S. (2005b) Relationship between spontaneous speech and speech made with effort during therapy by individuals with dysarthria. *The Japan Journal of Logopedics and Phoniatrics* 46, 237–244.

Nishio, M. and Niimi S. (2006) Comparison of speaking rate, articulation rate and alternating motion rate in dysarthric speakers. *Folia Phoniatrica et Logopaedica* 58, 114–131.

Nishio, M., Tanaka, Y., Abe, N., Shimano, A. and Yamaji, H. (2007) Efficacy of speech therapy for dysarthria. *The Japan Journal of Logopedics and Phoniatrics* 48, 215–224.

Nishio, M., Tanaka, T., Sakabibara, C. and Abe, N. (2011) Effective clinical management of patients with dysarthria: Use of speech rate-conversion software. *The Journal of Communication Research* 2, 1–12.

Ozawa, Y., Shiromoto, O., Ishizaki, F., Hasegawa, J., Nishimura, H. and Watamori, T. (2003) Word intelligibility testing using phonetic contrasts for Japanese speakers with articulation disorders. *The Japan Journal of Logopedics and Phoniatrics* 44, 119–1303.

Pike, K.L. (1947) *Phonemics: A Technique for Reducing Languages to Writing*. Ann Arbor, MI: The University of Michigan Press.

Sasai, H., Watanabe, Y., Muta, H. and Kubo, T. (2004) Level of satisfaction for treatments of spasmodic dysphonia. *The Japan Journal of Logopedics and Phoniatrics* 45, 8–12.

Sasanuma, S. (1971) Speech characteristics of a patient with apraxia of speech – A preliminary case report. *Annual Bulletin, Research Institute of Logopedics and Phoniatrics* 5, 85–89.

Sawashima, M. (1968) Movements of the larynx in articulation of Japanese consonants. *Annual Bulletin, Research Institute of Logopedics and Phoniatrics* 2, 11–20.

Sugishita, M. and Konno, K. (1985) Phonetical analysis of two cases with pure word dumbness. *Higher Brain Function Research* 5, 42–53.

Tachimura, T., Koh, H., Yoneda, M., Hara, H., Wada, T., Yoneyama, S. and Hayashi, K. (1998) Changes in velopharyngeal function of a stroke patients in association with continuous usage of a palatal lift prosthesis. *The Japan Journal of Logopedics and Phoniatrics* 39, 16–23.

Tanaka, Y. and Nishio, M. (2008) An approach of the practical use of the portable pacing board for a speaker with hypokinetic dysarthria. *Sogo Rehabilitation* 36, 593–597.

Tani, T., Izuka, Y. and Araki, R. (2002) Analysis of articulation errors and change of prosody in a case of apraxia of speech. *Higher Brain Function Research* 22, 280–291.

Watamori, T. (1984) Aphasia. In Y. Fukisako, M. Ithoh and S. Sasanuma (eds) *Manual for Speech-Language Therapy* (pp. 49–79). Tokyo: Ishiyaku.

World Health Organization (2001) *International Classification of Functioning, Disability and Health*. Geneva: World Health Organization.

Yamamoto, H. (1996) The efficiency of DAF in Parkinsonian dysarthria. *The Japan Journal of Logopedics and Phoniatrics* 37, 190–195.

Yorkston, K.M. and Beukelman, D.R. (1981) *Assessment of Intelligibility of Dysarthric Speech*. Austin, TX: Pro-Ed.

Yorkston, K.M., Beukelman, D.R., Minifie, F.D. and Sapir, S. (1984) Assessment of stress patterning. In M.R. MacNeil, J.C. Rosenbek and A.E. Aronson (eds) *The Dysarthrias: Physiology, Acoustics, Perception, Management* (pp. 131–162). San Diego, CA: College-Hill Press.

Yoshino, K.M. and Kawamura, M. (1993) A longitudinal study of speech in a case of pure apraxia of speech. *The Japanese Journal of Communication Disorders* 10, 110–119.

Yuasa, R. (1979) A communication device for patients with amyotrophic lateral sclerosis by a letter plate. In *Annual Report on Health and Welfare, The Ministry of Health and Welfare* (pp. 29–30). Tokyo: Japanese Ministry of Health and Welfare.

# 16 The Nature, Assessment and Treatment of Dysarthria and Apraxia of Speech in Portuguese

Karin Zazo Ortiz, Maysa Luchesi Cera and Simone dos Santos Barreto

This chapter opens with an overview of the phonetic and phonological features of Portuguese spoken in Brazil, and then goes on to describe some central studies of apraxia of speech (AOS) and dysarthria in speakers of Brazilian Portuguese (BP).

## The Speech Sound System of Brazilian Portuguese: Phonetic and Phonologic Features

Portuguese is one of the 10 most spoken languages in the world and has around 240 million speakers (Niskier, 2011). The language has one variant, BP, which is spoken by approximately 190 million speakers in Brazil (Instituto Brasileiro de Geografia e Estatística [Brazilian Institute of Geography and Statistics], 2010). It has 19 consonant phonemes (/p, b, t, d, k, g, f, v, s, z, ʃ, ʒ, m, n, ɲ, l, ʎ, R, r/) (Yavas *et al.*, 2002), 2 semivowels (/y/ and /w/) and 7 oral vocalic segments (/i, e, ɛ, a, ɔ, o, e, u) in stressed positions (Guimarães, 2005; Silva, 2009). Variants of the phonetic inventory of Portuguese occur by region in Brazil. In some regions, such as the majority of the south-east, the phonetic inventory is characterised by the palatalization of the phonemes /t/ and /d/ when preceding the vowel /i/, transforming these into the allophones [tʃ] and [dʒ] (Barbosa & Albano, 2004).

Based on articulatory phonetics, the consonants of Portuguese are classified according to the categories: manner of articulation (plosive, fricative, affricate, nasal and liquid), place of articulation (labial, dento-alveolar, palatal and velar) and voicing (voiced and voiceless) (Yavas *et al.*, 2002). Not all manner of articulation occurs at all places of articulation (there is no velar nasal phoneme for instance). In addition, restrictions exist regarding the occurrence of phonemes in certain positions in words (e.g. the phoneme /r/ never occurs at the beginning of words while the phoneme /λ/ has a very low frequency of occurrence in the initial position of words). The vowels are classified based on the criteria: tongue height and backness, and lip rounding (Silva, 2009).

On the distinctive features matrix of Chomsky and Halle (1968) (see Yavas *et al.*, 2002), BP exhibits the following features: sonorant, syllabic, consonantal, continuant, strident, delayed release, nasal, lateral, anterior, coronal, low, posterior and voiced.

Regarding the syllabic structure of BP, all syllables contain at least one vowel which constitutes the syllable nucleus. The minimum syllabic structure is V and the maximum $C_1 C_2 V C_3 C_4$ (Silva, 2009), with the CV structure being the most frequent (V = vowel; C = consonant). Lexical stress can fall in final, penultimate or antepenultimate positions, penultimate being the most frequent pattern. Recent studies indicate that BP has a mixed rhythmic pattern: syllabic and accentual (Barbosa, 2000; Barbosa & Albano, 2004).

The ensuing text outlines studies on AOS and dysarthria conducted in speakers of BP and also discusses the importance of taking into account the phonetic and phonological aspects of the language under study when proposing and/or adapting instruments for assessing speech motor disorders and in applying therapeutic strategies.

## Assessing motor speech disorders in Brazil

No single protocol for assessing motor speech disorders validated for use in the Brazilian population is yet available. However, the protocols published to date in Brazil exploring specific aspects of production of speech and providing a more comprehensive assessment of AOS and dysarthria will now be described. These protocols were first published in 2004 and 2006 and are currently being reviewed and updated.

### Apraxia of speech

In 2004, Martins and Ortiz proposed an assessment protocol for diagnosing AOS in any brain-damaged individual, even those with concomitant aphasia and dysarthria (Appendix A). The protocol is divided into two parts: assessment of non-verbal oral apraxia and assessment of AOS. The protocol was devised based on standard tasks in the international literature for assessing speech and non-verbal apraxias. The verbal stimuli of the protocol were adapted for the Portuguese language. The variables that influence the speech output of AOS patients were used to select the verbal stimuli. These variables include: word length (Canter *et al.*, 1985; Johns & Darley, 1970; Kent & Rosenbek, 1983), frequency of words (Duffy,

1995), frequency of phonemes in the language (Cera & Ortiz, 2009) and words that require rapid alternation between place of articulation (Freed, 2000; Ogar et al., 2006).

The verbal protocol included all oral output tasks (word repetition; phrase repetition; speech that is more automatic-reactive, e.g. counting numbers, months and days of the week; spontaneous speech and reading aloud). Developing a phonetically balanced protocol with regard to the frequency of the phoneme in the language and all variables that can interfere with speech production remains an important goal for future Brazilian studies on AOS. A qualitative and quantitative analysis of the errors provides an accurate diagnosis of disease severity and presumably a differential diagnosis and also helps guide the therapeutic process (Martins & Ortiz, 2004). There are no Brazilian studies available analyzing differences in phonetic and phonemic errors between apraxic and aphasic patients. However, studies on this subject have been conducted in speakers of other languages (Canter et al., 1985; Romani et al., 2002) showing that many questions remain open regarding the phonetic and phonemic error characteristics in apraxic and aphasic speakers.

## Dysarthria

The protocol for assessing individuals with suspected dysarthria initially proposed by Ortiz (2006) and recently republished (Ortiz, 2010), is the result of a compilation of several tasks from other published protocols (Drummond, 1993; Freed, 2000; Mayo Clinic, 1998). Comprising seven sections, the protocol employs perceptual assessment to evaluate: (i) phonoarticulatory structures; (ii) the five motor processes of speech: respiration, phonation, resonance, articulation and prosody; and (iii) orofacial sensitivity. The assessment includes the collection of both qualitative and quantitative data on the motor acts related to speech production and yields information on potential deficits in the functioning of the motor processes of speech.

The aspects investigated in the dysarthria assessment protocol are the same as those evaluated by the majority of the assessment instruments used in other languages/countries, including tasks such as: aspects of facial musculature, of the tongue and soft palate at rest, respiratory type and rate, maximum phonation time, voice type, vocal attack, loudness, pitch, vocal instability, nasal emission and type of resonance. Moreover, we carried out a subjective evaluation of strength, range and rate from velar, lip, jaw and tongue movements in verbal motor tasks. This protocol includes items for the assessment of non-verbal movement of the articulators. It is only applied when dysarthria is suspected. Verbal motor tasks comprise individual phonemes (e.g. production of the vowel /a/ in a sequence separated by pauses for assessing velar movement) or syllable sequences. In the last section, the protocol encompasses an assessment of orofacial tactile sensation.

Conversely, aspects of speech production whose analysis entails connected speech tasks are evaluated by stimuli which are similar to those used in assessment protocols developed in English (words, phrases and text), including tests assessing the number of words per breath group, intelligibility of speech and prosodic aspects (lexical stress, intonation, pauses and speech rate). A specific test was devised to assess speech intelligibility in dysarthric speakers of BP. This test entails the repetition of phonetically balanced words and sentences by the assessed speakers. The speech samples are used to produce sound recordings which are later played back to listeners who orthographically transcribe what they hear (Alexandre *et al.*, 2011; Barreto & Ortiz, 2010a).

A comparison of studies carried out in various countries reveals differences and similarities in assessment parameters adopted. Studies conducted in Brazil have demonstrated different normative values for maximum phonation time (Behlau & Pontes, 1995) and speech rate (Oliveira *et al.*, 2004). On the other hand, similar values have been found for phonoarticulatory diadochokinetic rates (Padovani *et al.*, 2009) compared to studies involving the English language. However, it is not possible to claim that differences between studies are specifically due to differences between languages, since methodologies differ among such studies. In addition, findings from linguistic studies in Brazil point to the importance of taking into account dialect variants in the dysarthric assessment process, especially concerning analysis of prosodic changes. Speakers of the *Mineiro* dialect (from Minas Gerais state) have a higher speech rate and a greater tendency to reduce the medial post-stressed vowel than speakers of the *Paulista* dialect do (from São Paulo city) (Meireles & Barbosa, 2009; Meireles *et al.*, 2010). These studies indicate a vast unexplored field of investigation involving the assessment of dysarthric speech that considers the specificities of BP and its dialect variants.

## Apraxia of speech: Brazilian studies

To address this topic, studies in Brazilian-speaking subjects with AOS will be examined to identify the phonetic and phonological similarities and differences compared to the English language.

Cera and Ortiz (2009) carried out an analysis of consonant production of 20 patients with AOS and aphasia. The study used a phonetic transcription of patients' responses on tasks from the Martins and Ortiz protocol. The phonetic transcription was performed by two academically trained transcribers. In the event of no consensus being reached between the two, a third speech-language pathologist provided the decisive assessment. The authors found that some phonemes of BP most susceptible to errors are not the same as those reported by studies involving speakers of English.

In Portuguese, the phonemes substituted (use of one phoneme in the matrix to replace another in the perceptual analysis) in over 5% of cases involved consonant segments: /b/ 6.9%, /g/ 9.2%, /v/ 5.2%, /ʃ/ 5.5%, /ʒ/ 12.2%, /ʎ/ 20%; in coda (final consonant): /r/ 5.8%; consonant cluster: /l/ 25.9%. The main difference observed is: substitution of the phonemes /b/, /ʎ/ and /ʒ/ was highly frequent in this sample of BP-speaking patients (Cera & Ortiz, 2009). It is important to note the differences in the methodologies used for classifying errors in AOS. Odell *et al.* (1990) included the distortion error type in their data analysis. The group observed 14 types of distortion, the most common of which was prolongation, followed by devoicing. In a study by Cera and Ortiz (2009), errors such as devoiced, voiced and labialized were considered substitution rather than distortion errors as classified by Odell *et al.* (1990).

The authors also discussed the places and manner of articulation involved in the most frequently occurring substitution errors in the sample studied. With regard to articulation manner, the differences between these authors' findings vs the results in other languages (predominantly English) were related to the affricate consonants of BP: /tʃ/ and /dʒ/ (these phonemes were not more susceptible to error in this Brazilian study). The results found by Cera and Ortiz (2009) for fricative consonants, in consonant clusters and liquid consonants, with the exception of the phoneme /ʎ/, were in line with international studies. In terms of fricative and liquid phonemes however, a Brazilian study on developmental apraxia showed a higher error rate (Rechia *et al.*, 2009). The phoneme /ʎ/, frequently produced erroneously by speakers of BP with AOS, is rarely used in the language, a fact which may increase susceptibility to error. Since this phoneme is not part of the phonetic inventory of standard English, one cannot of course compare this to English speaker productions.

Concerning substitution errors, Cera and Ortiz (2009) observed a different pattern of errors compared to studies in speakers of other languages. The bilabial consonant /b/ and the palatals /ʎ/ and /ʒ/ were produced with a high rate of errors. In contrast to /ʎ/, the phoneme /ʒ/ is part of the phonetic inventory of English where it is classified as a palatal consonant, and likewise in BP. As shown by the authors, although this phoneme has not been described in other studies investigating the consonants affected by AOS (most likely as /ʒ/ is a rare sound in English with a very restricted distribution), previous reports have found the palatal place of articulation to be frequently compromised in this disorder (Cera & Ortiz, 2009).

In relation to omission-type errors (production of a phoneme is perceived to be dropped), the results of the study by Cera and Ortiz (2009) were similar to those of international studies in that errors generally occurred in phonemes in consonant clusters and in the phonemes /R/ and /r/ (Johns & Darley, 1970). In addition, the phonemes in coda also showed a high frequency of omission in the study by Cera and Ortiz (2009).

The Brazilian study by Cera and Ortiz (2010) phonologically analysed the distinctive features involved in substitution, the most common error type affecting speech in their group of patients analysed. The impaired features were voiced, continuant, low, anterior, coronal and posterior. The high frequency of devoicing had been reported previously in earlier studies in speakers of the English language. Odell *et al.* (1990) reported that devoicing was one of the most frequent errors in the cited study. While Cera and Ortiz (2010) considered devoicing as a substitution (because the marked phoneme was perceived as substituted by an unmarked phoneme), Odell *et al.* (1990) classified the error as distortion. However, 'the mean substitution of the marked to unmarked feature was statistically higher that the reverse' (Cera & Ortiz, 2010: 60). The authors ascribed this finding to a higher frequency of errors with the increasing complexity of motor adjustment required by the articulation. Devoicing represents a phoneme switch (when the analysis is based on perceptual transcriptions) or distortion (when the instrumental analysis reveals instability of voice onset time).

Regarding the types and frequencies of errors of speech in AOS patients, the Brazilian study by Cera *et al.* (2010) showed that differences in studies involving speakers of other languages are centred on omission- and addition-type errors. The authors analyzed the types and frequency of errors produced by 20 patients with AOS. This study used the same methodology applied by Cera and Ortiz (2009). According to the authors, addition errors (when a phoneme or a syllable is perceived to be introduced into the word, e.g. /ˈpia/ → /ˈpiλa/), which presented a lower mean in this Brazilian study, may have been more attributable to alterations in language or praxis among the subjects assessed. The results of this Brazilian study corroborated the findings of other studies involving phonological analysis of phonemic paraphasia committed by aphasics (Canter *et al.*, 1985; Halpern *et al.*, 1976; Romani *et al.*, 2002). Differences in omission errors, the second most common error in this Brazilian sample, may stem from differences in the methodology used for classifying error types. Johns and Darley (1970) for example, included omissive substitutions under the classification of error substitution (such as *peat* for *pleat*) whereas omissive substitutions were considered omissions in the Brazilian study. These findings were similar to those of the study by Cera *et al.* (2012) analyzing the manifestations of AOS present in the speech output of Brazilian-speaking patients with Alzheimer's disease, supporting the theory that the difference found between speakers of Portuguese and other languages may be related not only to the methodology employed but also to differences in the phonetic and phonological features of the languages.

It is fundamental to take the interference of phonetic and phonological aspects into account when assessing the performance of patients with AOS, since each language has its own specific corpus, combinations and frequency of use of phonemes. This is especially true in the case of speech therapy, in which the variables impacting production performance in this group of patients must be considered. Despite the advances in the studies on AOS in BP, there were limitations in the differential diagnosis between errors derived from linguistic planning (phonemic paraphasias) and motor planning (AOS). The proposed four-level framework of speech sensorimotor control was depicted by Van der Merwe (2009) with the different phases: linguistic-symbolic planning, motor planning, motor programming and execution. Linguistic-symbolic planning involves phonological planning, which entails the selection and sequential combination of phonemes in accordance with the phonotactic rules of the languages, and it is portrayed as a linguistic-symbolic function in the proposed framework (Van der Merwe, 2009). McNeil *et al.* (2009) highlighted that speech errors (linguistic or motor) like perseverative, anticipatory or metathetic errors that without phonetic or motoric distortions are more consistent with the assignment of a phonological error. McNeil *et al.* (2009) have reported studies that had used kinematic measures and fine-grained perceptual measures of movement and speech and deficits in relative timing, amplitude and phase were found. Thus, these deficits are more distorted movements than substitutions (McNeil *et al.*, 2009).

According to Van der Merwe (2009), motor planning entails formulating a plan of action by specifying motor goals. In this phase, motor planning difficulty may impact on motor programming and also cause sound distortion (as a secondary sign). These aspects should be considered in future research on AOS in BP speakers. Moreover, the use of a standardised classification of types of errors is crucial to facilitate the comparison of findings in several languages and contribute to the selection of therapeutic strategies. No studies on the rehabilitation of AOS specific to BP speakers were found in the literature.

## Dysarthria: Brazilian studies

The results of a literature search of the SciELO, LILACS, MEDLINE, Web of Science and CINAHL databases, for national studies in dysarthric speakers are outlined below. In line with the proposal by Yorkston (2007), the studies retrieved were classified into the following categories: basic descriptions, clinical management (assessment and treatment) and psychosocial aspects of dysarthria.

The majority of the studies belonged to the basic description category, predominantly investigating the perceptual and/or acoustic characteristics of dysarthric speech (Azevedo *et al.*, 2003a; Barreto *et al.*, 2009; Brabo *et al.*, 2010; Busanello *et al.*, 2007; Carrilo & Ortiz, 2007; Feijó *et al.*, 2004; Knopp *et al.*, 2002; Ortiz & Carrilo, 2008). Two studies involved analyses of the outcomes of pharmacological or surgical interventions for

Parkinson's disease (PD), including the effect of levodopa on prosody (Azevedo *et al.*, 2003b) and of unilateral posteroventral pallidotomy on voice (Mourão *et al.*, 2005). Several studies investigated other correlates of dysarthria, such as its relationship with dysphagia (Furquim *et al.*, 1998) and the demographic and clinical variables of specific dysarthric populations (Palermo *et al.*, 2009; Ribeiro & Ortiz, 2009). A retrospective study by Talarico *et al.* (2011) reported a 33% prevalence of dysarthric disorders in a cohort of 244 patients who attended at the outpatient clinic for acquired neurological speech and language disorders of the Federal University of São Paulo over a five-year period.

With regard to clinical management, two studies focused on assessment. Depret (2005) confirmed that the rate of oral diadochokinesis (syllables per second) was the most sensitive measure for distinguishing between people with dysarthria from different types of neurologic diseases and healthy speakers. In another study, Barreto and Ortiz (2010b) verified the influence of predictability of sentences on intelligibility scores in dysarthric speakers. Regarding treatment, a Phase I study employing the palatal lift prosthesis for dysarthric speech yielded positive results (Ribeiro *et al.*, 2003). Two Phase II studies had also been carried out; the first demonstrated the efficacy of the Lee Silverman method for treating dysarthria in PD (Dias & Limongi, 2003) while the second study suggested the efficacy of speech therapy carried out in groups, according to a subjective evaluation made by patients together with a formal reappraisal conducted by researchers after treatment (Miranda *et al.*, 2005).

Only one study sought to investigate the psychosocial impact of dysarthria in the Brazilian population using the Quality of Life and Voice Questionnaire (Veiga *et al.*, 2006). The results of the study found a negative impact of dysarthria on quality of life.

Overall, considering the differences in methodology, the results of the studies cited mirror the findings of research carried out in English, where the differences found so far cannot be conclusively attributed to phonetic or phonological differences between languages. Nevertheless, language studies conducted in Brazil have made a valuable contribution to our understanding of some characteristics of dysarthric speech (Iliovitz, 2004, 2006; Vieira *et al.*, 2004). Data from the study by Iliovitz (2006) for instance, indicated that the use of the segmental phonological process of syllable degemination (omission of the first syllable in a sequence of two unstressed syllables, whose consonants are /t/ or /d/) by dysarthric speakers can improve perception of rhythm of speech and intelligibility. Speakers with severe dysarthria tend to use this process, while speakers with mild dysarthria tend not to use it. Further work on this line of investigation could yield valuable knowledge for refining assessment instruments and therapeutic strategies which specifically consider the language of the speaker.

# Final Considerations

The data outlined in this chapter highlight the importance of considering the phonetic and phonological aspects of the language for evaluation and particularly for rehabilitation of acquired neurological speech disorders (for instance, affricate phonemes are often produced erroneously by speakers of English with AOS, a phenomenon not seen in BP). The aspects described in this chapter concerning the differences between Brazilian studies and similar investigations involving other languages, should be considered in the clinical management of patients with AOS or dysarthria in BP speakers.

# Appendix A

Some examples of tasks from the Speech and Orofacial Apraxia Assessment Protocol (Martins & Ortiz, 2004).

Word repetition task

Pipa; Bebê; Sapo / Sapato / Sapateiro; Pedra / Pedreiro / Pedregulho

Sentence repetition task

A garota bonita está dançando; O estranho andou ao longo da estrada

Automatic production: 1–20; months of the year

Spontaneous speech: The 'Cookie Theft' figure from the Boston Diagnostic Aphasia Examination was used to elicit spontaneous speech production (Goodglass & Kaplan, 1983)

Oral reading aloud: Pão; Gol; Zebra; Caderno; Motorista; Felicidade; O seu time de futebol ganhou no domingo.

# References

Alexandre, E., Barreto, S.S. and Ortiz, K.Z. (2011) Predictability of sentences used in the Assessment of Intelligibility of Speech in dysarthria. *Jornal da Sociedade Brasileira de Fonoaudiologia* 23, 119–123.

Azevedo, L.L., Cardoso, F. and Reis, C. (2003a) Análise acústica da prosódia em mulheres com doença de Parkinson: comparação com controles normais [Acoustic analysis of prosody in females with Parkinson's disease: Comparison with normal controls]. *Arquivos de Neuro-Psiquiatria* 61, 999–1003.

Azevedo, L.L., Cardoso, F. and Reis, C. (2003b) Análise acústica da prosódia em mulheres com doença de Parkinson: efeito da levodopa [Acoustic analysis of prosody in females with Parkinson's disease: Effect of L-dopa]. *Arquivos de Neuro-Psiquiatria* 61, 995–998.

Barbosa, P.A. (2000) Syllable-timing in Brazilian Portuguese: uma crítica a Roy Major. *Documentação de Estudos em Linguística Teórica e Aplicada* 16, 369–402.

Barbosa, P.A. and Albano, E.C. (2004) Brazilian Portuguese. *Journal of the International Phonetic Association* 34, 227–232.

Barreto, S.S., Nagaoka, J.M., Martins, F.C. and Ortiz, K.Z. (2009) Spinocerebellar ataxia: Perceptual and acoustic analysis of speech in three cases. *Pró-Fono Revista de Atualização Científica* 21, 167–170.

Barreto, S.S. and Ortiz, K.Z. (2010a) Intelligibility: Effects of transcription analysis and speech stimulus. *Pró-Fono Revista de Atualização Científica* 22, 125–130.

Barreto, S.S. and Ortiz, K.Z. (2010b) Speech intelligibility in dysarthric speakers: Analysis of intelligibility scores in sentences. Paper presented at the 39th Annual Convention International Association of Orofacial Myology, São Paulo, SP.

Behlau, M. and Pontes, P. (eds) (1995) *Avaliação e tratamento das disfonias [Assessment and Treatment of Dysphonias]*. São Paulo: Lovise.

Brabo, N.C., Cera, M.L., Barreto, S.S. and Ortiz, K.Z. (2010) Disartria na doença de Wilson: análise de dois casos em fases distintas [Dysarthria in Wilson's disease: Analysis of two cases in different stages]. *Revista CEFAC* 12, 509–515.

Busanello, A.R., Castro, S.A.F.N. and Rosa, A.A.A. (2007) Disartria e doença de Machado-Joseph: relato de caso [Dysarthria in Machado-Joseph disease: Case report]. *Revista da Sociedade Brasileira de Fonoaudiologia* 12, 247–251.

Canter, G.J., Trost, J.E. and Burns, M.S. (1985) Contrasting speech patterns in apraxia of speech and phonemic paraphasia. *Brain and Language* 24, 204–222.

Carrilo, L. and Ortiz, K.Z. (2007) Vocal analysis (auditory–perceptual and acoustic) in dysarthrias. *Pró-Fono Revista de Atualização Científica* 19, 381–386.

Cera, M.L. and Ortiz, K.Z. (2009) Phonological error analysis of acquired speech apraxia. *Pró-Fono Revista de Atualização Científica* 21, 143–148.

Cera, M.L. and Ortiz, K.Z. (2010) Phonological analysis of substitution errors of patients with apraxia of speech. *Dementia and Neuropsychologia* 4, 58–62.

Cera, M.L., Minett, T.S.C. and Ortiz, K.Z. (2010) Analysis of error type and frequency in apraxia of speech among Portuguese speakers. *Dementia and Neuropsychologia* 4, 98–103.

Cera, M.L., Ortiz, K.Z., Bertolucci, P.H.F. and Minett, T.S.C. (2012) Manifestações da apraxia de fala na doença de Alzheimer [Manifestations of apraxia of speech in Alzheimer's disease]. *Revista da Sociedade Brasileira de Fonoaudiologia* 16, 337–343.

Darley, F.L., Aronson, A. and Brown, J.R. (eds) (1975) *Motor Speech Disorders*. Philadelphia, London, Toronto: Saunders.

Depret, M.M.P. (2005) Análise da diadococinesia articulatória e laríngea em indivíduos com ou sem transtornos neurológicos [Articulatory and glottal alternative motion rate (AMR) in subjects with and without neurological disorders]. Master's thesis, Federal University of São Paulo.

Dias, A.E. and Limongi, J.C.P. (2003) Tratamento dos distúrbios da voz na doença de Parkinson: o método Lee Silverman [Treatment of vocal symptoms in Parkinson's disease: The Lee Silverman method]. *Arquivos de Neuro-Psiquiatria* 61, 61–66.

Drummond, S.S. (ed.) (1993) *Dysarthria Examination Battery*. Tucson, AZ: Communication Skill Builders.

Duffy, J. (ed.) (1995) *Motor Speech Disorders*. St. Louis, MO: Mosby.

Feijó, A.V., Parente, M.A., Behlau, M., Haussen, S., De Veccino, M.C. and Martignago, B.C.F. (2004) Acoustic analysis of voice in multiple sclerosis patients. *Journal of Voice* 18, 341–347.

Freed, D. (ed.) (2000) *Motor Speech Disorders: Diagnosis and Treatment*. San Diego, CA: Singular Publishing Group.

Furquim, A.M., Pela, S., Manrique, S. and Perissinoto, J. (1998) Disfagia e disartrofonia pós-AVCi: relato de um caso [Dysphagia and dysarthrophonia post-cerebral vascular stroke: Case report]. *Pró-Fono Revista de Atualização Científica* 10, 3–7.

Goodglas, H. and Kaplan, E.F. (1983) *The Assessment of Aphasia and Related Disorders*. Philadelphia, PA: Lea & Febiger.

Guimarães, E. (2005) A língua portuguesa no Brasil [The Portuguese language in Brazil]. *Ciência e Cultura* 57, 24–28.

Halpern, H., Keith, R.L. and Darley, F.L. (1976) Phonemic behavior of aphasic subjects without dysarthria or apraxia of speech. *Cortex* 12, 365–372.

Iliovitz, E.R. (2004) VOT e disartria: alguns resultados preliminares [VOT and dysarthria: Some preliminary results]. *Estudos Linguísticos (São Paulo)* XXXIII, 1329–1334.

Iliovitz, E.R. (2006) Ritmo linguístico na fala disártrica [Rhythm of language in dysarthric speech]. *Estudos Linguísticos (São Paulo)* XXXV, 743–748.

Instituto Brasileiro de Geografia e Estatística [Brazilian Institute of Geography and Statistics] (2010) Censo Demográfico 2010. See http://www.ibge.gov.br/home/estatistica/populacao/censo2010/default.shtm (accessed September 2011).

Johns, D. and Darley, F. (1970) Phonemic variability of apraxia of speech. *Journal of Speech and Hearing Research* 13, 556–583.

Kent, R.D. and Rosenbek, J.C. (1983) Acoustic patterns of apraxia of speech. *Journal of Speech and Hearing Research* 26, 231–249.

Knopp, D.B., Barsottini, O.G.P. and Ferraz, H.B. (2002) Avaliação fonoaudiológica na atrofia de múltiplos sistemas: estudo com cinco pacientes [Multiple system atrophy speech assessment: Study of five cases]. *Arquivos de Neuro-Psiquiatria* 60, 619–623.

Martins, F.C. and Ortiz, K.Z. (2004) Proposta de protocolo para avaliação da apraxia de fala [Proposal of protocol for the evaluation of apraxia of speech]. *Fono Atual* 30, 53–61.

Mayo Clinic (ed.) (1998) *Mayo Clinic Examinations in Neurology*. Rochester, NY: Mosby.

McNeil, M.R., Robin, D.A. and Schmidt, R.A. (1997) Apraxia of speech: Definition, differentiation, and treatment. In M.R. McNeil (ed.) *Clinical Management of Sensorimotor Speech Disorders* (pp. 311–344). New York: Thieme.

McNeil, M.R., Robin, D.A. and Schmidt, R.A. (2009) Apraxia of speech. In M.R. McNeil (ed.) *Clinical Management of Sensorimotor Speech Disorders* (pp. 249–268). New York: Thieme.

Meireles, A.R. and Barbosa, P.A. (2009) Speech rate effects on linguistic change. In *10th Annual Conference of the International Speech Communication Association 2009 (INTERSPEECH 2009)* (pp. 2939–2942). Curran Associates, New York: USA.

Meireles, A.R., Tozetti, J.P. and Borges, R.R. (2010) Speech rate and rhythmic variation in Brazilian Portuguese. In *Proceedings of the Fifth International Conference on Speech Prosody*, Chicago, IL. See http://speechprosody2010.illinois.edu/stylefiles.php (accessed March 2014).

Miranda, C.S., Soares, E.C.S. and Ortiz, K.Z. (2005) Eficácia do processo terapêutico fonoaudiológico em grupo para disartria [Efficacy of group speech therapy in dysarthric patients]. *Fono Atual* 8, 32–39.

Mourão, L., Aguiar, P.M.C., Ferraz, F.A.P., Behlau, M.S. and Ferraz, H.B. (2005) Acoustic voice assessment in Parkinson's disease patients submitted to posteroventral pallidotomy. *Arquivos de Neuro-Psiquiatria* 63, 20–25.

Niskier, A. (2011) A língua do futuro. *Correio Braziliense*. See http://www.academia.org.br/abl/cgi/cgilua.exe/sys/start.htm?sid=772&from_info_index=31 (accessed March 2011).

Odell, K., McNeil, M.R., Rosenbek, J.C. and Hunter, L. (1990) Perceptual characteristics of consonant production by apraxic speakers. *Journal Speech Hearing Disorders* 55, 345–359.

Ogar, J., Slama, H., Dronkers, N., Amici, S. and Gorno-Tempini, M.L. (2006) Clinical and anatomical correlates of apraxia of speech. *Brain and Language* 97, 343–350.

Oliveira, C.R., Ortiz, K.Z. and Vieira, M.M. (2004) Disartria: um estudo da velocidade de fala [Dysarthria: A speech rate study]. *Pró-Fono Revista de Atualização Científica* 16, 39–48.

Ortiz, K.Z. (2010) Avaliação das disartrias [Evaluation of dysarthrias]. In K.Z. Ortiz (ed.) *Distúrbios neurológicos adquiridos: fala e deglutição* (pp. 73–96). São Paulo: Manole. (Original work published 2006.)

Ortiz, K.Z. and Carrilo, L. (2008) Comparação entre as análises auditiva e acústica nas disartrias [Comparison between auditory-perceptual and acoustic analyses in dysarthrias]. *Revista da Sociedade Brasileira de Fonoaudiologia* 13, 325–331.

Padovani, M., Gielow, I. and Behlau, M. (2009) Phonoarticulatory diadochokinesis in young and elderly individuals. *Arquivos de Neuro-Psiquiatria* 67, 58–61.

Palermo, S., Basto, I.C.C., Mendes, M.F.X., Tavares, E.F., Santo, D.C.L. and Ribeiro, A.F.C. (2009) Avaliação e intervenção fonoaudiológica na doença de Parkinson: análise clínica-epidemiológica de 32 pacientes [Phonoaudiology assessment and intervention in Parkinson's: Clinical-epidemiological analysis of 32 patients]. *Revista Brasileira de Neurologia* 45, 17–24.

Rechia, I.C., Souza, A.P.R., Mezzomo, C.L. and Moro, M.P. (2009) Processos de substituição e variabilidade articulatória na fala de sujeitos com dispraxia verbal [Substitution processes and articulatory variability in the speech of subjects with verbal dyspraxia]. *Revista da Sociedade Brasileira de Fonoaudiologia* 14, 547–552.

Ribeiro, A.C., Pegoraro-Krook, M.I., Vieira, J.M., Teles-Magalhães, L.C., Fonseca, C.B.F. and Padovani, C.R. (2003) Efeito da prótese de palato na análise acústica vocal de pacientes disártricos [The effect of palatal lift in the vocal acoustic analysis of dysarthric patients]. *Pró-Fono Revista de Atualização Científica* 15, 45–54.

Ribeiro, A.F. and Ortiz, K.Z. (2009) Perfil populacional de pacientes com disartria atendidos em hospitais terciários [Population profile of dysarthric patients attended at a tertiary hospital]. *Revista da Sociedade Brasileira de Fonoaudiologia* 14, 446–453.

Romani, C., Olson, A., Semenza, C. and Granà, A. (2002) Patterns of phonological errors as a function of a phonological versus an articulatory locus of impairment. *Cortex* 38, 541–567.

Silva, T.C. (ed.) (2009) *Fonética e fonologia do português: roteiro de estudos e guia de exercícios* [Phonetics and Phonology of Portuguese: Study Guide and Exercises]. São Paulo: Contexto.

Talarico, T.R., Venegas, M.J. and Ortiz, K.Z. (2011) Perfil populacional de pacientes com distúrbios da comunicação decorrentes de lesão cerebral, assistidos em hospital terciário [Population profile of patients with human communication disorders after brain injury, attended at a tertiary hospital]. *Revista CEFAC* 13, 330–339.

Van der Merwe, A. (2009) A theoretical framework for the characterization of pathological speech sensorimotor control. In M.R. McNeil (ed.) *Clinical Management of Sensorimotor Speech Disorders* (pp. 3–18). New York: Thieme.

Veiga, L.A.P., Costa, T.C., Juliano, Y. and Oliveira, M.F.R. (2006) Impacto da disartrofonia na qualidade de vida de pacientes com lesão encefálica adquirida [Impact of dysarthria on quality of life of patients with acquired brain injury]. *Medicina de Reabilitação* 25, 71–74.

Vieira, J.M., Barbosa, P.A. and Pegoraro-Krook, M.I. (2004) A pausa na produção da fala com comprometimento neurológico [A pause in production of speech in neurologic impairment]. *Revista de Estudos da Linguagem* 12, 181–191.

Yavas, M., Hernandorena, C.L.M. and Lamprecht, R.R. (eds) (2002) *Avaliação Fonológica da criança: reeducação e terapia* [Phonological Assessment of Children: Reeducation and Therapy]. Porto Alegre: Artmed.

Yorkston, K.M. (2007) The degenerative dysarthrias: A window into critical clinical and research issues. *Folia Phoniatrica et Logopaedica* 59, 107–117.

# 17 The Nature, Assessment and Treatment of Dysarthria and Apraxia of Speech in Spanish

Natalia Melle,
María-Teresa Martín-Aragoneses
and Carlos Gallego

This chapter begins with a review of some of the central aspects of the distinctive sound system of Spanish, including the segmental and suprasegmental aspects and the relationship to components of morphology and syntax. Next, methods, procedures, tools and techniques for assessment and intervention are described, highlighting clinical findings and their contribution to normal and pathological models, with an emphasis on the differences between Spanish and English. Finally, future research lines to improve the assessment and intervention of motor speech disorders in Spanish speakers are identified.

## The Spanish Sound System and its Relationships with Other Components of Language

Bearing in mind that there are some distinct contrasts in the different forms of Spanish not just across the Atlantic but also within regions either side, the general number of phonemes in Spanish is 23 (5 vowels and 18 consonants), or 24 if one considers two coronal units (/s/' and /θ/ as in Castilian). In the present description, we use features of articulation based on feature geometry.

### The vowels

The vowel phonemes are /i/, /e/, /a/, /o/ and /u/. For spoken language, the relative frequency of occurrence of vowel phonemes in Spanish is 48.13%, with the most frequent vowels being /e/ and /a/ (15.12% and 12.27%, respectively; Moreno Sandoval *et al.*, 2006). Certain variations in the position of the articulators can be observed with three of these phonemes (/e/, /o/, /a/); however, these are not considered allophones, since the variations are not in complementary distribution, but free variation (i.e. the variations of the vowel phoneme can appear in the same phonetic context). Given this, the phonetic execution of vowels in Spanish is much more stable than in English, where the phonetic context affects production more closely.

As in other languages, Spanish vowels are [– consonantal], [+ sonorant], [+ continuant] and [+ voiced]. The vowels can be articulated differently on the basis of the degree of openness (high, medium and low) and place of articulation (front, central and back). Nasality and duration are not considered distinctive – though see below regarding phonetic-level descriptions.

It is important to note that in Spanish the labial feature is not distinctive since labialization is only observed in back vowels (/o/ and /u/), which are pronounced through lip rounding, whereas central and frontal vowels are always unrounded (/a/, /i/ and /e/).

The five vowel phonemes have different phonetic realisations depending on the phonetic context in which they appear. These allophones include five primary vowels ([i, e, a, o, u]) and five nasalized vowels ([ĩ, ẽ, ã, õ, ũ]). The latter occur in complementary distribution to oral vowel allophones when the vowel is placed between two nasal consonants (e.g. 'm**a**nta'; *blanket* in English) or when it is in word initial position followed by a nasal consonant (e.g. '**a**nda'; *walk* in English).

In Spanish, it is possible to find sequences of vowel phonemes in the same syllable or in different syllables. In a single syllable, vowels may form *diphthongs* or *triphthongs* (i.e. a low or mid vowel with one or two high vowel/s, or vice versa; e.g. 'h**oy**' and 'b**uey**', *today* and *ox*). In different sylla-bles, it forms a *hiatus* (i.e. two non-high vowels, or a low or mid unstressed vowel and high stressed one, such as '**le**o' or '**oí**', *(I) read* and *(I) heard*). In the case of diphthongs or triphthongs, one vowel constitutes a syllable nucleus and the other vowels are marginal vowels or glides. In Spanish, there are only two glides and these are considered to be allophones of their corresponding vowels (/i/ and /u/). In the case of a hiatus, each vowel represents a syllabic nucleus. At times, especially when speech is fast or less formal (Navarro, 1991; Quilis, 1993), the phonetic-acoustic realisation of these sequences may vary, since a tendency to pronounce vowel groups in a simplified way has been observed in Spanish (similar to the English 'our' being pronounced as one or two syllables).

## The consonants

The 19 phonemes are /p/, /b/, /t/, /d/, /k/, /g/, /ʧ/, /f/, /θ/, /s/, /x/, /ʝ/, /m/, /n/, /ɲ/, /l/, /ʎ/, /ɾ/ and /r̄/. Taken together, the relative frequency of consonant phonemes – around 51.87% – is slightly higher than that of vowel phonemes. The individual frequency of consonant phonemes is lower than that of vowel phonemes, the most frequent being /s/ and /n/ (8.11% and 7.05%, respectively; Moreno Sandoval *et al.*, 2006).

Consonant phonemes may be phonologically described according to the following articulatory features. The root features are: [+ consonantal] and [± sonorant]. The laryngeal feature: [± voiced]. The supralaryngeal features can be divided by manner: [± continuant], [± strident], [± lateral], [± nasal] and place: [± round] for labial; [± anterior], [± distributed] for coronal; y [± high] and [± back] for dorsal (Real Academia Española, 2011).

Some phonemes have more than one phonetic realisation depending on their phonetic context. The articulatory features used to describe these allophones are the same as for English, i.e. manner and place of articulation, vibration of the vocal folds (voiced or voiceless) and action of the soft palate (oral or nasal). There is no agreement on how many consonant allophones there are in Spanish.

## The syllable

Syllable structure is simpler in Spanish than in English. Open syllables predominate. The most common syllable pattern in Spanish is consonant-vowel (CV), followed by consonant-vowel-consonant (CVC), while more complex structures such as consonant-consonant-vowel-consonant-consonant (CCVCC) rarely occur. Consonant clusters are formed by a labial, labiodental or velar consonant and a liquid consonant (/pr, br, pl, bl, fr, fl, gr, gl, kl, kr/) or a dental consonant and a rhotic consonant (/dr, tr/), and they can appear both inside and at the beginning of a word, but always in prenuclear syllabic position. The syllable types and their relative frequencies, according to the study by Moreno Sandoval *et al.* (2006), are presented in Table 17.1.

**Table 17.1** Frequency of syllable types in Spanish

| Syllabic structure | Relative frequencies |
| --- | --- |
| .CV. | 51.35 |
| .CVC. | 18.03 |
| .V. | 10.75 |
| .VC. | 8.60 |
| .CVV. | 3.37 |
| .CVVC. | 3.31 |
| .CCV. | 2.96 |
| .CCVC. | 0.88 |

Source: Moreno Sandoval *et al.* (2006)

## Suprasegmental features: Accent, intonation and rhythm

### Accent

Spanish is a language with free accent. Stress can appear on any syllable, and can be conveyed by means of an increase in pitch (mainly), loudness and duration so that one syllable of a word is stressed against the others (stress vs unstressed). At the word level, it allows the distinction of phonologically identical sequences such as 'medico' which can either mean *doctor* or *medicated* in English. At the sentence level, accent guides the listener to the important information, i.e. the stressed (or tonic) syllables tend to occur in words carrying lexical information (verbs, nouns, tonic pronouns, etc.), whereas the unstressed (or atonic) syllables are associated with grammatical function words (e.g. prepositions, conjunctions, determiners) (Quilis, 2003).

Each word can only contain one stressed syllable occupying any position in the last three syllables. The only words that carry two stressed syllables are adverbs ending in -mente (-*ly* in English; e.g. 'felizmente', *happily*). Table 17.2 gives the lexical accentual patterns and their frequencies in spoken language. As can be seen in Table 17.2, the *paroxytone* is the most frequent scheme, followed by the *oxytone* and the *proparoxytone* (Quilis, 1993). In addition, the *superproparoxytone* is another pattern that arises when the word contains atonic enclitic pronouns (e.g. 'tráemela'; *bring it to me* in English).

**Table 17.2** Spanish lexical accentual patterns and their frequencies in spoken language

| | Lexical accentual patterns | Frequency in spoken language (%) | Examples |
|---|---|---|---|
| Oxytone | ◜ | 17.68 | Calce**tín** (*sock*) |
| Paroxytone | ◜ | 79.50 | A**mi**go (*friend*) |
| Proparoxytone | ◜ | 2.76 | **Cír**culo (*circle*) |
| Supraproparoxytone | ◜ | | Al**cán**zamelo (*catch it for me*) |

Source: Quilis (1993)

### Intonation

Intonation is acoustically marked by variations in fundamental frequency resulting from the integration of the accent and the melody. As with accent, these variations also modify the intensity and the duration of the utterance.

Methods of analysis and the study of the characteristics of intonation in Spanish have changed dramatically in the last decade. Traditional descriptions followed the analysis system developed by the British school, a configuration-based approach that almost exclusively considers the melodic structure of the sentence (i.e. level, rising or falling tonemes), without taking into account stressing aspects. Recently, analysis by levels taken from the North American school has gained increasing weight in the study of intonation in Spanish. The work of this approach has been developed mainly within autosegmental metrical theory. Initially, four pitch accents were described for the Spanish prosodic system, three of them being bitonal and one tonal (Table 17.3). Several researchers have included three other pitch accents (last three rows in Table 17.3) to explain other observed structures. Following this, seven types of contrastive tonal accents are described in Spanish (Aguilar *et al.*, 2009) (Table 17.3).

**Table 17.3** Description of the proposed pitch accents for Spanish language

| Pitch accent | Description | Example |
|---|---|---|
| L*+H | Bitonal: rising tone from the stressed syllable (in low tone) to the post-tonic syllable (in high tone). The F0 peak is aligned in the stressed syllable. | ¿Le **die**ron el número de vuelo? (*Did you get the flight number?*) |
| L+H* | Bitonal: rising tone from pre-tonic syllable (in low tone) to the stressed syllable (in high tone). | No, no, de li**mo**nes! (*No, no, of lemons!*) |
| H+L* | Bitonal: falling tone from the pre-tonic syllable (in high tone) to the stressed syllable (in low tone). | ¿Es María quién **vie**ne? (*Is it Mary who's coming?*) |
| H* | Monotonal: small rise in tone without a prior low tone, employed in cases not identifiable as any of the other three accents. | ¿Cuándo lo ha**rás**? (*When will you do (it)?*) |
| L+>H | Bitonal: rising tone from stressed syllable (in low tone) to the post-tonic syllable (in high tone) with F0 peak shifted. | La **ni**ña morena come mandarinas (*The dark-haired girl is eating tangerines*) |
| L* | Monotonal. In the case where there is a progressive decrease in F0. | Bebe una limo**na**da *She/he is drinking lemonade* |
| L+H!* | Bitonal. Indicates an upstep, for example, in an exclamatory partially, interrogative sentence. | ¿**Ma**rina? ¿Estás seguro? *Marina?? Are you sure?* |

Source: Hugalde (2003); Vilaplana and Prieto (2008); Face and Prieto (2007); Aguilar *et al.* (2009)
H: high tone; L: low tone; *: stressed syllable; +: adding another tone.

Referring to boundary tones, various tones have been proposed according to the level of the prosodic phase. As in English, two levels of phrase are considered: an intonational phrase, which is marked with boundary tones by the symbol '%' (H%, M%, L%), and the intermediate phrase marked with phrase accent using the symbol '-' (H-, M-, L-). In Spanish, it is unclear whether a single level is enough or both levels are necessary, and both views have their supporters and opponents (Hugalde, 2002; Sosa, 1999, respectively). Vilaplana and Prieto (2008) have considered it relevant to establish two levels of prosodic domain for Spanish, but they have argued that a phrase accent to outline the intermediate phrase level is not necessary, since the same could be done with combinations of boundary tones in the form of bitonal or tritonal tones. In this sense, Aguilar *et al.* (2009) have identified seven types of boundary tones in Spanish: two monotonal tones (L% and M%), four bitonal tones (HH%, LH%, HL% and LM%) and a tritonal tone (LHL%). Finally, 19 different nuclear configurations formed by the combination of pitch accents and boundary tones are described in Spanish. All of these configurations, as well as those indicated above, may be reviewed in more detail in Aguilar *et al.* (2009). This reference constitutes a useful tool for looking up accent schemes, tonal configurations, examples of labelled utterances with intonational meaning and samples from audio data with examples of a spectrogram and oscillogram using the SpToBI system (Spanish Tones and Break Indices).

### Rhythm

Traditionally, Spanish has been considered as syllable timed. Accordingly, it is characterised by syllabic production at regular intervals, a lack of perceptual contrast in vowel duration (i.e. there is a contextual and intrinsic but not phonemic decrease in duration), a simple phonotactic structure (i.e. CV structures are most frequently) and an accent with a weak temporal prominence compared to unstressed segments (Ramus, 1999; Ramus *et al.*, 1999; White & Mattys, 2007). This has been confirmed acoustically. Specifically, Spanish rhythmic characteristics can be described phonologically as follows: a higher value of the proportion of intervocalic intervals (%V); a lower value of the index of variability of vocalic intervals in pairs (Ramus *et al.*, 1999; Toledo, 2010; White & Mattys, 2007).

# Relations with other components of the system: Morphology and syntax

The Spanish morphological system is more complex than English. One morpheme can be realised in different ways, as different *allomorphs*, depending on the constraints imposed by the phonological, morphological or syntactic properties of its contexts. Morphophonological alternations in Spanish are few and their level of productivity is also low. Phonologically conditioned allomorphy affects the verbal and nominal flexion, the composition, and, to a greater extent, derivation (Martín, 2001).

Examples of phonologically conditioned allomorphy are, similar to English, the negative morpheme 'in-', whose nasal sound varies according to the phonetic context exhibiting different phonetic variants, and number marking which has three phonological allomorphs in Spanish: '-s, -es, -0' depending on the final phoneme of the word to which the morpheme will be attached (e.g. 'coche→coches', 'cajón→cajones' and 'análisis→análisis', respectively).

Another example present in verbal inflectional morphology is the alternation between diphthongs and mid vowels (/e-ie, o-ue/) or between high and mid vowels (/i-e, u-o/), that is conditioned by phonological stress. In the former case, although there are exceptions, all verbs that have *ie* or *ue* in their root show these diphthongs only in those forms of the paradigm where the root receives the stress, and have a simple vowel in those forms where the stress is on the suffix (infinitive – 'pen's-ar', to *think*; present indicative *vs* 'piens-o', *I think*; preterite – 'pen's-e', *I thought*. In these examples, the apostrophe indicates the accented syllable and the midline indicates the division between the root and the morpheme). In the last case (/i-e, u-o/), the alternation between high and mid vowels is restricted to third conjugation verbs (infinitive in –ir). The vowels roots are mid vowel, /e/ or /o/, when the following syllable has the vowel /i/ (e.g. 'serv-ir' or 'podr-ido') and are high vowel, /i/ or /u/, when the following syllable has a different vowel or a diphthong (e.g. 'sirv-o' or 'pudr-o'). Some verbs show both phenomena: vowel alternation and diphthongization (e.g. 'dorm-ir', *to sleep* in English; 'durm-amos', *we sleep* in English; 'duerm-o', *I sleep* in English). It's possible to find a similar alternation, mid vowel/diphthong, in derivational morphology (e.g. 'diente – dental'; *tooth-dental* in English) although not all suffixes trigger a reduction of diphthongs (i.e. diminutive maintains the diphthong: 'diente – dientecito', *tooth – small tooth* in English) (Hualde, 2005).

At the phonosyntactic level, the concurrence of homologous phonemes, which are part of different words, resyllabification and syllable contraction across word boundaries, are present in Spanish. In relation to the concurrence of homologous consonant phonemes across word boundaries (e.g. 'el loro' – [el:óro]; *the parrot*), there is a tendency to produce only one of them when there are two similar alveolar sounds (voiceless fricative, nasal, rhotic and lateral) or two similar voiced dental sounds. In the case of the voiceless fricative sounds, the most frequent realisation is a consonant of the same type, whose duration is the same as the one intervocalic (e.g. 'las salas' – [lasálas]; *the rooms*). The same is true for the nasal and lateral consonants, but their production is somewhat longer during formal speech (e.g. 'con nada' – [kon:áða] and 'el lado' – [el:áðo], respectively; *with nothing* and *the side*). On the other hand, rhotic sounds are performed as an intervocalic rhotic sound and dental sounds are produced as a dental fricative sound (e.g. in the utterance 'cantar regional', [kaṇtá r̄exionál]; *regional song*). In the case of two identical vowels across word boundaries (with or without lexical stress), they may be reduced to the duration of a single vowel (e.g. in the utterance 'te esperamos', [tesperámos]; *we await you*) (Hualde, 2005; Quilis, 1993).

Resyllabification is the link of the final consonant of a word with the initial vowel of the following word, when both of them belong to the same phonic group. In Spanish, this phonological process is influenced by a particular tendency towards open syllable, replacing VC-V sequences with V-CV structures (e.g. in the phrase 'por ejemplo', [po-re-xém-plo]; *for example*). In the case of word-initial glides, these are considered as consonants, not as vowels. Thus, there is no resyllabification of word-final consonants before word-initial glides (e.g. 'las hierbas', [laz j'erβas]; *the herbs*) (Hualde, 2005).

Another process is syllable contraction across word boundaries. This is the case in glides that are grouped in a syllable across word boundaries when a word ending in an unstressed vowel is followed by another word beginning with an unstressed vowel. This affects sequences containing unstressed vowels, /i, u/+/a e o/ (e.g. 'mi hermano', [miermáno], *my brother*; 'tu abuelo', [tuaβuélo], *your grandfather*) and also sequences of /a e o/ (e.g. 'no entiendo', [noentiéndo]; *I don't understand*) (Hualde, 2005; Irribarren, 2005).

Finally Spanish intonation performs a distinctive grammatical role. This function assigns different stable configurations depending on intonational mode (neutral declarative, neutral exclamatory or neutral yes/no questions) without requiring any other grammatical elements to it, unlike in English that usually requires modifications to the order of the words or use different morphemes to indicate such variations (RAE, 2011).

So, in summary, the chief contrasts found between the English and Spanish sound systems are: in English there is a greater quantity and variety of vowels; the length of the vowel is not significant in distinguishing between words in Spanish and its phonetic execution is much more stable than in English; syllabic structure is more complex in English, with longer consonant sequences in onset and coda positions; although the two languages show free stress, in Spanish the stressed syllable has a window of three syllables; English is a stress-timed language while Spanish is a syllable-timed language; both languages have different pitch accents, boundary tones and nuclear configurations and, in Spanish, it is proposed to employ combinations of boundary tones instead of phrase accents in intermediate phrases; morphophonology presents more complex patterns of variation in Spanish than in English; and, finally, Spanish intonation can act as the only mark to differentiate between types of grammatical sentence, without changes in word order.

The following section presents a review of the methods, procedures, tools and techniques used for the assessment and intervention of motor speech disorders in Spanish-speaking people and, finally, it identifies future lines of enquiry in this regard.

## Assessment: Methods, Procedures, Tools and Techniques

Over the past decade, methods of assessment in motor speech disorders, and more specifically dysarthria, have been defined in a more precise and multidimensional way in Spain. This is not the case for apraxia of speech, however. Clinical and scientific research on apraxia of speech is rare in Spanish-speaking populations, where it is unclear which diagnostic criteria are being applied, and the assessment is usually carried out using ad hoc tasks – basically, techniques of syllable repetition (isolated and/or in sequences of identical or different syllables), repetition of words and phrases with different lengths and complexities, and production of automatic and spontaneous speech. The interpretation of performance though follows criteria employed in other languages without firm evidence of their application in Spanish (Melle & Gallego, 2012; Melle et al., 2012).

In the case of dysarthria, a comprehensive assessment that includes a case history, interview, perceptual analysis using the Grade, Roughness, Breathiness, Asthenia, Strain (GRBAS) scales (Hirano, 1981), acoustic evaluation of voice (by MedivozCaptura, WPvox, and the like), neurophysiological testing of phonoarticulatory mechanisms and the evaluation of the impact of motor speech disorder on daily activities (e.g. Voice Handicap Index [Núñez-Batalla et al., 2007]; and ad hoc scales) are the methods adopted. This assessment protocol has been applied to both degenerative and stable/recovering dysarthria, achieving similar findings to those observed for other languages (Gamboa et al., 2001; Godino-Llorente et al., 2006; Melle, 2003, 2007; Melle & Gallego, 2012; Melle et al., 2012; Núñez-Batalla et al., 2011; Velasco et al., 2009).

For intelligibility, it is worth mentioning the word pairs test applied by Fraas (2003) to 11 patients with a diagnosis of Parkinson's disease. The test, which incorporates principles proposed by Kent et al. (1989) and Whitehill and Ciocca (2000), assesses 17 phonetic contrasts, all of them identified as altered in English-speaking dysarthric patients. For almost all acoustic features, except for formant transitions, the results were similar to those obtained for English, but not with respect to the factors that most affect the degree of intelligibility in English (i.e. voice onset time [VOT], distribution of vowels in the vowel space and formant transitions in CV sequences). Regarding these factors, only VOT of /p/ correlated with the degree of intelligibility measured by native Spanish speakers, explaining 61% of the variance. It is possible that the impairment in the distribution of vowels in the vowel space has a less clearly marked effect on intelligibility in Spanish due to the size and distribution of its vowel repertoire, to differences in the severity of the disorder and/or to the type of words used for this Intelligibility Test. Kim *et al.* (2011) note that vowel space alone is not sufficient to address vowel characteristics and their relation to intelligibility. They conclude that the degree of overlap among vowels is a better predictor of a speaker's overall intelligibility. It is possible that differences in the disorder severity and/or in the size and distribution of Spanish vowel space may influence the degree of overlap between registered Spanish vowels in Fraas's study. It is possible that, in these cases, the degree of overlap present in Spanish vowels is smaller than in English studies. In regard to the type of words used in the Intelligibility Test, it was not controlled for word frequency or the number of possible lexical neighbours. Furthermore, Fraas (2003) suggested the variability in disease severity or factors such as the type of medication prescribed and the time of its administration as an explanation for the absence of significant differences between groups (i.e. pathological and control) in formant transitions as well as the lack of predictive value of the formant transition on intelligibility. Kim *et al.* (2011) propose that perhaps another type of measure, e.g. time-varying formant changes, could be used to study the possible relations among dysarthria and intelligibility.

## Clinical Findings in Spanish Speakers and Their Contributions to Models of Pathology and Normality

As elsewhere, the taxonomy of motor speech disorders in Spain has been strongly influenced by Darley *et al.* (1975). Studies carried out with Spanish-speaking populations are fewer compared to those with English speakers, both in terms of numbers and in terms of the diversity of pathologies considered. Most of them have focused on the analysis of degenerative motor speech disorders, finding results similar to those obtained in English (e.g. Velasco *et al.* [2009] in Huntington's chorea; Gamboa *et al.* [1998] in essential tremor; Brancal *et al.* [1998] in Friedreich's ataxia). However, studies of apraxia of speech and orofacial apraxia when their origin is non-degenerative have also been conducted in Spanish speakers (e.g. Briera *et al.*, 2003; Infante *et al.*, 2000; Martí *et al.*, 2001; Melle & Gallego, 2012).

Despite similarities, some small differences from results observed for English speakers have been documented. For example, during laryngeal examination of the characteristics of hypokinetic dysarthria in Parkinson's patients, Jiménez-Jiménez *et al.* (1997) and Gamboa *et al.* (1997) found no defect in the glottis closure as seen in English-speaking patients (Smith *et al.*, 1995). The authors suggested differences in the methods of examination used and the severity/duration of disease as an explanation for this mismatch, requiring further research on this aspect with more control over these factors.

A similar case is that of Melle and Gallego (2012). Studying the acoustic features of patients with spastic dysarthria after acquired brain injury, the authors confirmed results found in studies with non-Spanish speakers, except for the magnitude of the F2 variation in sequencing tasks for vowels [i-u]. Bradlow (1995) found that English vowels are articulated with a fronted tongue position relative to Spanish vowels; therefore, English vowels are significantly higher in the F2 dimension than their Spanish counterparts. According to the author, this cross-linguistic difference in precise phonetic realisations is due to different base-of-articulation of each language. Furthermore, the F2 of the two English vowels are more closely spaced than those of Spanish vowels. The absence of significant differences to formant centralisation in Spanish could be explained here by differences between languages. Thus, it is possible that Spanish requires more severe alterations of tongue mobility to observe significant differences in the F2 dimension compared to English.

## Intervention: Methods, Procedures and Techniques

Compared to the lack of work on assessment in Spanish, several works describing intervention in Spanish speakers with neurological damage have been published from medical, speech therapy and social participatory approaches (e.g. Donesteve & Fuente, 1995; Melle, 2007a, 2007b; Núñez-Batalla et al., 2011). These largely reflect procedures and techniques developed for speakers of other languages to describe methods of intervention for each of the mechanisms involved in speech as well as pragmatic and communicative aspects.

Thus, Donasteve et al. (1995) present different exercises for speech subsystems following the principles outlined by Dworkin (1991), based on his highly non-verbal, part-task principles that have not found strong support in recent years. Melle (2007a, 2007b) expands on the notions of intervention based on the World Health Organisation International Classification of Function to target changes on different levels of impairment, activity limitation and participation restriction. From a purely medical point of view, Núñez-Batalla et al. (2011) offer specific laryngological treatments in the area of neurological voice disorders (e.g. use of botulinum toxin injection and lidocain).

Other works are concerned with treatment programmes for specific disorders. So, for instance, Real et al. (2010) outline an intensive treatment programme for respiration for people with multiple sclerosis. Carrión et al. (2001) described intervention in a case of spastic dysarthria. The regime worked through the different speech subsystems and employed motor techniques such as inspiratory checking, voice accent method and integral stimulation (audio, visual and imitative) to achieve tone power and coordination of movement. Other intervention studies have covered for instance an intervention programme in a case of ataxic dysarthria (Galarza, 1988) and in patients with severe apraxia of speech (González *et al.*, 2007). All these studies claimed significant improvement in articulation after intensive, long-term treatment.

## The Way Forward

The progress made in recent years regarding the methodology and procedures for assessment and intervention in motor speech disorders has led to improvements in the care of people affected by these pathologies in Spain. However, many issues still remain.

In this sense, it would be necessary to develop new testing tools to cover unexplored areas in the assessment of people with motor speech disorders in Spain. Some of these needs would be: protocols to validly and reliably differentially diagnose apraxic and dysarthric problems; scales to estimate the impact of these disorders on daily living for patients, both from the point of view of reliable informants and self-evaluation by the patient. Valid and reliable tests to determine the degree of severity and intelligibility levels, using phonetic contrasts or significant acoustic variables for Spanish speakers would also be a priority.

Advances in the autosegmental system-based normative knowledge of Spanish prosodic features are also considered a relevant issue by the authors of this chapter, as these data can better characterise deviations present in motor speech disorders, thereby providing a better understanding of disorders as well as their diagnosis and intervention.

Finally, in the field of intervention it would be necessary to improve certain methodological aspects such as the operationalisation of intervention variables, establishing well-documented baselines, conducting studies on the comparative effectiveness between techniques or the effect of their implementation order, determining the frequency for practice, the type of stimuli, the reinforcing system and the type of feedback.

## References

Aguilar, L., De-la-Mota, C. and Prieto, P. (2009) Sp_ToBI Training Materials. See http://prosodia.upf.edu/sp_tobi/ (accessed March 2014).

Bradlow, A. (1995) A comparative acoustic study of English and Spanish vowels. *Journal of the Acoustic Society of America* 97, 1916–1924.

Brancal, M. and Ferrer, A. (1998) Análisis perceptual de las características del habla en personas afectas de ataxias hereditarias. *Revista de Logopedia, Foniatría y Audiología* 4, 213–224.

Briera, L., Begué, R., Trejo, A. and Martín, M. (2003) Apraxia bucofacial cruzada. *Medicina Clínica (Barcelona)* 120, 717–719.

Carrión, J., Viñals, A., Vega, D. and Domínguez-Morales, M. (2001) Disartria espástica: rehabilitación de la fonación de un paciente con traumatismo cráneo-encefálico. *Revista Española de Neuropsicología* 3, 34–45.

Darley, F., Aronson, A. and Brown, J. (1975) *Motor Speech Disorders*. Philadelphia, PA: W.B. Saunders.

Donesteve, J. and Fuente, M. (1995) Metodologías específicas para el tratamiento de las disartrias. *Revista Española de Foniatría* 8, 79–90.

Face, T. and Prieto, P. (2007) Rising accents in Castilian Spanish: A revision of Sp_ToBi. *Journal of Portuguese Linguistics (Special Issue on Prosody of Iberian Languages)* 6 (1), 117–146.

Fraas, M.R. (2003) Towards intelligibility testing in dysarthria: A study of motor speech deficits in native Spanish speakers with Parkinson's disease. University of Cincinnati. See http://rave.ohiolink.edu/etdc/view?acc_num=ucin1051723241 (accessed March 2014).

Galarza, I. (1988) Disartria cerebelosa: tratamiento logopédico. *Revista de Logopedia, Foniatría y Audiología* VIII, 84–87.

Gamboa, J., Jiménez-Jiménez, F., Nieto, A., Montojo, J., Ortí-Pareja, M., Molina, J., García-Albea, E. and Cobeta, I. (1997) Acoustic voice analysis in patients with Parkinson's disease treated with dopaminergic drugs. *Journal of Voice* 11, 314–320.

Gamboa, J., Jiménez-Jiménez, F., Nieto, A., Cobeta, I., Vegas, A., Ortí-Pareja, M., Gasalla, T., Molina, J. and García-Albea, E. (1998) Acoustic voice analysis in patients with essential tremor. *Journal of Voice* 12, 444–452.

Gamboa, J., Jiménez-Jiménez, F., Mate, M. and Cobeta, I. (2001) Alteraciones de la voz causadas por enfermedades neurológicas. *Revista de Neurología* 33, 156–168.

Godino-Llorente, J., Sáenz-Lechón, N., Osma-Ruíz, V., Aguilera-Navarro, S. and Gómez-Vilda, P. (2006) An integrated tool for the diagnosis of voice disorders. *Medical Engineering and Physics* 28, 276–289.

González, M., Armenteros, N., García, E., Casabona, E. and Real, Y. (2007) Aproximación terapéutica basada en la evidencia para contrarrestar apraxia total del habla en pacientes afásicos. *Revista Mexicana de Medicina Física y Rehabilitación* 19, 56–62.

Hirano, M. (1981) *Clinical Examination of Voice*. New York: Springer-Verlag.

Hualde, J.I. (2005) *The Sounds of Spanish*. Cambridge: Cambridge University Press.

Hugalde, J. (2002) Intonation in Spanish and the other Ibero-Romance languages: Overview and status questions. In C. Wiltshire and J. Camps (eds) *Romance Phonology and Variation: Selected Papers from the 30th Linguistic Symposium on Romance Languages* (pp. 101–116). Gainsville, FL; Amsterdam: John Benjamins.

Hugalde, J. (2003) El modelo métrico-autosegmental. In P. Prieto (ed.) *Teorías de la entonación* (pp. 155–184). Barcelona: Ariel.

Infante, J., Sánchez, M., Polo, J., Carril, J., Berciano, J. and Oterino, A. (2000) Anartria progresiva: a propósito de un caso sin apraxia lingual. *Neurología* 15, 208–210.

Iribarren, M. (2005) *Fonética y fonología españolas*. Madrid: Síntesis.

Jiménez-Jiménez, F., Gamboa, J., Nieto, A., Guerrero, J., Ortí-Pareja, M., Molina, J., García-Albea, E. and Cobeta, I. (1997) Acoustic voice analysis in untreated patients with Parkinson's disease. *Parkinsonism & Related Disorders* 3, 111–116.

Kent, R., Welsmer, G., Kent, J. and Duffy, J. (1989) Towards explanatory intelligibility testing in dysarthria. *Journal of Speech and Hearing Disorders* 54, 482–499.

Kim, H., Hasegawa-Johnson, M. and Perlman, A. (2011) Vowel contrast and speech intelligibility in dysarthria. *Folia Phoniatrica et Logopaedica* 63, 187–194.

Martí, I., Moreno, F., Mendioroz, M. and Martí, J. (2001) Apraxia bucofacial cruzada. *Neurología* 16, 322–324.

Melle, N. (2003) Disartria en el daño cerebral adquirido: hacia un método global de evaluación. *Revista de Logopedia, Fonatría y Audiología* 23, 20–29.

Melle, N. (2007a) *Guía de intervención logopédica en la disartria.* Madrid: Editorial Síntesis.

Melle, N. (2007b) Intervención logopédica en la disartria. *Revista de Logopedia, Foniatría y Audiología* 27, 187–197.

Melle, N. and Gallego, C. (2012) Differential diagnosis between apraxia and dysarthria based on acoustic analysis. *The Spanish Journal of Psychology* 15, 495–504.

Melle, N., Martín-Aragoneses, Mª.T. and Gallego, C. (2012) La atención en el sistema asistencial español a los trastornos motores del habla de origen neurológico: epidemiología y diagnóstico en el marco de la CIF. In AELFA (ed.) *Libro de Actas XXVIII Congreso Internacional Asociación Española de Logopedia, Foniatría y Audiología* (pp. 341–355). Madrid: AELFA.

Moreno Sandoval, A., Torre, D., Curto, N. and de la Torre, R. (2006) Inventario de frecuencias fonémicas y silábicas del castellano espontáneo y escrito. In L. Buera, E. Lleida, A. Miguel and A. Ortega (eds) *IV Jornadas en Tecnología del Habla* (pp. 77–81). Zaragoza: Universidad de Zaragoza – Red Temática en Tecnologías del Habla. See http://www.lllf.uam.es/ESP/Publicaciones/LLI-UAM-4JTH.pdf (accessed March 2014).

Navarro, T. (1991) *Manual de pronunciación española.* Madrid: Consejo Superior de Investigaciones Científicas.

Núñez-Batalla, F., Corte-Santos, P., Señaris-González, B., Llorente-Pendás, J., Górriz-Gil, C. and Suárez-Nieto, C. (2007) Adaptación y validación del índice de incapacidad vocal (VHI-30) y su versión abreviada (VHI-10) al español. *Acta de Otorrinolaringología Española* 58, 386–392.

Núñez-Batalla, F., Díaz-Molina, J., Costales-Marcos, M., Moreno, C. and Suárez-Nieto, C. (2011) Neurolaringología. *Acta Otorrinolaringológica Española* 63, 132–140.

Quilis, A. (1993) *Tratado de fonética y fonología españolas.* Madrid: Editorial Gredos.

Quilis, A. (2003) *Principios de fonética y fonología.* Madrid: Arco/Libros.

Quilis, A. and Esgueva, M. (1980) Frecuencia de fonemas en Español hablado. *Lingüística Española Actual* II, 1–25.

Quilis, A. and Fernández, J. (1985) *Curso de fonética y fonología españolas para estudiantes angloamericanos.* Madrid: C.S.I.C.

Ramus, F. (1999) *Rythme des langues et acquisition du langage.* Paris: École des Hautes Études en Sciences Sociales.

Ramus, F., Nespor, M. and Mehler, J. (1999) Correlates of linguistic rhythm in speech. *Cognition* 73, 265–292.

Real Academia de la Lengua (RAE) (2011) *Nueva gramática de la lengua española. Fonética y fonología.* Barcelona: Espasa Libros.

Real, Y., López, M., Díaz, R. and Cabrera, J. (2010) Efectividad de un programa de rehabilitación respiratoria en pacientes con esclerosis múltiple. *Revista Cubana de Salud Pública* 3, 12–18.

Smith, M., Ramig, L., Dromey, C., Pérez, K. and Samandari, R. (1995) Intensive voice treatment in Parkinson's disease: Laryngostroboscopic findings. *Journal of Voice* 9, 453–459.

Sosa, J. (1999) *La entonación del Español.* Madrid: Cátedra.

Toledo, G. (2010) Métricas rítmicas en tres dialectos Amper-España. *Estudios Filológicos* 45, 110–120.

Velasco, M., Cobeta, I., Martín, G., Alonso-Navarro, H. and Jimenez-Jimenez, F. (2009) Acoustic analysis of voice in Huntington's disease patients. *Journal of Voice* 25, 208–217.

Vilaplana, E. and Prieto, P. (2008) La notación prosódica del español: una revisión del Sp_ToBI. *Estudios de Fonética Experimental* XVII, 263–283.

White, L. and Mattys, S. (2007) Rhythmic typology and variation in first and second languages. In P. Prieto, J. Mascaró and M.J. Solé (eds) *Segmental and Prosodic Issues in Romance Phonology, Current Issues in Linguistic. Theory Series* (pp. 237–257). Amsterdam; Philadelphia, PA: John Benjamins.

Whitehill, T. and Ciocca, V. (2000) Perceptual-phonetics predictors of single-word intelligibility: A study of Cantonese dysarthria. *Journal of Speech, Language, and Hearing Research* 43, 1451–1465.

# 18 The Nature, Assessment and Treatment of Dysarthria and Apraxia of Speech in Swedish

## Ellika Schalling

## The Swedish Sound System

The opening section briefly describes the Swedish sound system, consisting of 17 contrasting vowels and 18 consonants. Phonotactics, tone, stress and rhythm in Swedish are also outlined. The second section looks at Swedish assessment materials for motor speech disorders before giving an overview of the few descriptive and treatment studies focusing on dysarthria in Swedish.

### Vowels

Swedish has a relatively large inventory of vowels consisting of 17 contrasting vowels, nine long and eight short, /iː eː ɛː ɑː oː uː ʉː yː øː ɪ ɛ a ɔ ʊ ɵ ʏ œ/, as illustrated in Table 18.1. The short vowels are more centred and lax. The front vowels appear in rounded and unrounded pairs. There is a rounded high front vowel in Swedish /yː/. There is also a more central rounded vowel /ʉː/. The /y/ is articulated with protruded lips, whereas the /ʉː/ is articulated with compressed lips. The vowels /ɛ/ and /ø/ have a lower quality and are realised as /æ/ and /œ/ when preceding /r/ and the retroflex consonants ([ ɖ, ɭ, ɳ, ʂ, ʈ ]). Unstressed /ɛ/ is realised as [ə], the schwa vowel.

In some Swedish dialects, long vowels are realised as diphthongs. For example, in southern regions of Sweden /ʉː/ and /ɑː/ are realised as rising diphthongs [eʉ] and [aɑ].

### Consonants

There are 18 consonants in Swedish, as displayed in Table 18.2: three unvoiced and three homorganic voiced plosives, /p, t, k/ and /b, d, g/, the five unvoiced and two voiced fricatives /f, s, ç, ɧ, h/ and /v, j/, three nasals /m, n, ŋ/, the trill /r/ and the approximant /l/. The unvoiced plosives are

**Table 18.1** Swedish vowels

| | Front | | | | Central | | Back | | |
| | Unrounded Long | Unrounded Short | Rounded Long | Rounded Short | Rounded Long | Unrounded Short | Rounded Long | Short | Unrounded Short |
|---|---|---|---|---|---|---|---|---|---|
| High | iː | ɪ | yː | ʏ | ʉː | | uː | ʊ | |
| Mid high | eː | ɛ | /øː/ | | | | oː | | |
| Mid low | ɛː | ɛ | œ | | | ɵ | ɔ | | |
| Low | æː | æ | œ̈ː | œ̈ː | | | ɑː | | a |

**Table 18.2** Swedish consonants

|  | Bilabial | Labiodental | Dental | Retroflex | Palatal | Velar | Glottal |
|---|---|---|---|---|---|---|---|
| Plosive | p b |  | t d | ʈ ɖ |  | k g |  |
| Approximant |  |  | l | ɭ |  |  |  |
| Fricative |  | f v | s | ʂ | ç j | ɧ | h |
| Tremulant |  |  | r |  |  |  |  |
| Nasal | m |  | n | ɳ |  | ŋ |  |

aspirated in initial position except after /s/ and the voiced plosives are unaspirated in Swedish. Finally, there are five retroflex consonants in Swedish: [ɖ, ɭ, ɳ, ʂ, ʈ].

The velar fricative /ɧ/ can also be produced as a post/palato-alveolar fricative [ʃ], which may be considered an allophone. Many Swedish speakers consistently use one of these variants, but they may also be used in complementary distribution. The Swedish velar fricative includes double articulations, although there is no agreement as to the exact place of articulation for this phoneme. There are further regional differences in the production of the trill /r/. In middle and northern Sweden, the speech sound is commonly produced as an alveolar trill [r], in central Sweden it may be pronounced as a fricative [z̺], whereas in southern regions of Sweden /r/ is produced as a uvular trill [R] (Engstrand, 2004).

## Phonotactics

Closed syllables are common in Swedish. Clusters can consist of two or three consonants both in initial and final position (Elert, 1970). The following structure is therefore possible in Swedish: (C) (C) (C) (V) (C) (C) (C).

There are six possible three-consonant clusters in initial position: /skr, skv, spj, spl, spr, str/, but as many as 31 possible two-consonant clusters. In final position, the number of possible two-consonant clusters is as high as 62. In compound nouns, long combinations of consecutive consonants are possible e.g. in the word 'sandstrand' ('sand beach'). Adding inflections to final clusters can result in long consonant combinations, e.g. in the word 'västkustskt', which consists of 'västkust' ('west coast') with the adjective suffix -sk and the neuter suffix -t. This is unusual and has to be considered as an exception from the general rule.

## Tone, Stress and Rhythm

Words can be differentiated by tone in Swedish. There are two word accents, the acute and grave accents. There are regional differences in the realisation of these accents. In standard Swedish, words with an acute accent have a rising or high tone on the first stressed syllable followed by a falling or low tone on the second syllable ['ãndèn] (the duck). Words with a grave accent have a falling tone on the first stressed syllable, followed by a high falling tone again on the second syllable ['ãndên] (the spirit) (Engstrand, 2004). Like English, Swedish is considered a stress-timed language, meaning that intervals between stressed syllables are isochronous. This results in syllables having varying duration, which is partly achieved through vowel reduction.

# Swedish Studies of Dysarthria

There are a limited number of studies on Swedish speakers with motor speech disorders. The main focus has been on describing the nature and prevalence of speech deficits in some neurological disorders; additionally, a few treatment studies have been performed.

## Swedish studies of prevalence and the nature of motor speech disorders

Hartelius and Svensson (1994), studied the prevalence of speech and swallowing disorders in Parkinson's disease and multiple sclerosis (MS). Seventy percent of individuals with Parkinson's and 44% of individuals with MS reported speech and voice symptoms following disease onset. The prevalence and characteristics of speech symptoms were further studied in 77 individuals drawn from a cohort of patients with MS and in this group the prevalence of mild–severe dysarthria was 51%, with mixed dysarthria the most common type of dysarthria (both ataxic and spastic speech signs). There were deficits in all components of speech production: respiration, phonation, prosody, articulation and nasality (Hartelius et al., 2000a). The acoustic characteristics of dysarthria in MS were also studied by Hartelius et al. (1997a). Acoustic measures of long-term phonatory instability differentiated between subjects with MS and matched healthy speakers. In addition, non-dysarthric speakers with MS were also differentiated from healthy controls using the same measures, indicating that there are subclinical speech signs.

Hartelius et al. (2000b) studied the temporal-prosodic aspects of speech in 14 individuals with MS and ataxic dysarthria and 15 healthy controls. Significantly increased syllable equalization (more isochrony for syllables) in combination with increased inter-stress variability (less isochrony for inter-stress intervals) was shown for speakers with MS and ataxic dysarthria compared to healthy speakers. This study did not include comparisons with speakers of other languages.

In an attempt to compare perceptual assessments of speech between Australian and Swedish speakers with dysarthria, 10 Swedish speakers with MS were closely matched (for age and gender as well as type and severity of dysarthria) with 10 Australian subjects with MS. Four experienced speech and language pathologists (two Australian and two Swedish) were recruited for perceptual assessments of speech samples using a protocol including 33 speech parameters. Results showed, not surprisingly, that basically the same perceptual parameters were most prevalent in both Australian and Swedish speakers (imprecise consonants, harshness and glottal fry, reduced speech rate, pitch level and loudness). These findings were, in principle, the same as the speech characteristics found in previous studies of dysarthria secondary to MS in both English- and Swedish-speaking populations. In addition, it was also found that the same perceptual parameters were identified by both pairs of judges regardless of whether the listeners rated a speaker of a known or an unknown language (Australian raters did not know Swedish), although Swedish raters were generally more critical and assessed more dimensions as being deviant. For the more prevalent speech parameters such as precision of consonants, pitch and loudness level and rate, it seemed more difficult to agree on the degree of deviation. For example, deviations in stress pattern and phoneme length were among the dimensions with the highest number of disagreements between raters and thus seemed somewhat more difficult to assess, possibly indicating that prosodic dimensions are harder to rate in an unfamiliar than a known language (Hartelius et al., 2003).

Speech symptoms in spinocerebellar ataxia (SCA) were studied using perceptual and acoustic methods by Schalling and Hartelius (2004), Schalling et al. (2007) and Schalling and Hartelius (2013). The speech parameters 'imprecise consonants' and 'imprecise vowels', 'equalized stress', 'monotony', 'stereotypic intonation', 'inappropriate silences', 'prolonged intervals' and 'speech rate' were rated significantly more deviant in a group of 21 subjects with SCA compared to 21 matched control subjects. A factor analysis resulted in two main factors, one related to articulation and timing and the other related to voice quality. The acoustic findings supported perceptual results.

The progression of speech and voice symptoms was followed in nine subjects with SCA over close to three years and it was found that perceptual characteristics related to articulation and prosody were more severely affected than perceptual characteristics related to vocal quality. Acoustic analysis showed statistically significant reductions in speech rate over time and also significant changes in some of the measures of duration and variability. In addition, there was a statistically significant change in the dysarthria test score over the 33 months between the first and third assessment. Changes were more pronounced over time in subjects with early disease onset (Schalling et al., 2008).

Speech symptoms were studied in a group of 19 individuals with mild and moderate Huntington's disease. There were deviations in all areas of speech production with the most pronounced deviations in phonation, oral motor function and prosody (Hartelius et al., 2003a).

There have been no studies specifically addressing the breakdown of the tone system in Swedish. However, one of the classic studies of foreign accent syndrome (Moen, 2006; Monrad-Krohn, 1947) concerned a speaker of Norwegian, which has a tone system very similar to some Swedish dialects. The apparent foreign accent that was heard by listeners was interpreted to lead back to her difficulty signaling the correct pitch accents in her speech.

# Swedish Materials for Assessment of Motor Speech Disorders

## Standardised test materials

There is one standardised test for the assessment of dysarthria in Sweden called 'Dysartritest' ('Dysarthria test') (Hartelius & Svensson, 1990). The test assesses function related to respiration, phonation, oral-motor skills, articulation, prosody and intelligibility. Ratings of each task are made on a five-point scale from 0 to 4 (0 = normal or not significantly deviating function, 4 = severe deviation or no function). The test gives an overall test score (mean test score) which indicates the severity of impairment (ranging from 0 to 4). A test profile that gives an overview of the most prominent features of the speech disorder is also included in the summary of test findings (Hartelius & Svensson, 1990).

## Intelligibility

The assessment of intelligibility in the Swedish dysarthria test is done by the transcription of words and sentences that the patient reads from randomly drawn stimulus cards (10 one-syllable words, 10 two-syllable words and 10 sentences). A subjective rating of intelligibility in spontaneous speech and text reading is also done by the speech and language pathologist as an indication of communicative effectiveness. As in many other materials for the assessment of intelligibility with a closed set of test items, familiarity with the speech material may become a problem when the test is frequently used. Therefore, the Swedish Intelligibility Assessment (SWINT) was developed by Lillvik et al. (1999). SWINT is a computerised assessment procedure including words and sentences. The word section includes words with 22 different phonetic contrasts. The test items are randomly selected from a lexicon comprising approximately 1500 words using a computerised procedure and there is a multiple-choice answering format. Nonsense sentences are used in the sentence section (sentences that are syntactically correct but semantically impossible), thus no semantic contextual cues are given. Using a computerised procedure, sentences are also randomly generated from a word pool of nouns, verbs and adjectives (100 words in each category). For each assessment list, 12 sentences are generated: two practice sentences and 10 test items. The patient reads the sentences that are subsequently transcribed by the listener.

## Subjective experiences of communication difficulties

In order to capture subjective experiences of living with motor speech disorders, a self-report questionnaire was developed by Hartelius *et al.* (2008) called 'Självsvarsformulär Om Förvärvade Talstörningar' (SOFT; 'Self-report form on acquired speech deficits'). It consists of three sections. Section A includes questions related to the individual's perception of his/ her speech function; section B questions relate to communicative activity/ participation; and section C to personal and environmental factors influencing communication. The questionnaire also has a section where general background information can be documented. In total, SOFT includes 30 statements and the individual has to indicate how well each statement applies to her/him at the present time by selecting one of four alternative (not correct at all, sometimes correct, mostly correct and exactly correct).

## Perceptual assessment

Perceptual assessment of speech has been used in a structured and systematic way in several Swedish studies of dysarthria. The methods used are based on the Stockholm Voice Evaluation Approach (SVEA), which is a procedure for the audio-perceptual assessment of voice function developed by researchers at Karolinska Institutet in Stockholm. SVEA aims to systematise perceptual terminology and use valid scales; it has been used in a number of studies of dysphonia (Hammarberg, 2000). A similar methodology was used in several studies for the assessment of speech deficits in dysarthria after adapting the protocol to also include speech parameters relevant to capture articulatory and prosodic aspects of speech (Johansson *et al.*, 2011; Schalling *et al.*, 2007, 2008).

## Assessment of apraxia of speech

There is no standardized Swedish test for the assessment of apraxia of speech. A pilot version of a test has recently been developed with test items selected based on international research on apraxia of speech. The test items include repetition of words (with and without change of articulatory position), repetition of articulatory complex words, repetition of nonsense words, tasks for the assessment of articulation rate and speech rate as well as tasks contrasting automatised and non-automatised speech. The pilot version has only been used on 50 healthy speakers to collect normative data (Albinsson & Berglund, 2010). Based on this study, a slightly revised version of the test was recently tested on eight participants with apraxia of speech, eight participants with dysarthria and six healthy control speakers. Preliminary results indicate the test could differentiate the groups and no further problems related to the administration of the test in a disordered population were noted. The authors suggest further work on the validation and development of norms (Lindau & Zachariassen, 2013).

In the absence of standardised tests, the current assessment of apraxia of speech in clinical praxis is generally done by combining some speech tasks from the dysarthria test (for example the task for alternating and sequential motion rates) with speech tasks suggested in the literature and from clinical experience to be sensitive to apraxic symptoms such as repetition of words of increasing length, articulatory complex words and so-called tongue twisters, nonsense words – notwithstanding the authors' awareness that at least some of these symptoms are currently under debate.

## Treatment studies

The positive effects of a speech-language pathology intervention program was shown in a treatment study focusing on dysarthria in MS. Seven individuals with MS were consecutively enrolled and the program focused on vocal efficiency, effective use of contrastive stress and optimising verbal repair strategies. Five of the seven individuals with MS improved their speech after intervention based on perceptual assessments by independent judges (Hartelius et al., 1997b).

In recent years, some treatment pilot studies have been performed as master's theses in speech and language pathology. In a treatment study with a single-subject design repeated across three subjects, positive perceptual and acoustic changes were shown following intensive voice treatment (Lee Silverman Voice Treatment [LSVT®]) in three individuals with ataxic dysarthria (Kärrholt & Lindblad, 2009). The effects of biofeedback in the treatment of Parkinson's has also been studied. Norrlinder and Olsson (2009) showed positive effects of visual feedback during intensive voice treatment for subjects with Parkinson's in three case studies. Bulukin Wilén and Gustafsson (2011) also showed positive effects of biofeedback regarding voice intensity in patients with Parkinson's administered with a newly developed Swedish portable phonation monitor. This ambulatory phonation monitor, based on a voice accumulator, monitors sound pressure level, fundamental frequency and phonation time. Similar positive effects of biofeedback on sound pressure levels in patients with Parkinson's using a portable phonation monitor have also been shown in a study by Schalling et al. (2013).

The effects of repetitive transcranial magnetic stimulation (rTMS) on speech and voice in 10 individuals with Parkinson's were assessed by Hartelius *et al.* (2010). Speech samples included maximum fricative duration /s:/, sustained vowel duration /a:/, alternating and sequential syllable repetitions, intelligibility test sentences and text reading. The rTMS did not have an effect on speech and voice in the subjects in the study; however, a placebo effect was shown with acoustic analysis, indicating a reduction in fundamental frequency (F0) variation, pitch period perturbation, amplitude period perturbation, noise-to-harmonics ratio and coefficient of variation in F0 between recordings before compared to after the sham condition.

Another recently pursued area of research concerns investigations of the effects of respiratory treatment on patients with neurological disease or injury. Johansson *et al.* (2011) studied glossopharyngeal breathing training in seven subjects with cervical spinal cord injuries (CSCI), and found improvements in the areas of voice intensity, vocal stability and phrase length following the intervention. The same technique has also been applied to subjects with impaired speech and voice function secondary to MS, and marked positive changes have been reported in a case report of a tetraplegic man with severe MS (Johansson *et al.*, 2012).

## Cross-language studies

The only Swedish study to date directly comparing speakers with dysarthria with different native languages is the comparison by Hartelius *et al.* (2003b) between Swedish and Australian speakers with MS (including comparisons between perceptual ratings by clinicians with different linguistic backgrounds), as detailed above. Some characteristics of the Swedish language could theoretically result in more pronounced speech deficits for individuals with motor speech disorders compared to speakers of other languages. Swedish has a relatively large inventory of vowels (with close articulatory proximity differentiating vowels). Vowel distortions (e.g. in ataxic dysarthria) could possibly be more prominent in Swedish speakers. The large inventory of consonant clusters is another example where one could speculate that Swedish speakers could be more prone to reduced articulatory precision compared to speakers of languages with more limited repertoires of clusters. In fact, the perceptual parameter 'imprecision of consonants' was noted in 92% of patients in a Swedish population of speakers with MS (Hartelius *et al.*, 2000a), but was only noted in 52% of speakers with MS in a similar Australian study (Theodoros *et al.*, 2000). There are also a number of word pairs in Swedish that are differentiated by acute and grave accents, yet another language-specific feature that theoretically could lead to more difficulties in Swedish individuals with impaired prosody compared to speakers of other languages without contrasting tone.

To date, there are only a limited number of descriptive studies of motor speech disorders in Swedish, only one cross-language comparison and very few treatment studies, so there is no basis for any statements about language-specific effects in this area. Possible effects of language-specific features, such as for example tone or stress or features related specifically to the sound system in Swedish compared to other languages in individuals with dysarthria or apraxia of speech remain to be further investigated in future studies.

## References

Albinsson, S. and Berglund, J. (2010) A test battery for apraxia of speech – development and pilot norms. Unpublished master's thesis, Uppsala University.

Bulukin Wilén, F. and Gustafsson, J. (2011) Voice use and effect of biofeedback in patients with Parkinson's disease studied with a voice accumulator, VoxLog. Unpublished thesis, Karolinska Institutet.

Elert, C-C. (1970) *Ljud och ord i svenskan*. Stockholm: Almqvist och Wiksell.

Engstrand, O. (2004) *Fonetikens grunder*. Lund: Studentlitteratur.

Hammarberg, B. (2000) Voice research and clinical needs. *Folia Phoniatrica* 52, 92–102.

Hartelius, L. and Svensson, P. (1990) *Dysartritest*. Stockholm: Psykologiförlaget AB.

Hartelius, L. and Svensson, P. (1994) Speech and swallowing symptoms associated with Parkinson's disease and multiple sclerosis: A survey. *Folia Phoniatrica* 46, 9–17.

Hartelius, L., Buder, E.H. and Strand, E.A. (1997a) Long-term phonatory instability in individuals with multiple sclerosis. *Journal of Speech, Language and Hearing Research* 40, 1056–1072.

Hartelius, L., Wising, C. and Nord, L. (1997b) Speech modification in dysarthria associated with multiple sclerosis; an intervention based on vocal efficiency, contrastive stress and verbal repair strategies. *Journal of Medical Speech-Language Pathology* 5, 113–140.

Hartelius, L., Runmarker, B. and Andersen, O. (2000a) Prevalence and characteristics of dysarthria in a multiple-sclerosis incidence cohort: Relation to neurological data. *Folia Phoniatrica* 52, 160–177.

Hartelius, L., Runmarker, B., Anderson, O. and Nord, L. (2000b) Temporal speech characteristics of individuals with multiple sclerosis and ataxic dysarthria: 'Scanning speech' revisited. *Folia Phoniatrica* 52, 228–238.

Hartelius, L., Carlstedt, A., Ytterberg, M., Lillvik, M. and Laakso, K. (2003a) Speech disorders in mild and moderate Huntington disease: Results of dysarthria assessment of 19 individuals. *Journal of Medical Speech-Language Pathology* 11, 1–14.

Hartelius, L., Theodoros, D., Cahill, L. and Lillvik, M. (2003b) Comparability of perceptual analysis of speech characteristics in Australian and Swedish speakers with multiple sclerosis. *Folia Phoniatrica* 55, 177–188.

Hartelius, L., Elmberg, M., Holm, R., Lövberg, A-S. and Nikolaidis, S. (2008) Living with dysarthria: Evaluation of a self-report questionnaire. *Folia Phoniatrica* 60, 11–19.

Hartelius, L., Svantesson, P., Hedlund, A., Holmberg, B., Revesz, D. and Thorlin, T. (2010) Short-term effects of repetitive transcranial magnetic stimulation on speech and voice in individuals with Parkinson's disease. *Folia Phoniatrica* 62, 104–109.

Johansson, K., Nygren-Bonnier, M., Klefbeck, B. and Schalling, E. (2011) Effects of glossopharyngeal breathing on voice and speech in individuals with cervical spinal cord injury. *International Journal of Therapy and Rehabilitation* 18, 501–510.

Johansson, K., Nygren-Bonnier, M. and Schalling, E. (2012) Effects of glossopharyngeal breathing on speech in multiple sclerosis: A case report. *Multiple Sclerosis Journal* 18, 905–908.

Kärrholt, A. and Lindblad, P. (2009) Effects of treatment with intensive voice treatment (the Lee Silverman Voice Treatment, LSVT, on voice and speech in patients with ataxic dysarthria. Unpublished thesis, Karolinska Institutet.

Lillvik, M., Allemark, E., Karlström, P. and Hartelius, L. (1999) Intelligibility of dysarthric speech in words and sentences: Development of a computerized assessment procedure in Swedish. *Logopedics Phoniatrics Vocology* 24, 107–119.

Moen, I. (2006) Analysis of a case of the foreign accent syndrome in terms of the framework of gestural phonology. *Journal of Neurolinguistics* 19, 410–423.

Monrad-Krohn, G. (1947) Dysprosody or altered melody of language. *Brain* 70, 405–415.

Norrlinder, K. and Olsson, L. (2009) Phonetogram as visual feedback in intensive voice therapy for 3 patients with Parkinson's disease. Unpublished thesis, Karolinska Institutet.

Schalling, E. and Hartelius, L. (2004) Acoustic analysis of speech tasks performed by three individuals with spinocerebellar ataxia (SCA). *Folia Phoniatrica* 56, 367–380.

Schalling, E., Hammarberg, B. and Hartelius, L. (2007) Perceptual and acoustic analysis of speech in individuals with spinocerebellar ataxia. *Logopedics Phoniatrics Vocology* 32, 31–46.

Schalling, E., Hammarberg, B. and Hartelius, L. (2008) A longitudinal study of dysarthria in spinocerebellar ataxia – aspects of articulation, prosody and voice. *Journal Medical Speech and Language Pathology* 16, 103–117.

Schalling, E., Gustafsson, J., Ternström, S., Bulukin Wilén, F. and Södersten, M. (2013) Effects of tactile feedback by a portable voice accumulator on voice sound level in speakers with Parkinson's disease. *Journal of Voice* 27(6), 729–737.

Schalling, E. and Hartelius, L. (2013) Speech in spinocerebellar ataxia. *Brain and Language* 127, 317–322.

Theodoros, D., Murdoch, B. and Ward, E. (2000) Perceptual features of dysarthria in multiple sclerosis. In B.E. Murdoch and D.G. Theodoros (eds) *Speech and Language Disorders in Multiple Sclerosis* (pp. 15–29). London: Whurr.

Zachariassen, H. and Lindau, D. (2013) Further development of a test for apraxia of speech evaluated on groups with apraxia of speech and dysarthria. Unpublished thesis, Karolinska Institutet.

# 19 Conclusion

## Anja Lowit and Nick Miller

## Where are We Now?

The starting point for creating this book was a desire to take a cross-language look at motor speech disorders (MSDs) from two angles. The first aim was to highlight what is known about universal aspects of speech output and speech breakdown from the point of view of features of sound systems, elements of design as well as the execution of sound systems that are common to all human spoken languages. The aspiration was that such a view would facilitate an examination of underlying regularities across languages for how speech sound systems break down in the face of damage to the central and peripheral nervous systems. In turn, this would address issues around the development of assessment approaches, devising intervention materials and testing out treatment techniques that relate to basic design features of speech output organisation and control and so should be generalisable across languages.

The second aim of the book then was to counter, or at least weigh up the suspicion that theories and practices developed around MSDs are potentially not generalisable outside of the narrow English/related languages context in which the majority of research has taken place to date. Exposition of the issues in Chapter 2 pointed out ways in which similar underlying neuromuscular or planning disorders may be exhibited differently across languages, dependent on the characteristics of the sound inventory, phonotactics, sound contrasts and suprasegmental dimensions of any given language. It highlighted some existing examples of cross-language divergences in the perception and classification of MSDs.

These aspirations underscored the potential power of cross-language studies in the field of MSDs. Examples of this potential arise in all chapters. The chapters also illustrate, however, that in many respects we have a long way to travel yet in fully exploiting these possibilities.

In locating authors for chapters on individual languages, it was apparent that very few people worldwide currently work specifically along cross-language lines in MSDs. More discouraging was the fact that for most languages, including some major world languages such as Arabic and Hindi, there are no or very few studies of MSDs. In other languages, clinical tools seem to have at least been developed, but closer scrutiny divulges that these are often adapted from English into that language, without questioning the suitability of the resulting materials.

At the same time, there is active, high-quality work under way in many widely spoken languages. This is amply demonstrated in the individual language chapters in the book. New assessments are being devised based on language-specific criteria. Examinations of many different MSDs have been completed using materials devised for the particular studies rather than lifted inappropriately from English language work. Treatment efficacy studies are being conducted to ascertain if findings from English language studies are realised in a different context. On a further positive note, the state of play indicates that much work is underway, and background facts and figures are already in place and growing in multiple areas that provide a firm basis for cross-language exploits.

Nevertheless, the individual language chapters are unanimous in highlighting that much work remains to be completed within languages and all the chapters point out the absence of cross-language verification of findings or the instigation of cross-language studies addressing theory, speech output universals, as well as clinical and psychosocial issues.

## Where Do We Go Next?

The field is open for extensive and fruitful investigation. An expansion of the number of languages in which people are actively investigating MSDs would be a desirable step. Systematic comparisons across languages of key issues in MSD impairment and classification would yield important findings, e.g. what perceptual features are prominent in types of dysarthria associated with different lesion sites in languages with contrasting centrality of nasality, stress and intonation patterns, syllable structure and so forth?; what are the common denominators in speech disintegration in apraxia of speech across similarly distinct languages?; how are ataxia or the dysfluencies of spasmodic dysphonia manifest in languages of radically diverging sound system properties? The same would be applicable to therapy studies. Do loudness/intensity therapies have similar outcomes across languages?; what are the effects of rate control on intelligibility across different languages?; do metric therapies result in the same improvements irrespective of the rhythmic structure of a language?

Programmes of research need to examine not just the content and structure of therapies. Important gains would emerge from how programmes need to be modified to adapt to the service delivery and psychosocial challenges across diverse cultures. It cannot be assumed that one size fits all when it comes to methods of delivery.

The chapters in this book highlight too the need to develop much more dedicated assessment and intervention materials. In this respect there appears to be a role for education away from the too frequent misguided simple translation of assessments or materials and the unquestioning acceptance of findings on treatment or diagnosis from one language to another.

In sum, many of the suppositions regarding cross-language variations in the manifestation of MSDs await confirmation. The field of study is rife for exploitation. If essential differences transpire, then these will offer important issues in our understanding of speech motor control, speech output and speech perception and MSDs. They will also have key consequences for the assessment and management of MSDs in different languages and comparisons across languages. These lessons will be able to guide the development of assessments and treatment exercises for different languages. In a world where the number of bi- and multilingual speakers is ever increasing, cross-language studies will deliver significant insights into the evaluation and treatment of changes in their languages.